High Dose Chemotherapy

High Dose Chemotherapy
Principles and Practice

Edited by

Paul Lorigan MB FRCP
Senior Lecturer in Medical Oncology
Department of Clinical Oncology
Weston Park Hospital
Sheffield, UK

Elisabeth Vandenberghe PhD MB MRCP MRCPath
Consultant Haematologist
Haematology Department
St James's Hospital
Dublin, Ireland

MARTIN DUNITZ

First published in the United Kingdom in 2002 by Martin Dunitz Ltd, The Livery House, 7-9 Pratt Street, London NW1 0AE

Tel: +44 (0) 20 7482 2202
Fax: +44 (0) 20 7267 0159
E-mail: info@dunitz.co.uk
Webiste: http://www.dunitz.co.uk

Although every effort has been made to ensure that the drug doses and other information are presented accurately in this publication, the ultimate responsibility rests with the prescribing physician. Neither the publishers nor the author can be held responsible for errors or any other consequences arising from the use of information contained herein.

A CIP record for this book is available from the British Library.

ISBN 90-5823-232-8

Although every effort has been made to ensure that all owners of copyright material have been acknowledged in this publication, we would be glad to acknowledge in subsequent reprints or editions any omissions brought to our attention.

Distributed in the USA by
Fulfilment Center
Taylor & Francis
7625 Empire Drive
Florence, KY 41042, USA
Toll Free Tel: +1 800 634 7064
E-mail: cserve@routledge_ny.com

Distributed in Canada by
Taylor & Francis
74 Rolark Drive
Scarborough, Ontario M1R 4G2, Canada
Toll Free Tel: +1 877 226 2237
E-mail: tal_fran@istar.ca

Distributed in the rest of the world by
ITPS Limited
Cheriton House
North Way
Andover, Hampshire SP10 5BE, UK
Tel: +44 (0)1264 332424
E-mail: reception@itps.co.uk

The front cover design incorporates a photograph of "Field" by Hugh Lorigan.
"Field" derives from the idea of an area of activity, study or exploration: in medicine this would be oncology; in art it would be ceramics. Use of this term in the visual arts would be as a colour field, a scattering or placement of objects on an area which itself becomes the matrix or field. On the cover of this book these pieces have different connotations from those they might have in a gallery. Lorigan Ceramics, Old Buttermarket, Shandon Craft Centre, Shandon, Cork, Ireland. Tel: +353 (0) 21 439 9022; email: hughlorigan@eircom.net

Composition by Wearset Ltd, Boldon, Tyne and Wear
Printed and bound in Great Britain by Biddles Ltd

Contents

Contributors

Stephen Beard MSc
RT1 Health Solutions
Research Triangle Institute
Williams House
Manchester
UK

Germana Beltrami MD
Division of Hematology and Stem Cell
Transplantation Unit
Casa Sollievo della Sofferenza – IRCCS
San Giovanni Rotondo, Foggia
Italy

Rhada Bhaskaran MB
Cancer Research UK Department of Medical
Oncology
Christie Hospital
Manchester
UK

Paul Burt MB FRCR FRCP
Cancer Research UK Department of Medical
Oncology
Christie Hospital
Manchester
UK

Angelo Michele Carella MD
Division of Hematology and Stem Cell
Transplantation Unit
Casa Sollievo della Sofferenza – IRCCS
San Giovanni Rotondo, Foggia
Italy

Rajesh Chopra PhD MB MRCPath MRCP
Stem and Leukaemia Cell Biology Group
Paterson Institute for Cancer Research
Christie Hospital
Manchester
UK

Bertrand Coiffier MD
Service D'Hématologie
Centre Hospitalier Lyon-Sud
Hospices Civils de Lyon
Pierre-Bénite
France

Maria Teresa Corsetti MD
Division of Hematology and Stem Cell
Transplantation Unit
Casa Sollievo della Sofferenza – IRCCS
San Giovanni Rotondo, Foggia
Italy

Rainer F Storb MD
Fred Hutchinson Cancer Research Center
Seattle WA
USA

Ron Stout MB FRCP FRCR
Cancer Research UK Department of Medical
Oncology
Christie Hospital
Manchester
UK

John W Sweetenham MB DM FRCP
Cancer Research UK Wessex Medical Oncology
Unit
Southampton General Hospital
Southampton
UK

Nydia G Testa MD
Kay Kendall Laboratory
Patterson Institute for Cancer Research
Christie Hospital
Manchester
UK

Nicholas Thatcher MB FRCP DMRT DCH Eng
Cancer Research UK Department of Medical
Oncology
Christie Hospital
Manchester
UK

**Elisabeth Vandenberghe PhD MB MRCP
MRCPath**
Haematology Department
St James's Hospital
Dublin
Ireland

Jaap Verweij PhD MD
Department of Medical Oncology
Rotterdam Cancer Institute
Daniel den Hoed Kliniek and University
Hospital
Rotterdam
The Netherlands

Preface

High dose therapy has changed enormously over the last 10 years. The early 1990s saw the cautious introduction of stem cell-supported high dose therapy in clinical trials as salvage therapy for rare tumour types. It quickly became apparent that stem cell-supported ablative therapy was associated with more rapid haematological recovery than bone marrow-supported treatment, translating into lower transplant-related morbidity and mortality. This procedure was extended to a number of common, chemosensitive tumours, initially as salvage therapy in advanced disease but then as adjuvant therapy. The reports from the European Bone Marrow Transplantation Registry catalogue a year-on-year increase in the use of this technology from 1990 until 1998. Initial enthusiasm was subsequently tempered by a number of large negative trials in breast cancer, targeted therapy in chronic myeloid leukaemia and the development of non-myeloablative allogeneic transplantation. At present, the estimated use of high dose therapy is one in 2000 persons per 10 years.

The late 1990s were characterized by a more cautious application of this technology, not least because of stricter control of resources by health care commissioners. Hand in hand with this was a realization that self-regulation using accreditation standards was vital to ensure clinical quality. We also saw further scientific and technological developments, with the appreciation that modulation of the immune system in allogeneic-supported procedures could maximize the therapeutic benefit whilst reducing the morbidity of myeloablative procedures.

Our aim in *High Dose Chemotherapy: Principles and Practice* has been to summarize the current state of the art in high dose therapy and to indicate the direction it may take in the next few years. This text is designed for haematologists and oncologists in training, or accredited specialists not working in this field. It is an educational text rather than a reference book. With this in mind, we asked the leading authorities to write an overview of their area of expertise. We felt it was important to cover a number of areas, including the rationale behind this treatment, day-to-day clinical management of high dose therapy patients and the disease-related chapters, to inform the many trainees and oncologists who will be exposed to these patients during their careers. We also felt it important to take a forward perspective, and have asked authors to predict how stem cell transplantation may develop in the future.

We are grateful to all our expert contributors for their hard work, dedication and patience; you are in good company.

PL
EV

Part 1
Scientific basis of high dose chemotherapy

1

Haemopoiesis and isolation of stem cells

Erika A de Wynter, T Michael Dexter and Nydia G Testa

CONTENTS • **Introduction** • **Haemopoiesis** • **Isolation of stem and progenitor cells**

INTRODUCTION

Our knowledge of the regulation and function of the haemopoietic system has progressed enormously, due to the variety of experimental assays that allow precise definition of developmental stages. These assays permitted the discovery of an array of regulatory cytokines, many of which have already been incorporated into clinical practice. The haemopoietic tissue offers a system in which physiological differentiation, proliferation and senescence can be investigated. This has led to the demand for purified or enriched populations of specific haemopoietic cells for clinical applications, gene therapy and stem cell research. Current work centres on new treatment for elimination of malignant cells, ex vivo manipulation of primitive haemopoietic cells and better prevention of graft-versus-host disease (GVHD). In this chapter we will consider some aspects of haemopoiesis including the structure and development of the tissue, the haemopoietic system and regulation of cell production, followed by identification and methods for isolation of primitive haemopoietic cells.

HAEMOPOIESIS

Haemopoiesis is the process by which mature blood cells are generated. The mature cells recognizable in the blood as erythrocytes, granulocytes (neutrophils, basophils, eosinophils), monocytes, platelets, and T and B lymphocytes arise from a small number of stem cells present in the bone marrow. The scale of production of the blood cells is vast, with a daily turnover of 2.2×10^{11} erythrocytes and 10^{11} neutrophils, which means that the haemopoietic tissue generates around 3×10^{11} blood cells each day to replace those cells which are lost in natural wastage and senescence. In addition to these steady-state requirements, cell production must be adjusted in response to increased demand, for example during stress situations caused by infection, bleeding, decreased oxygen availability, abnormal cell destruction, or following damage due to radiation and/or chemotherapy.

Development of haemopoietic tissue

During early fetal development, the fetal liver is the main site of haemopoiesis, with erythropoiesis starting as dominant and granulopoiesis developing later. The spleen is also haemopoietic until about the time of birth, although making a smaller contribution than the liver. From week 20 of gestation, the bone marrow becomes increasingly important and it becomes the main haemopoietic organ. During the first 2–3 years of life, part of the active marrow found in all organs is gradually replaced by inactive fatty marrow. In the adult, active marrow is only found in the epiphyses of long bones and in trabecular bone, and in the sternum, ribs, cranium, vertebra and pelvis. There is no further expansion of the tissue after infancy, but there may be a decrease in older people.

The liver and spleen, however, conserve the capacity to sustain extramedullar haemopoiesis through life and may be recolonized if required (for example, in patients with haemolytic anaemia) by stem cells from the bone marrow that have migrated via the circulation. It follows from this that stem cells are found in peripheral blood, albeit in very low numbers, in normal individuals. It is noteworthy that at the time of birth, there are still large numbers of primitive cells in the cord blood, numbers similar to those in adult bone marrow.[1] Although the number of primitive cells in blood falls rapidly after birth, by administration of cytokines it can be increased to a magnitude that makes blood a viable alternative to bone marrow as a source of cells for transplantation.

The haemopoietic system

The haemopoietic system belongs, with gut and skin, to the hierarchical tissues of the body, where short-lived differentiated end cells are continuously replaced through processes of proliferation, differentiation and maturation starting at the level of stem cells. The pluripotent stem cells give rise to more developmentally restricted progeny, the progenitor cells, and the progeny of these progenitor cells in any particular lineage are the maturing cells. Figure 1.1 provides a scheme of haemopoiesis divided broadly into three compartments: the stem cell, progenitor cell and maturing cell compartments. Although depicted as separate compartments,

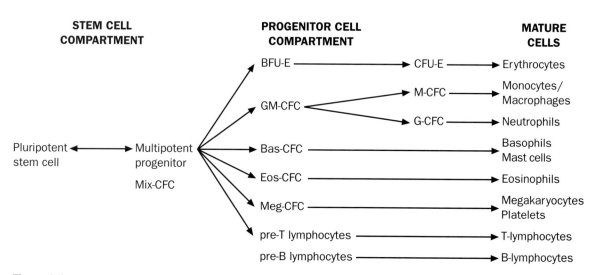

Figure 1.1

Scheme of haemopoiesis. Bas-CFC, basophil colony forming cell; BFU-E, burst forming unit–erythroid colony forming cell; CFU-E, colony forming unit–erythroid; Eos-CFC, eosinophil colony forming cell; G-CFC, granulocyte colony forming cell; GM-CFC, granulocyte–macrophage colony forming cell; M-CFC, macrophage colony forming cell; Meg-CFC, megakaryocyte colony forming cell; Mix-CFC, multipotent colony forming cell–mixed.

the process is essentially a continuum with cells proceeding irreversibly towards maturation.

Stem cells comprise between 0.01 and 0.05% of the total marrow population and are generally quiescent under steady-state conditions, most being in a G_0 state of the cell cycle. They are only reluctantly induced to divide as seen by their relative resistance to cell cycle active agents such as 5-fluorouracil. Indeed, even after in vivo cytotoxic injury, about 48 h are required before primitive populations of quiescent cells are recruited into cell cycle and enter its S phase.[2,3] Stem cells are classically defined as those cells which have the ability to generate all the lymphoid and myeloid lineages, have extensive proliferation potential and have the capacity to self-renew.

The progenitor cells may be regarded as transitory cells which under the appropriate stimuli will divide, differentiate and progress down their developmental pathways. As the progenitor cells move towards maturation, their proliferative and differentiation potential is gradually diminished. It is generally agreed that the decision to enter a particular differentiation lineage distinguishes the progenitor from the stem cell populations. The commitment to differentiation appears to be irreversible: for example, erythroid progenitors manipulated to express receptors for macrophage colony stimulating factor (M-CSF, which has an important role in macrophage development) still develop into erythroid cells when exposed to this cytokine.[4] Conversely, macrophage progenitor cells manipulated to express erythropoietin (Epo) receptors develop into macrophages and not into erythroid cells in response to Epo stimulation.[5] As development and maturation proceed, cells can be recognized morphologically by the use of appropriate staining techniques and eventually reach a stage where the recognizable mature cells are released into the circulatory system.

Assays for stem and progenitor cells

Stem cells are assessed experimentally by in vivo or in vitro methods, because they cannot be distinguished by any morphological criteria. A key property of stem cells is the ability to repopulate the haemopoietic tissue. Thus, experimentally, cells with the ability to regenerate haemopoiesis in lethally irradiated recipient animals for 6 or more months are defined as marrow repopulating cells (MRC). This assay is now regarded as a definitive measure of stem cells in the mouse. Human marrow repopulating cells may only be measured by experimental transplant assays of human cells using xenografts. The most commonly used involves immunosuppressed SCID or NOD/SCID mice which, when inoculated with human haemopoietic cells following sublethal irradiation, allow the establishment of active human haemopoiesis.[6–10] The cell responsible for initiating engraftment in these mice has been termed the SCID-repopulating cell or SRC. Although this assay is widely used, at present it is not fully understood: the numbers of cells required for successful transplantation are about an order of magnitude higher than the number of murine cells required to rescue mice from haemopoietic death following ablation. The reason for this low efficiency is not clear. Furthermore, there is a bias towards B cell differentiation and the numbers of human myeloid cells produced may be very small.

An alternative in vitro assay used frequently for detecting primitive cell populations is the long-term culture initiating cell (LTC-IC) assay. The human LTC-IC has been defined as a primitive haemopoietic cell responsible for the output of clonogenic progenitors (colony forming cells, CFC) after 5 weeks or more in culture on a haemopoietic supportive stroma.[11] To determine the absolute number of LTC-IC, limiting dilution assays are performed.[12] The murine LTC-IC cultures can regenerate haemopoiesis in an irradiated mouse, suggesting that they contain MRC,[13] but this property has not been demonstrated for human LTC-IC. A similar assay, the cobblestone area forming cell (CAFC), uses a direct visual end point, i.e. a phase-dark haemopoietic focus, rather than the generation of CFC.[14] When this is combined with limiting dilution analysis, it becomes possible to make an assessment of the absolute number of LTC-IC present in a population. Although LTC-ICs are thought to represent immature haemopoietic progenitors, they are still heterogeneous and a small percentage (c.10%) can give rise to large numbers of secondary CFC more than 60 days after seeding on competent stroma. These cells are termed extended-LTCIC (ELTCIC).[15]

There are a number of other in vitro assays currently in use, all of which measure some aspect of stem cell activity. The blast colony forming cell (blast CFC) assay allows formation of colonies with high secondary recloning capacity, self-renewal potential and the ability to generate multiple lineage committed progeny.[16] High proliferative potential colony forming cells (HPP-CFC) generate macroscopic colonies containing up to 50 000 cells when cultured in a semi-solid medium.[17] An in vitro colony forming assay, the CFU-A, which detects primitive cells of both murine and human origin in agar, was described by Lorimore.[18,19] It is likely that these assays identify similar or overlapping populations.

The detection of progenitor cell populations was aided by the development of in vitro clonogenic soft-gel systems.[20,21] In these assays the haemopoietic cells are immobilized in a soft-gel matrix (agar, agarose, methylcellulose or plasma clot) and cultured with an enriched or conditioned medium containing the appropriate growth stimuli. Under these conditions the clonogenic cells proliferate and form colonies of recognizable mature cells; the cells giving rise to colonies are termed colony forming cells (CFC). These assays have allowed identification of bipotent progenitors such as granulocyte–macrophage colony forming cells (GM-CFC) and multipotent progenitors, Mix-CFC (multipotent colony forming cell-mixed) or GEMM (granulocyte, erythroid, macrophage, megakaryocyte) which proliferate and mature into cells of the various lineages. As the progenitor cells become progressively more limited in their potential for differentiation and proliferation they become restricted to one lineage giving rise to small colonies containing less than 100 cells. The cell populations detected in clonogenic assays and their place in the scheme of haemopoiesis are illustrated in Fig. 1.1.

Regulation of cell production

To maintain steady-state haemopoiesis both positive and negative regulation is necessary, enabling the system to respond to stimulation and to avoid overproduction of cells. Haemopoietic cell proliferation is stimulated by specific regulatory factors. The first of these regulators was identified based on the ability to support the growth of distinct haemopoietic colonies in soft-gel assays.[22–24] They were termed colony stimulating factors (CSFs): multi-CSF (also known as interleukin-3 – IL-3), GM-CSF, G-CSF (granulocyte CSF) and M-CSF (macrophage CSF, also known as CSF-1). The genes coding for the CSFs, as well as many other cytokines, have been cloned and sequenced and large amounts of recombinant material can now be produced using a variety of expression systems.

It is appropriate here to clarify the varied terminology used for haemopoietic regulators, which developed using descriptive, response-related terminology. One example has already been given: the CSFs, which were defined by their capacity to stimulate in vitro colony growth. The interleukins were described as molecules produced by white blood cells, like T cells, able to exert their effect on other white cells. Later, it became apparent that the effects of interleukins were much wider and could be targeted on several tissues. For example, receptors for interleukins were shown to be present on fibroblasts, and endothelial and neural cells.[25] Table 1.1 lists the more relevant of these interleukins, the CSFs and their haemopoietic target cell populations. It is clear from Table 1.1 that the actions of individual haemopoietic regulators are not restricted to cells of a single lineage and that there is considerable overlap in the target cell populations. For example, granulocytic production may be stimulated by G-CSF, GM-CSF, IL-3, stem cell factor (SCF) or IL-6 and high doses of M-CSF.

Table 1.1 Haemopoietic growth factors and their haemopoietic target cells	
Growth factor	**Target CFC***
GM-CSF	HPP-CFC, Mix-CFC, GM-CFC, BFU-E, Eos-CFC, Meg-CFC
G-CSF	HPP-CFC, Mix-CFC, GM-CFC
M-CSF	HPP-CFC, GM-CFC
Erythropoietin	BFU-E, CFU-E,
SCF	HPP-CFC, Mix-CFC, GM-CFC, BFU-E, Bas-CFC
Flt-3 ligand	Mix-CFC, GM-CFC, BFU-E
IL-1	HPP-CFC
IL-3	HPP-CFC, Mix-CFC, GM-CFC, BFU-E, Eos-CFC, Bas-CFC, Meg-CFC
IL-4	GM-CFC, BFU-E, Bas-CFC
IL-5	Eos-CFC
IL-6	HPP-CFC, GM-CFC
IL-9	BFU-E
IL-11	GM-CFC, BFU-E, Meg-CFC
Thrombopoietin	Meg-CFC, BFU-E

*Bas-CFC, basophil colony forming cell; BFU-E, burst forming unit–erythroid; CFU-E, forming unit–erythroid; Eos-CFC, eosinophil colony forming cell; GM-CFC, granulocyte–macrophage colony forming cell; HPP-CFC, high proliferation potential colony forming cell; Meg-CFC, megakaryocyte colony forming cell; Mix-CFC, multipotent colony forming cell–mixed.

An expanding group of cytokines called chemokines (chemotactic cytokines) was originally defined by their property of exerting chemotactic effects on cells involved in inflammatory processes. It is now known that many of the more than 50 chemokines described also exert effects on the regulation of haemopoietic cell production or function.[26]

Several general properties are ascribed to cytokines: they may be produced by a variety of cells, they tend to have a variety of effects on different (or even on the same) target cells, and different cytokines may synergize when acting on the same cells. This synergy may be expressed in different ways: for example, one CFC may produce larger progeny and/or more

CFC may be recruited by the action of several cytokines when acting in unison.[27] In addition, cytokines may modulate the expression of receptors for other cytokines, increasing or decreasing the number of receptors. They may also influence signalling by receptors for another cytokine.

Clearly, there is a high degree of complexity in the regulation of the haemopoietic system where deficiencies in production of a cytokine will not necessarily result in cessation of a specific maturation pathway.

Inhibitors of haemopoiesis have also been described and perhaps need to be postulated as ways of avoiding fluctuations in the numbers of cells produced and also as a means of preventing overproduction once an exceptional need for cells has been satisfied. The two most commonly described are macrophage inflammatory protein 1-α (MIP-1α) and transforming growth factor-beta (TGF-β). They fulfil the characteristics of inhibitors in that they are not toxic and their actions are reversible. Primitive haemopoietic cells exposed to MIP-1α do not enter DNA synthesis (S phase) of the cell cycle. This effect is seen in primitive cells (in this context, MIP-1α was originally described as a stem cell inhibitor), but MIP-1α may also exert a stimulatory action on some of the more mature subpopulations of CFC.[28,29] The action of TGF-β on the proliferation of early and late progenitor cells is similar. Other molecules, such as the pentapeptide (pEEDCK; Glu-Glu-Asp-Cys-Lys) and tetrapeptide (AcSDKP; Acetyl-N-Ser-Asp-Lys-Pro) also have a reversible action, inhibiting cell progress into S phase of the cycle. A number of other suppressor molecules have been reported [e.g. prostaglandins, lactoferritin, isoferritins, negative regulatory protein (NRP), platelet factor 4 and interferon-inducible protein] but in many cases their effects may be indirect and complex and, in some cases, are controversial.

Phenotype of stem and progenitor cells

In conjunction with biological assays, progress has also been made in determining the phenotype of primitive haemopoietic cells. This allows purification of discrete cell subpopulations, or even the isolation of single cells, which may be characterized further by biological assays. Defining the expression of certain epitopes as a function of maturation and/or lineage commitment is essential for better separation of subpopulations of primitive cells.

One of the most useful markers characterized is the CD34 antigen, which is a membrane glycoprotein present on 1–4% of human bone marrow cells.[30] CD34 is expressed at high levels on almost all stem and progenitor cells, though expression declines as cells mature. Although no function has been unequivocally assigned to

this molecule, it may act as a regulator of haemopoietic cell adhesion in the bone marrow microenvironment and may also be involved in the maintenance of the haemopoietic stem/progenitor phenotype and function.[31,32] When CD34+ selected cells were re-infused into patients following myeloablative chemotherapy, haemopoiesis was completely reconstituted, indicating that the cells responsible for engraftment reside within the CD34+ compartment.[33] In steady-state peripheral blood the percentage of CD34+ cells is normally about 0.02–0.10% but this can be increased dramatically if bone marrow cells are mobilized into the blood with growth factors, chemotherapy or both.[34,35] After mobilization, the cells harvested from the circulation (peripheral blood progenitor cells or PBPC) contain large numbers of CD34+ cells, the committed progenitors of various lineages and a small proportion consisting of primitive progenitors and stem cells. The presence of CD34+ cells in haemopoietic samples is now used routinely in the clinic as a marker of stem and progenitor cells.

The CD34+ cell population is heterogeneous, so by itself the CD34 marker cannot distinguish stem cells from progenitor cells. However, using a judicious combination of various other cell surface markers, primitive haemopoietic cells can be classified by their expression – or lack of expression – from the more differentiated progenitors. Some of these markers are listed in Table 1.2 and include the recently reported AC133 antigen (now CD133) that is expressed on human cells highly enriched in SRC and LTC-IC.[29]

The value of the CD34 antigen as a marker for human stem cells has been challenged by work aimed at identification of a homogeneous population of stem cells. Distinct populations of cells have been identified which are enriched in long-term repopulating activity but lack the CD34 marker.[36–38] As the presence of the CD34 marker varies with the functional status of the cells, it is possible to detect stem cells which are CD34−.[39] However, for practical purposes, the CD34 marker is present on the majority of stem cells.

Table 1.2 Phenotype of human stem and progenitor cells

	LTRC	LTC-IC	Progenitors (early)	Progenitors (late)
CD34	+	+	+	+
CD33	–	–	–	+
CD38	–		+	+
CD45RA	?	–	Low	+
CD71	–	–	Low/+	+
CD90 (Thy 1)	Low		Low	
CD117 (c-kit)	Low	?		+
Lin (lineage)	–	–		
HLA-DR	–	–		+
AC133	+	+	+/–	
Rhodamine	–	Low	+	

LTRC, long term repopulating cell; LTC-IC, long term culture initiating cell.

ISOLATION OF STEM AND PROGENITOR CELLS

Historically, enriched populations of stem and/or progenitor cells were separated based on physical properties such as cell size and buoyant density, using density gradient centrifugation or counterflow elutriation. Cell surface markers characteristic of primitive cells were identified and, with the development of monoclonal antibodies and their specificity for defined epitopes, this led to new purification strategies. By combining flow cytometry with dyes that stain the nucleic acid content of the cell, populations of stem and progenitor cells can be distinguished.[40,41] In addition, immunoadsorption systems are now available for analytical purposes, as well as larger devices for clinical use. These latter systems are usually based on the use of ferromagnetic beads or affinity columns and allow easy access to highly enriched immature cell populations.

Flow cytometry

Flow cytometry is a process in which individual cells pass in single file in a fluid stream, which passes a light beam. This light beam usually originates in a laser and sensors or detectors register the light pulses emitted by each passing cell. The detectors measure physical characteristics such as the size and granularity (or nuclear to cytoplasmic ratio) of the cells as well as the fluorescence intensity generated by fluorochromes. In practice, a monoclonal antibody is conjugated to a fluorochrome and bound to the target cell. As the cell passes through the laser light beam the fluorochrome emits light which is measured and recorded. Several cell surface markers may be bound simultaneously to a cell provided each marker is conjugated to a different fluorochrome. In this manner, it is possible to perform detailed analysis of individual cells by combining information obtained on both the physical and fluorescent parameters. Cell sorting developed from flow cytometry and allows separation and collection of cells of

Table 1.3 Stem and progenitor cell separation using stains and dyes

Dyes and stains	References
BODIPY aminoacetaldehyde (BAAA) fluorescent substrate for aldehyde dehydrogenase (enzyme high in primitive cells)	Storms et al.[49]
Merocyanine 540 (MC540) to distinguish quiescent and metabolically active cells	Pyatt et al.[50]
Hoechst/rhodamine	Leemhuis et al.[51]
Rhodamine 123	Udomsakdi et al.[52]
Hoechst	Gothot et al.[42]

interest displaying defined characteristics. In the past, there were some limitations on the use of the flow cytometer for handling large clinical samples, as the speed of cell sorting was low, generally less than 3000 cells/s. This has been overcome as instruments with sorting rates of >25 000 cells/s have been developed, eliminating the tedium of sorting for rare events or sorting samples with large cell numbers.

A variety of fluorescent stains and dyes may also be used in flow cytometry to analyse primitive cell populations as outlined in Table 1.3. Dyes such as Hoechst 33342, which stains the cellular content of DNA, have long been used to identify cells in different phases of the cell cycle (G0/G1 and G2/S + M). A combination of Hoechst and Pyronin Y, which stains the RNA content of the cell, now allow sorting and collection of viable cells in the G0 or G1 phase of the cycle.[42] One procedure based on the ability of primitive cells to efflux Hoechst 33342 has recently been used to identify an extremely small and homogeneous population of cells highly enriched in LTC-IC.[37] By exploiting the intrinsic properties of primitive cells, such as quiescence, metabolic inactivity and high concentrations of specific enzymes, enriched populations of stem and progenitor cells can be obtained.

Immunoadsorption techniques

Positive and negative selection
Positive or negative selection is generally performed using ferromagnetic beads. For CD34+ cell isolation, positive selection is generally less expensive as only one antibody is required. A second advantage is speed of isolation compared with negative selection, which may require multiple cycles before target cells are sufficiently enriched. Cells are labelled by a direct or indirect method. In the direct method, mononuclear cells are incubated with paramagnetic beads coupled to antigen specific antibodies. The labelled cell population can then be isolated directly from the complex mixture of cells. Indirect methods involve addition of antigen specific primary antibody to the cell suspension to label the target cells. After incubation, excess primary antibody is removed and the labelled cells identified by a secondary antibody. The indirect method is preferred if only low affinity primary antibodies are available.

Some antibodies can cause cells to transmit signals across the membrane, i.e. antigen activation. To avoid isolation of activated cells, negative selection is preferable. In negative selection, all unwanted cell types are removed from the sample so that the enriched cells obtained will not have bound antibody at any time during the purification procedure. This method is obligatory where there is no specific antibody for the cells required, though in general yield and purity are lower than for positive isolation. In practice, a panel of monoclonal antibodies recognizing specific lineage markers for myeloid, lymphoid and erythroid cells are used to deplete the mononuclear cell population and to obtain CD34+ cells often referred to as CD34+Lin− cells.

Immunomagnetic beads and immunoaffinity columns

The beads are available in a range of sizes from 6 μm to 60 nm, i.e. from cell size to submicroscopic particle size. In the direct method, mononuclear cells and paramagnetic beads coupled to CD34 antibodies are incubated together. The target cells are then isolated by application of a magnetic field. Alternatively, CD34+ cells may be labelled with a biotinylated or unconjugated CD34 antibody. Labelled cells are subsequently bound to paramagnetic beads coated with streptavidin or anti-mouse antibodies. The target cells are then captured in a magnetic field.

The basis of the immunoaffinity column system is the strong affinity between biotin and avidin. A biotin-conjugated CD34 antibody binds to CD34+ cells in a cell suspension, after which the cells are passed through a column that contains avidin-coated beads. This results in specific capture of the target cells. The attached biotinylated antibody bind to the avidin-coated beads in the column while unwanted cells flow through the system. Because the cells are continuously flowing through the column, non-specific binding is kept to an absolute minimum. Purified cells are then released from the column by gentle agitation and washing.

All of the systems yield enriched populations, though in general column techniques are preferred because they are quick, relatively easy and give good results in a short time. There have been a number of reports examining and comparing the performance of the different CD34+ cell selection systems.[43–46]

Clinical applications for isolated cells

Two main factors influence the long-term outcome of autologous stem cell transplanted patients: (1) the lack of GVL effect and (2) minimal residual disease reinfused with the graft persisting after the conditioning regime and contributing to relapse.[47,48] This second issue may at least in part be addressed by 'purging' techniques. The possibility of selecting the haemopoietic cells able to engraft and sustain haemopoiesis appears to be a rational strategy of purging. Although the clinical value of purging still has to be established, the positive selection of haemopoietic progenitors appears an alternative to other forms of purging by negative selection.

The rationale for the use of CD34+ selected cells is to reduce the tumour cell contamination by 2–4 log in the autologous setting or the T cell load by 3–4 log in the case of allogeneic transplantation. As a result of preclinical studies demonstrating that CD34+ cells were able to reconstitute the haemopoietic system after myeloablation, a number of CD34 selection systems were developed for clinical use. Those currently available are closed and almost completely automated systems that guarantee a sterile procedure and are based on the beads and column methods described above.

Allogeneic bone marrow transplantation is currently the treatment of choice for some malignant haematological disorders. As matched unrelated donors or mismatched related donors are frequently used, this procedure is accompanied by a significant high risk of graft failure and GVHD. The presence of T cells in the graft may in part be responsible for this, and different strategies of T cell purging have been employed. Selection of CD34+ cells enables a high level of T cell depletion to be achieved. Although this has already been used clinically, the clinical usefulness of the method is not universally accepted.

The incidence of LTC-IC in PBPC after G-CSF administration is 1 in 10^4 to 2 in 10^4 mononuclear cells and 1 in 200 CD34+ cells. The purification of LTC-IC is actively pursued in many laboratories using CD34 and other markers, in attempts to isolate, characterize and manipulate where appropriate these cells as targets for gene transfer. Gene therapy for inherited diseases will in many instances require treatment early in life or even in utero. In this context, umbilical cord blood is being considered as a source of target cells for genetic manipulation, as the incidence of CD34+ cells and of colony forming cells in normal cord blood is equivalent to that in bone marrow and is even higher in the cord blood of premature infants.

The selection of CD34+ cells also offers the opportunity of isolating target populations for short-term progenitor expansion and gene manipulation. Ex vivo expanded CD34+ cells can be used to transplant larger numbers of progenitors to further accelerate recovery. Specific clinical situations may take advantage of this procedure, for example patients with heavily pretreated marrow or if cord blood is intended for transplantation of adult patients. Studies are accumulating which demonstrate maintenance of transplantation potential of CD34+ cells expanded ex vivo using combinations of growth factors. However, the usefulness of this approach awaits vigorous demonstration.

CONCLUSIONS

Haemopoietic stem cell transplantation has progressed from a highly experimental procedure to being accepted as the preferred form of treatment for a variety of diseases. Research on composition, content and behaviour of the graft should lead to steady improvement in solving the problems that are still associated with transplantation.

REFERENCES

1. Broxmeyer HE, Douglas GW, Hangoc G et al. Human umbilical cord blood as a potential source of transplantable hematopoietic stem/progenitor cells. Proc Natl Acad Sci USA 1989;86:3828–32.

2. Lahiri SK, van Putten LM. Location of the G0-phase in the cell cycle of the mouse haemopoietic spleen colony forming cells. Cell Tissue Kinetics 1972;5:365–9.
3. Testa NG, de Wynter EA, Weaver A. The study of haemopoietic stem cells in patients: concepts, approaches and cautionary tales. Ann Oncol 1996;7:5–8.
4. McArthur GA, Rohrschneider LR, Johnson GR. Induced expression of c-fms in normal hematopoietic cells shows evidence for both conservation and lineage restriction of signal transduction in response to macrophage colony-stimulating factor. Blood 1994;83:972–81.
5. McArthur GA, Longmore GD, Klingler K, Johnson GR. Lineage-restricted recruitment of immature hematopoietic progenitor cells in response to Epo after normal hematopoietic cell transfection with EpoR. Exp Hematol 1995;23:645–54.
6. McCune JM, Namikawa R, Kaneshima H, Shultz LD, Lieberman M, Weissman IL. The SCID-hu mouse: murine model for the analysis of human hematolymphoid differentiation and function. Science 1988;241:1632–9.
7. Lapidot T, Pflumio F, Doedens M, Murdoch B, Williams DE, Dick JE. Cytokine stimulation of multilineage hematopoiesis from immature human cells engrafted in SCID mice. Science 1992;255:1137–41.
8. Nolta JA, Hanley MB, Kohn DB. Sustained human hematopoiesis in immunodeficient mice by cotransplantation of marrow stroma expressing human interleukin-3: analysis of gene transduction of long-lived progenitors. Blood 1994;83:3041–51.
9. Larochelle A, Vormoor J, Hanenberg H. Identification of primitive human hematopoietic cells capable of repopulating NOD/SCID mouse bone marrow: implications for gene therapy. Nature Med 1996;2:1329–37.
10. Wang JCY, Doedens M, Dick JE. Primitive human hematopoietic cells are enriched in cord blood compared with adult bone marrow or mobilised peripheral blood as measured by the quantitative in vivo SCID-repopulating cell assay. Blood 1997;89:3919–24.
11. Sutherland H, Eaves C, Eaves A. Characterisation and partial purification of human marrow cells capable of initiating long-term hematopoiesis in vitro. Blood 1989; 74:1563–9.
12. Sutherland HJ, Lansdorp PM, Henkelman DH,

Eaves AC, Eaves CJ. Functional characterization of individual human hematopoietic stem cells cultured at limiting dilution on supportive marrow stromal layers. Proc Natl Acad Sci USA 1990;87:3584–88.

13. Ploemacher RE, van der Sluijs JP, van Beurden AJ, Baert MRM, Chan PL. Use of limiting-dilution type long-term marrow cultures in frequency analysis of marrow-repopulating and spleen colony-forming hematopoietic stem cells in the mouse. Blood 1991;78:2527–33.

14. Breems DA, Blokland EAW, Neben S, Ploemacher RE. Frequency analysis of human primitive haematopoietic stem cell subsets using a cobblestone area forming cell assay. Leukemia 1994;8:1095–104.

15. Hao QL, Shah AJ, Thiemann FT, Smorgorzewska EM, Crooks GM. Extended long-term culture reveals a highly quiescent and primitive human haemopoietic progenitor population. Blood 1996;88:3306–13.

16. Nakahata T, Ogawa M. Identification in culture of a class of hemopoietic colony-forming units with extensive capacity to self-renew and generate multipotential hemopoietic colonies. Proc Natl Acad Sci USA 1982;79:3843–7.

17. Bradley TR, Hodgson GS. Detection of primitive macrophage progenitor cells in mouse bone marrow. Blood 1979;54:1446–50.

18. Lorimore SA, Eckmann L, Pragnell IB, Wright EG. Synergistic interactions allow colony formation in vitro by murine haemopoietic stem cells. Leuk Res 1990;14:481–9.

19. Graham GJ, Freshney MG, Donaldson D, Pragnell IB. Purification and biochemical characterisation of human and murine stem cell inhibitors (SCI). Growth Factors 1992;7:151–60.

20. Pluznik DH, Sachs L. The cloning of mast cells in tissue culture. J Cell Physiol 1965;6:319–24.

21. Bradley TR, Metcalf D. The growth of mouse bone marrow cells in vitro. Aust J Exp Biol Med Sci 1966;44:287–300.

22. Metcalf D, Begley CG, Nicola NA, Johnson GR. Quantitative responsiveness of murine hemopoietic populations in vitro and in vivo to recombinant Multi-CSF (IL-3). Exp Hematol 1987;15:288–95.

23. Metcalf D, Nicola NA. Proliferative effects of purified granulocyte colony-stimulating factor (G-CSF) on normal mouse hematopoietic cells. J Cell Physiol 1983;116:198–206.

24. Metcalf D. The granulocyte–macrophage colony stimulating factors. Science 1985;229:16–22.

25. Collard R, Gearing A. The cytokine facts book. London: Academic Press, 1994.

26. Broxmeyer HE, Kim CH. Regulation of hematopoiesis in a sea of chemokine family members with a plethora of redundant activities. Exp Hematol 1999;27:1113–23.

27. Metcalf D. Haemopoietic regulators: redundancy or subtlety? Blood 1993;82:3515–23.

28. Broxmeyer HE, Sherry B, Cooper S et al. Comparative analysis of the human macrophage inflammatory protein family of cytokines (chemokines) on proliferation of human myeloid progenitor cells. J Immunol 1993;150:3448–58.

29. de Wynter EA, Durig J, Cross MA, Heyworth CM, Testa NG. Differential response of CD34+ cells isolated from cord blood and bone marrow to MIP-1α and the expression of MIP-1α receptors on these immature cells. Stem Cells 1998;16:349–56.

30. Civin CI, Strauss LC, Brovall V, Fackler MJ, Schwartz JF, Shaper JH. Antigenic analysis of hematopoiesis. III. A hematopoietic progenitor cell surface antigen defined by a monoclonal antibody raised against KG-1a cells. J Immunol 1984;133:157–65.

31. Fackler M, Krause DS, Smith OM, Civin CI, May WS. Full length but not truncated CD34 inhibits hematopoietic cell differentiation of M1 cells. Blood 1995;85:3040–7.

32. Healy L, May D, Grosveld F, Greaves M, Enver T. The stem cell antigen CD34 functions as a regulator of haemopoietic adhesion. Proc Natl Acad Sci USA 1995;92:12240–4.

33. Berenson RJ, Bensinger WI, Hill RS et al. Engraftment after infusion of CD34+ marrow cells in patients with breast cancer or neuroblastoma. Blood 1991;77:1717–22.

34. Gianni A, Siena S, Bregni M. Granulocyte-macrophage colony stimulating factor to harvest circulating haemopoietic stem cells for autotransplantation. Lancet 1989;2:580–5.

35. Siena S, Bregni M, Brando B. Circulation of CD34+ hematopoietic stem cells in the peripheral blood of high dose cyclophosphamide treated patients: Enhancement by intravenous recombinant human granulocyte–macrophage colony stimulating factor. Blood 1989;74:1905–14.

36. Bhatia M, Bonnet D, Murdoch B, Gan OI, Dick JE. A newly discovered class of human haemopoietic cells with SCID-repopulating activity. Nature Med 1998;4:1038–45.

37. Goodell MA, Rosenzweig M, Kim H et al. Dye efflux studies suggest that haemopoietic stem cells expressing low or undetectable levels of CD34 antigen exist in multiple species. Nature Med 1997;3:1337–45.

38. Zanjani ED, Almeida-Porada G, Livingston AG, Flake AW, Ogawa M. Human bone marrow CD34− cells engraft in vivo and undergo multi-lineage expression that includes giving rise to CD34+ cells. Exp Hematol 1998;26:353–60.

39. Sato T, Laver JH, Ogawa M. Reversible expression of CD34 by murine hematopoietic stem cells. Blood 1999;94:2548–54.

40. Visser JWM, Van Bekkum DW. Purification of pluripotent hemopoietic stem cells: past and present. Exp Hematol 1990;18:248–56.

41. Bertoncello I, Bradley TR, Hodgson GS, Dunlop JM. The resolution, enrichment, and organization of normal bone marrow high proliferative potential colony-forming cell subsets on the basis of rhodamine-123 fluorescence. Exp Hematol 1991;19:174–8.

42. Gothot A, Pyatt R, McMahel J, Rice S, Srour EF. Functional heterogeneity of human CD34+ cells isolated in subcompartments of the G0/G1 phase of the cell cycle. Blood 1997;90(11):4384–93.

43. de Wynter EA, Coutinho LH, Pei X-T et al. Comparison of purity and enrichment of CD34+ cells from bone marrow, umbilical cord and peripheral blood (primed for apheresis) using five separation systems. Stem Cells 1995;13:524–32.

44. Paulus U, Dreger P, Viehmann K, von Neuhoff N, Schmitz N. Purging peripheral blood progenitor cell grafts from lymphoma cells: quantitative comparison of immunomagnetic CD34+ selection systems. Stem Cells 1997;15:297–304.

45. Winslow JM, Liesveld JL, Ryan DH, Dipersio JF, Abboud CN. CD34+ progenitor cell isolation from blood and marrow: a comparison of techniques for small-scale selection. Bone Marrow Transplant 1994;14:265–71.

46. de Wynter EA, Ryder D, Lanza F et al. Multicentre European study comparing selection techniques for isolation of CD34+ cells. Bone Marrow Transplant 1999;23:1191–6.

47. Gribben JG, Freedman AS, Neuberg D et al. Immunologic purging of marrow assessed by PCR before autologous bone marrow transplantation for B-cell lymphoma. N Engl J Med 1991;325:1525–33.

48. Brenner MK, Rill DR, Moen RC et al. Gene-marking to trace origin of relapse after autologous bone-marrow transplantation. Lancet 1993;341:85–6.

49. Storms RW, Trujillo AP, Springer JB et al. Isolation of primitive human hematopoietic progenitors on the basis of aldehyde dehydrogenase activity. Proc Natl Acad Sci USA 1999;96:9118–23.

50. Pyatt RE, Jenski LL, Allen R et al. Use of merocyanine 540 for the isolation of quiescent, primitive human bone marrow hematopoietic progenitor cells. J Hematother 1999;8:189–98.

51. Leemhuis T, Yoder MC, Grigsby S, Aguero B, Eder P, Srour EF. Isolation of primitive human bone marrow hematopoietic progenitor cells using Hoechst 33342 and Rhodamine 123. Exp Hematol 1996;24:1215–24.

52. Udomsakdi C, Eaves CJ, Sutherland HJ, Lansdorp PM. Separation of functionally distinct subpopulations of primitive human hematopoietic cells using rhodamine-123. Exp Hematol 1991;19:338–42.

2

Pharmacology and principles of high dose chemotherapy

Miguel Hernández-Bronchud and Rhoda Molife

CONTENTS   Introduction • Pre-clinical and theoretical models • Pharmacokinetic and pharmacodynamic considerations • Agents commonly used in high dose setting • Commonly used regimens • Conclusion

INTRODUCTION

The advent of two new technologies in the field of chemotherapy has given impetus to the rapid growth of the use of high doses of chemotherapeutic agents in chemosensitive malignant disease.[1-4] The first is the clinical use of granulocyte and granulocyte–macrophage colony stimulating factors (G-CSF and GM-CSF, respectively) which enabled the use of higher than standard doses of chemotherapy by increasing the dose intensity.[5] The second is transplantation with previously mobilized peripheral blood stem cells (PBSC), permitting a faster time to haematological recovery following the administration of myelo-ablative doses of chemotherapy.[6] Furthermore, there has been a remarkable development in the supportive care of patients, making high dose therapy safer and more tolerable. In most centres, the treatment-related mortality has fallen from >20% to 2–5%.[7]

High dose chemotherapy (HDC) has now achieved widespread use in many oncology centres, with outpatient management of some parts of the procedure.[5] While it is too early to draw conclusions regarding the validity of this approach in terms of increased cure rates or survival, the considerable expense and not negligible treatment-related toxicities cannot have palliation of symptoms as their only goal. It would prove disappointing if their use did not result in some survival advantage.[8,9] This chapter will review the pharmacokinetic (PK) and pharmacodynamic (PD) aspects of HDC and will outline the regimens most commonly used.

PRE-CLINICAL AND THEORETICAL MODELS

The use of HDC derives from laboratory and clinical observations of tumour cell growth properties and the ability of chemotherapy agents to influence the growth of both replicating and non-replicating tumour populations.[7] The basic concepts are largely derived from work carried out by Skipper and Schabel using murine models exploring tumour cell growth and cell kill, dose, dose intensity, schedule and type of chemotherapy. These concepts have been established as Skipper's laws and are outlined below. They are not true 'natural laws' but empirical observations in experimental models.

The first of these laws is that the doubling time of proliferating cancer cells is constant,

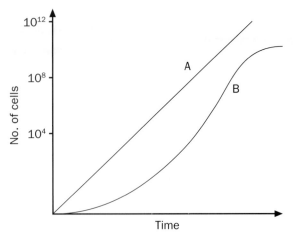

Figure 2.1
Two models of kinetics of tumour growth. In curve A the growth is exponential. In curve B there is progressive slowing of growth rate with increasing size, termed Gompertzian growth.[10]

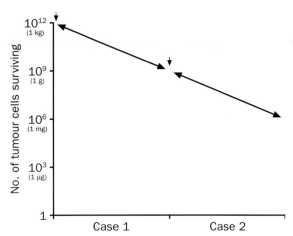

Figure 2.2
The 'fractional cell kill' hypothesis. In case 1, the drug dose (arrow indicates point at which drug is given) reduces the tumour from 10^{12} cells to 10^9 cells. In case 2 the same drug dose reduces 10^9 cells to 10^6 cells.[10]

forming a straight line on a semi-log plot (Fig. 2.1). The second law is that cell kill by drugs follows first order kinetics in that for a chemosensitive tumour, the same dose of a chemotherapy agent will kill the same fraction of tumour cells, independent of the tumour burden. Therefore, if a given dose of chemotherapeutic agent reduces 10^{12} cells to 10^9, the same dose applied against 10^9 cells will result in 10^6 cells surviving.[11] This concept is referred to as 'log cell kill' or 'fractional cell kill' (Fig. 2.2). For most drugs, the cell kill increases with increasing dose and, if two or more drugs are used, the cell kills are multiplicative.[11] If drug A at a given dose kills 90% of cells and drug B at a given dose kills 90%, A + B should kill 99% of the cells. Put another way, if A leaves 10^5 cells out of 10^6, and if treatment B alone does the same, then the combination should be able to reduce 10^6 cells to 10^4.

The principle of fractional cell kill suggests that the total cancer burden will soon become dose limiting for a given dose of chemotherapy. One way of overcoming this limitation is by substantially increasing the dose of chemother-

apeutic agent. The model used for demonstrating a dose–response effect from chemotherapy is again based on work by Skipper and Schabel using a murine L1210 leukaemia cell line. This has been reproduced using human cell lines.[12] Skipper and collaborators showed that most antineoplastic drugs, including alkylating agents, exhibit a steep dose–response curve. An exponential increase in cell kill followed small changes in drug dose. Therefore, doubling the dose may result in a 10-fold or more increase in tumour cell kill and thus potentially translates into an increased cure rate. These results form the basis of the laboratory rationale for dose intensification.

The relationship between drug dose and cell kill of human tumours follows a more complex pattern. Skipper's laws apply only to the proportion of cells within a tumour that are actively proliferating – the growth fraction. It is the proliferating cells that are responsible for the growth of a tumour, and that would be the ideal target for chemotherapy. Human tumours exhibit a Gompertzian growth pattern (see Fig. 2.1). There is a progressive decline in the rate of growth as the tumour increases in size. The Gompertzian growth curve is sigmoid in shape; cell numbers accumulate slowly initially because the number of proliferating cells is low. As the mass of the tumour increases, the diffusion of oxygen becomes insufficient to supply cells at the centre of the tumour and the rate of proliferation plateaus. As a tumour expands, it regularly outgrows its blood supply which lags behind the leading edge of the invading tumour. Small tumours have the largest growth fraction as their supply of nutrients and oxygen is maximal. Large tumours have a smaller growth fraction as the numbers of anoxic and necrotic cells are at a maximum. Norton and Simon constructed a cytokinetic model using the Gompertzian model to examine the relationship between tumour size and response to therapy.[13] They determined that tumour sensitivity to chemotherapeutic agent is directly related to its growth rate, which depends on its growth fraction and tumour volume. Maximum tumour sensitivity occurs when tumour size is 37% of its potential maximum size.[14] For tumours with Gompertzian kinetics where the rate of regrowth increases as the tumour shrinks, the level of therapy adequate to initiate regression or clinical response may not be able to sustain regression or produce cure as remaining cells enter the proliferation cycle and the tumour grows again.[14]

Drug resistance

Drug resistance may be inherent or acquired through mutations induced by prolonged drug exposure leading to the selection and proliferation of resistant clones.[14] There are multiple mechanisms of resistance, as listed in Table 2.1.

Most of these mechanisms of drug resistance are overcome by dose escalation;[14] data from drug resistance studies suggest that a five- to ten-fold increase in dose is necessary for a move into the curative range.[15] Referring again to Gompertzian kinetics, in some malignant lymphomas, regrowth of tumour is evident soon after achieving complete remission after

Table 2.1 Mechanisms of drug resistance
Decreased transport of drug across cells
Change in the level of activating or deactivating enzymes
Increased DNA repair
Use of alternative pathways for metabolites to circumvent the primary pathway that is the drug's target
Increased transport of drug out of cells
Gene amplification of enzyme target of drug
Decreased transport of drug into cells

induction therapy. The residual microscopic cancer often remains sensitive to chemotherapy but has somehow managed to survive the initial therapy. This suggests that resistance to chemotherapy may be due in part to cell growth kinetics rather than the aforementioned mechanisms of resistance. This regrowth of tumour may be overcome by initial intensive therapy.[14] Until recently, the accepted approach was to follow initial cytoreduction with conventional dose therapy with a single round of high dose therapy as consolidation. This strategy is termed late intensification therapy (see Chapter 12). Instead it seems more logical that in responsive tumours, intensive therapy be administered upfront.

Principles of drug selection

Most drug combinations used in the high dose setting are based on the following parameters:

- good activity as a single agent in conventional dose in that particular tumour type,
- evidence for a dose–response curve – the steeper the better,
- non cross resistance with other agents in combination,
- synergy between agents,

- haematological toxicity as the dose limiting toxicity, and
- non-additive non-haematological toxicities.[5,16]

Although most regimens were derived mainly on empirical grounds, several theoretical reasons exist for the inclusion of at least one alkylating agent. Alkylators show a steep dose–response curve to haematological and other malignancies. There is a lack of cross resistance among these agents and there is often in vitro and in vivo synergism.

Dose intensification will have the drawback of toxicity to normal cell populations. Myelosuppression is the dose-limiting side effect of many chemotherapeutic agents. With the use of autologous bone marrow transplantation (BMT) and PBSC transplantation to repopulate the marrow, this side effect can be overcome. Therefore, in the high dose setting, non-haematological toxicities have become more important.[17] Ototoxicity was strongly related to the cumulative carboplatin AUC (area under the concentration versus time curve) when high dose carboplatin was given in combination with cyclophosphamide and thiotepa.[18] For some drugs, where the metabolism/excretion of a certain drug is by a single pathway that can be easily measured, dosing of the drug can be individualized using biological parameters without relying on empirical weight/kilogram (wt/kg) or body surface area (BSA) dosing. An example is carboplatin, which is excreted almost exclusively by the kidneys. The dose or AUC can be individualized using the Calvert formula:

$$\text{Dose (mg)} = (\text{GFR(ml/min)} + 25)\, n,$$

where n is the desired target AUC. Therefore the dose required for a target AUC of 5 in a patient with a GFR of 125 is $(125 + 25) \times 5 = 750$ mg. Jones et al. showed that 53% of 38 patients treated with high dose cyclophosphamide, cisplatin and BCNU (carmustine) developed pulmonary injury – this was particularly associated with a BCNU AUC of >600 mg/ml/min.[19]

Table 2.2 lists some non-haematological dose limiting toxicities for drugs commonly used in the high dose setting.

PHARMACOKINETIC AND PHARMACODYNAMIC CONSIDERATIONS

The term pharmacokinetics (PK) refers to the handling of a drug within the body with respect to its absorption, distribution, metabolism and excretion. Pharmacodynamics (PD) refers to the biochemical and physiological effects of a drug, including the binding of the drug to cells, its uptake, its intracellular metabolism and its mode of action. Very few pharmacological studies have been conducted in HDC, although more recently there has been an increase in the interest in PK/PD analysis in relation to this field.[17] The lack of such information limits our understanding of the optimal combinations, optimal scheduling and PK interactions of chemo-therapeutic agents in this setting.

In theory, HDC should be effective because of the steep dose–response relationship in preclinical models.[22] In vitro studies using the MCF7 breast cancer cell line have illustrated a steep dose–response relationship for melphalan, thiotepa, cisplatin and cyclophosphamide.[23] Further information regarding the relationship between delivered dose and plasma drug exposure is derived from the AUC and the relationship between exposure and clinical anti-cancer efficacy. For most cytotoxic agents employed in intensive chemotherapy, the relationship between AUC and dose follows linear kinetics. However, there are some exceptions – for example, paclitaxel has a non-linear pattern where there is a threshold above which the AUC value increases more markedly. Hence, pharmacokinetic non-linearity becomes important in the selection of chemotherapeutic agents in high dose therapy.

The most commonly used agents for HDC exhibit wide individual pharmacokinetics and inter-patient exposure variability. For a given

Table 2.2 Extra-medullary toxicity characteristics of drugs used in high dose chemotherapy[14,20,21]

Drug*	Eye	Skin	CNS	GI tract	Renal or metabolic	Cardiac	Lung
Cyclo	–	–	–	–	SIADH	Haemorrhagic myocarditis	–
BCNU	–	–	–	–	HVOD	–	Fibrosis
Ara-C	Conjunctivitis	Rash	Cerebellar or cerebral dysfunction	Cholestatic jaundice	SIADH	–	Oedema
VP-16	–	–	–	Mucositis	–	–	–
Thio	–	–	–	Mucositis	–	–	–
Ifos	–	–	Encephalopathy	–	Haemorrhagic cystitis	–	–
Mel	–	Dermatitis	–	Mucositis	SIADH	–	Interstitial pneumonitis
Carbo	–	–	Ototoxicity	–	Nephrotoxicity	–	–
M-c	–	–	–	Enterocolitis Haemorrhagic pancreatitis	–	–	–
Bu	–	–	–	Mucositis	HVOD	–	Fibrosis
Cis	–	–	Ototoxicity Neurotoxicity	–	Nephrotoxicity	–	–
Mit	–	–	–	Mucositis	–	–	–

*Ara-C, cytosine arabinoside; BCNU, carmustine; Bu, busulphan; Carbo, carboplatin; Cis, cisplatin; Cyclo, cyclophosphamide; HVOD, hepatic veno-occlusive disease; Ifos, ifosfamide; M-c, mitomycin-c; Mel, melphalan; Mit, mitoxantrone; SIADH, syndrome of inappropriate anti-diuretic hormone secretion; Thio, thiotepa; VP-16, etoposide.

dose, some patients may be treated at sub-therapeutic doses, whilst others may be exposed to unacceptably high doses.[17] In HDC this is important because the risk of treatment-related death is increased in patients with a lower plasma clearance of cytotoxic compounds.

AGENTS COMMONLY USED IN THE HIGH DOSE SETTING

The commonly used alkylating agents and other drugs are outlined below.

Cyclophosphamide

This is widely used in the high dose setting. It is activated in hepatic microsomes to form 4-hydroxycyclophosphamide and aldophosphamide: acrolein is removed from aldophosphamide to form active phosphoramide mustard. Incubating cyclophosphamide with microsomal preparations has led to the observation that there are significant differences in the rate of conversion of cyclophosphamide to 4-hydroxycyclophosphamide and aldophosphamide.[24] This correlates with the wide interpatient PK variability of cyclophosphamide at high dose.[25] Cyclophosphamide is usually given as a total dose of 5–8 g/m^2 divided over 2–4 days. This dose pattern arose from observations that single large doses of the drug produced significant cardiotoxicity that was reduced when the dose was divided over several days.[26] High dose cyclophosphamide is usually given with mesna which combines with acrolein to reduce urothelial toxicity.

Ifosfamide

An isomer of cyclophosphamide, ifosfamide is also a pro-drug. Its rate of hydroxylation is slower resulting in lower peak levels of the active metabolite and a more prolonged production of mustard and acrolein. Ifosfamide is usually given as a continuous infusion. As with cyclophosphamide, ifosfamide is usually given with mesna.

Melphalan

This alkylates target tissue after formation of a mustard-type reactive intermediate. Although less than 15% of intact drug is renally excreted, severe renal failure delays drug excretion. The drug is usually given as a single rapid intravenous infusion. There is a three- to four-fold variability in the AUC of drug observed in patients when identical drug doses are given.[27]

Busulphan

Use of busulphan is limited by the lack of an intravenous preparation. It is given orally at a dose of 1 mg/kg every 6 h for 16 doses. Busulphan shows a clear-cut PD organ toxicity relationship at high dose, namely the risk of hepatic veno-occlusive disease (HVOD) with increasing drug exposure.[28] With PK guidance of busulphan dosage, both morbidity and mortality of busulphan-associated HVOD have been shown to be reduced.[28] Busulphan is a small molecule that may cross the blood–brain barrier, resulting in cerebral irritation; prophylactic anti-convulsants are usually given.

BCNU (carmustine)

Commonly, BCNU is given as a 2 h infusion. The drug undergoes spontaneous hydrolysis in intravenous solutions or plasma and this is potentiated by increasing temperature or light. In vivo, BCNU is hydrolysed to chlorethyliso-cyanate and a chlorethyl carbonium ion which are the cytotoxic agents.

Cisplatin

Hydrolysis activates cisplatin to produce a cis-diamine dihydroxy species that causes tissue alkylation. Nephrotoxicity and neurotoxicity are dose limiting and are exacerbated by low urinary flow or low urinary chloride concentration. In high dose therapy, cisplatin is administered as a 2- to 4- day continuous infusion. Urine flow is maintained above 200 ml/h during the infusion with chloride-rich intravenous fluid to avoid renal tubular toxicity.

Carboplatin

The substantial anti-tumour activity of carboplatin overlaps with cisplatin. Myelosuppression is the dose-limiting toxicity and this makes it ideal for high dose therapy. Like cisplatin, it is renally excreted. The creatinine clearance is predictive of drug elimination and can be used to predict the degree of thrombocytopaenia produced by a given dose of the drug.[29]

Thiotepa

This was one of the earliest alkylating agents developed. The dose-limiting toxicity is to the marrow allowing for huge dose escalations of 10- to 50-fold in high dose treatment. This drug also crosses the blood–brain barrier, and HVOD may occur when it is used in combination with other hepatotoxic chemotherapy agents.

Etoposide (VP-16)

This is the main non-alkylating agent used in HDC. It has good activity when combined with platinum-based compounds, as well as a high degree of single agent activity in lymphoma and testicular cancer.[30,31] It is renally excreted. Dose escalation is limited not only by mucosal toxicity but also by the need for prolonged infusion – the lipid vehicle used in the formulation results in hypotension.

Mitoxantrone

An anthraquinone, mitoxantrone's main dose-limiting toxicity is to the marrow. It can be escalated to three to five times the conventional dose before mucosal injury becomes limiting. It is less cardiotoxic than the related daunorubicin and doxorubicin. It is given in multiple doses divided over a number of days.

Cytosine arabinoside (Ara-C)

This is a cell cycle phase-specific drug and therefore the duration of cell exposure to drug is an important determinant of fraction of cells killed. A single bolus of $4\,g/m^2$ can be relatively well tolerated by patients whereas a continuous infusion of $1\,g/m^2$ over 48 h can lead to severe myelosuppression. Gastrointestinal toxicity can make parenteral nutrition necessary. In older patients, high dose Ara-C is limited by gastrointestinal and CNS toxicity, particularly when it is used in combination with other drugs.

COMMONLY USED REGIMENS

Single agent plus total body irradiation

Cyclophosphamide plus total body irradiation (TBI – Cyclo/TBI; Table 2.3) is probably the combination most widely used in the world, and extensive experience has accumulated since its introduction in the early 1960s by pioneers such as ED Thomas. The first regimen used in the leukaemias comprised radiotherapy alone; however, it soon became evident that the rate of leukaemic relapse was unacceptably high. To reduce it, cyclophosphamide was added to the regimen prior to TBI. This resulted in a striking decrease in the rate of recurrent leukaemia and became the basis of the Cyclo/TBI regimens. In general, Cyclo/TBI does not produce serious adverse additive toxicity and is of proven efficacy, particularly in the acute leukaemias. There is no single protocol for TBI.

Table 2.3 Single agent plus total body irradiation (TBI) regimens

Acronym	Drugs and doses	Indication	Notes
Cyclo/TBI	Cyclophosphamide 90–200 mg/kg TBI 500–1000 cGy in a single dose	Leukaemia and lymphoma	1200–1575 cGy TBI can be given in several fractions Little serious adverse toxicity
Mel/TBI	Melphalan 80–180 mg/m^2 TBI 500–1000 cGy in a single dose	Multiple myeloma	Nephrotoxicity and gastrointestinal complications increase markedly at melphalan doses $\geqslant$200 mg/m^2

Total body irradiation is also used in conjunction with melphalan (Mel/TBI) for patients with multiple myeloma who are fit, younger than 50–60 years of age and have experienced a good response to conventional cytoreductive chemotherapy. The main side effects of Mel/TBI are nephrotoxicity and gastrointestinal complications, including haemorrhagic diarrhoea and mucositis. These toxic effects increase markedly at doses of 200 mg/m^2 or more of melphalan.

Two-agent regimens

Classic two-agent regimens busulphan and cyclophosphamide (Bu/Cy) and busulphan and melphalan (Bu/Mel) have been used in acute leukaemias and solid tumours. Santos et al.[32] reported marrow transplantation for acute non-lymphocytic leukaemia after treatment with Bu/Cy. This proved an effective combination, and therapeutic results appeared comparable to Cyclo/TBI regimens. The dose of cyclophosphamide was later reduced to reduce toxicities (BuCy2).[33] At present, there is no evidence to suggest that the addition of any other drugs to Bu/Cy is more effective than this combination alone. Although one comparative study of Cyclo/TBI versus Bu/Cy suggested some superiority of the TBI regimen, other studies have so far failed to do so. Other two-agent regimens have been reported and are summarized in Table 2.4.

Three-agent regimens

Three-agent regimens have been extensively studied in breast cancer. The Dana Farber Cancer Institute group have evaluated the STAMP 5 protocol,[36] which consists of cyclophosphamide, thiotepa and carboplatin. This regimen had been criticized for the low dose of carboplatin, in the light of its shallower dose–response curve compared with cisplatin.

Table 2.4 Two-agent regimens

Acronym	Drugs and doses	Indication	Notes	References
Bu/Cy	Busulphan 4 mg/kg daily for 4 days Cyclophosphamide 200 mg/kg	Acute and chronic leukaemia		Santos et al.[32]
Bu/Cy2	Busulphan as before Cyclophosphamide 120 mg/kg	Acute and chronic leukaemia	Cyclophosphamide dose decreased to reduce toxicity	Ozkaynak et al.[33]
Carbo/VP-16	Carboplatin 800–1200 mg/m² over 4–6 days Etoposide 600–800 mg/m² over 3–4 days	Lymphoma Germ cell tumours		Bronchund,[2] Buckner et al.,[34] Carella et al.[35]
Bu/VP-16	Busulphan 16 mg/kg Etoposide 60 mg/kg	Acute myeloid leukaemia	Severe mucositis, skin toxicity, hyperbilirubinaemia and HVOD	Bronchund,[2] Buckner et al.,[34] Carella et al.[35]
	Thiotepa 225 mg/m² for 3 days Cyclophosphamide 2.5 g/m² for 3 days	Breast cancer Ovarian cancer		Bronchund,[2] Buckner et al.,[34] Carella et al.[35]
	Thiotepa 200 mg/m² for 3 days Carboplatin 800–1200 mg/m² over 4–6 days	Breast cancer Ovarian cancer		Bronchund,[2] Buckner et al.,[34] Carella et al.[35]
Mel/VP-16	Melphalan 60 mg/m² over 3 days Etoposide 400–1200 mg/m² over 3 days	Breast cancer		Bronchund,[2] Buckner et al.,[34] Carella et al.[35]
Bu/Mel	Busulphan 16 mg/kg Melphalan 120–200 mg/m²	Acute leukaemia	Used when TBI cannot be given because of previous irradiation Severe mucositis and diarrhoea	Bronchund,[2] Buckner et al.,[34] Carella et al.[35]

The Duke University BMT Unit in North Carolina further developed this regimen to comprise cyclophosphamide, cisplatin and BCNU.[37] However, this regimen can have substantial neurotoxicity; the dose of BCNU is high, increasing the potential for hepatic and pulmonary toxicity and haemolytic–uraemic syndrome (HUS). Several centres use slightly modified versions of these schedules.

Cyclophosphamide, BCNU, and VP-16 (CBV) is one of the most commonly used three-agent regimens in HD and NHL. It was first described by Jagganath et al.[38] and since this preliminary report, CBV has been used (with or without minor modifications) with significantly increased response rates. The combination of cyclophosphamide, VP-16 and melphalan (CEM) is another popular three-agent regimen.[39] These and other combinations are described in Table 2.5.

Four-agent regimens

Several four-agent regimens have been introduced. The most widely used are the BEAM and BEAC regimens used in a variety of solid tumours but most often in the lymphomas. These combinations are outlined in Table 2.6. The exact dosages and schedules are subject to variation between centres.

CONCLUSION

In recent years, there has been a rapid growth in the use of HDC, fuelled by the advent of the CSFs and PBSC transplantation. This chapter has outlined the scientific rationale behind the use of this therapeutic approach in chemosensitive disease and described the drug regimens most commonly used. Despite the availability of sound evidence, there have been few pharmacological studies into HDC, and as a result, our understanding of the optimal combinations, schedules and interactions is limited. There is, however, increasing interest in PK/PD analysis in relation to this field. Despite a rapid output

of novel combinations of three-agent regimens, it is difficult to prove clear-cut differences in their anti-tumour efficacy; prospective comparative studies in well-defined populations of patients are required. While a further increase in the number of cytotoxic agents (to five or more agents) might enhance anti-tumour effects, this approach has proven difficult primarily because current regimens already have a marginal therapeutic index. Haematological and non-haematological toxicities can not only be severe, but may be fatal. These toxicities might increase with the addition of further agents or might require a decrease in the doses of other agents in the combination.[44] Despite the importance of these toxicities, clinical outcomes, disease-free survival (DFS) and complete response rates remain the more important endpoints. There are promising potential future developments in the field which may supersede the present practice of initial cytoreduction followed by single-cycle consolidation HDC. Firstly, there is the possibility of including some of the newer active drugs such as the taxanes into existing regimens. Other strategies may include alternating HDC with such new effective drug regimens, and alternating schedules of HDC as up-front therapy.[7] If there is only minimal disease left after a course of HDC, this may be eradicated by immune manipulation.[5] Several groups are investigating the use of immunotherapy following intensive therapy, with strategies aimed at exploiting the graft versus tumour (host) effect of high intensity treatment.[5] It is possible to generate a graft-versus-host disease situation in the autologous setting with cyclosporin A; other immunomodulators that are being investigated include interleukin-2 (IL-2) and interferon.[5] Novel drugs which act on targets outside the nucleus are also being evaluated, and preliminary results with the anti-CD20 antibody rituximab appear promising.

Good evidence from large randomized controlled trials will determine which of these new approaches will be more effective than current practice. Finally, the biased media attention at the 1999 ASCO annual meeting on the use of

Table 2.5 Three-agent regimens

Acronym	Drugs and doses	Indications	Notes	References
CBV	Cyclophosphamide 6 g/m^2 BCNU 300 mg/m^2 Etoposide 750 mg/m^2 Etoposide 100 mg/m^2 every 12 h for 6 consecutive doses	Lymphoma	Numerous variations of the original are used	Jagganath et al.[38]
CEM	Cyclophosphamide 2 g/m^2 daily for 3 days Etoposide 2.5 g/m^2 over 1 day Melphalan 50 mg/m^2 daily for 2 days	Breast cancer Lymphoma Myeloma	Melphalan over 200 mg/m^2 total dose results in haemorrhagic mucositis	Moore et al.[39]
STAMP 25	Cyclophosphamide total dose 6 g/m^2 Thiotepa at 500 mg/m^2 Carboplatin 800 mg/m^2	Breast cancer		Antman et al.[36]
Duke regimen	Cyclophosphamide 1875 mg/m^2 as a 1-h infusion daily for 3 days Cisplatin 55 mg/m^2 as a continuous 72-h infusion over 3 days BCNU 600 mg/m^2 over 1 day	Breast cancer	Reasonably well tolerated Modified versions often used	Peters et al.[37]
	Carboplatin 1500 mg/m^2 Etoposide 1200 mg/m^2 Cyclophosphamide 5 g/m^2	Metastatic breast cancer		Kritz et al.[40]
	Busulphan 16 mg/m^2 Cyclophosphamide 120 mg/kg Etoposide 30 mg/kg	Haematological malignancies		Spitzer et al.[41]
TBC	Thiotepa 450–750 mg/m^2 Busulphan 10–12 mg/kg Cyclophosphamide 120–150 mg/kg	Leukaemia Myeloma Non-Hodgkins lymphoma	Regimen-related mortality at 6 weeks of 6%	Przepiorka et al.[42]
	VM-26 150 mg/m^2 daily for 5 days Ifosfamide 1500 mg/m^2/day over 5 days Carboplatin 200 mg/m^2/day over 5 days	Ovarian (stage IIIc–IV)	Considerable epithelial toxicity	Lotz et al.[43]

Table 2.6 Four-agent regimens

Acronym	Drugs and doses	Indications	Notes	References
BEAC	BCNU 300 mg/m^2 over 1 day Etoposide 100 mg/m^2/day for 3 days Ara-C 200 mg/m^2 12-hourly for 4 days Cyclophosphamide 1.5–2.5 g/m^2/day for 3 days	Lymphoma		Rosti et al.[44]
BEAM	As for BEAC but cyclophosphamide substituted by melphalan 120–180 mg/m^2 for 1 day	Lymphoma		Peters et al.[45]
BACT	BCNU 200 mg/m^2 over 1 day Ara-C 200 mg/m^2/day for 4 days Cyclophosphamide 50 mg/kg/day for 4 days Thioguanine 200 mg/m^2/day for 4 days	Lymphoma Leukaemia		Appelbaum et al[46]
BAVC	BCNU 600–800 mg/m^2 over 1 day Amsacrine 150 mg/m^2/day for 3 days Etoposide 150 mg/m^2/day for 3 days Cytosine arabinoside 300 mg/m^2/day for 3 days	Acute myeloid leukaemia		Meloni et al[47,48]

high-dose therapy in breast cancer should remind us that science is not conducted best in *The New York Times* or by NBC News. Conclusions on the relative merits of dose intensification in solid tumours can only be reached by mature review of data and careful scientific considerations.[45]

REFERENCES

1. Bronchund MH, Howell A, Crowther D et al. The use of granulocyte colony stimulating factor to increase the intensity of treatment with doxorubicin in patients with advanced breast and ovarian cancer. Br J Cancer 1989;60:121–5.
2. Bronchund MH. Care of the patient treated with intensive chemotherapy. Macclesfield: Gardiner-Caldwell Communications, 1993.

3. Gurney H, Dodwell D, Thatcher N, Tattersall MHN. Escalating drug delivery in cancer chemotherapy: a review of concepts and practice – Part 1. Ann Oncol 1993;4:23–34. Part 2 Ann Oncol 1993: 103–15.

4. Bronchund M, Henderson IC, Denis L, eds. The importance of dose in cancer chemotherapy: the role of haemopoietic growth factors 3rd edn. Macclesfield: Gardiner-Caldwell Communications, 2000.

5. Hornedo J, Cortes-Funes H. The role of high dose chemotherapy in adult solid tumours other than breast cancer. Ann Oncol 1996;7(suppl 2):23–30.

6. Kanz L, Brugger W, Mertelsman R. The use of haemopoietic growth factors for high dose chemotherapy and peripheral blood progenitor cell transplantation. Semin Oncol 1994;21(6) (suppl 16):10–18.

7. Bezwoda WR. High dose chemotherapy with haemopoietic rescue in breast cancer: from theory to practice. Cancer Chemother Pharmacol 1997;40 (suppl):79–87.

8. Frei E III. Curative cancer chemotherapy. Cancer Res 1985;45:6523–37.

9. Frei E III, Antman KH, Teicher B et al. Bone marrow auto-transplantation for solid tumours – prospects. J Clin Oncol 1989;7:515–26.

10. Souhami R, Tobias J. Biology of cancer. In: Cancer and its management, 3rd edn. Oxford: Blackwell Science, 1998: 23–40.

11. Norton L. The Norton Simon hypothesis. In: Perry MC, editor. The chemotherapy source book. Baltimore: Williams and Wilkins, 1992: 36–53.

12. Leonard, RCF. High-dose chemotherapy in solid tumours: breast cancer. In: Reiffers J, Goldman JM, Armitage JO, editors. Blood stem cell transplantation. London: Martin Dunitz, 1998.

13. Norton L, Simon R. Tumour size, sensitivity to therapy, and design of treatment schedules. Cancer Treat Rep 1977;61:1307–17.

14. Odaimi M, Ajani J. High-dose chemotherapy: concepts and strategies. Am J Clin Oncol 1987;10(2):123–32.

15. Saijo N. Chemotherapy: the more the better? Overview. Cancer Chemother Pharmacol 1997; 40(suppl):100–6.

16. Pinedo HM. Dose effect relationship in breast cancer. Ann Oncol 1993;4:351–7.

17. Sasaki Y. Pharmacological considerations in high dose chemotherapy. Cancer Chemother Pharmacol 1997;40(suppl):115–18.

18. Warmerdam LC van, Rodenhuis SR, van der Wall E et al. Pharmacokinetics and pharmacodynamics of carboplatin in a high dose combination regimen with thiotepa, cyclophosphamide and peripheral stem-cell support. Br J Cancer 1996;73:979.

19. Jones RB, Matthes S, Shpall EJ et al. Acute lung injury following treatment with high dose cyclophosphamide, cisplatin, and carmustine: pharmacodynamic evaluation of carmustine. J Natl Cancer Inst 1993;85:640–7.

20. Livingston RB. High dose cancer therapy without stem cell support – human solid tumours. In: Armitage JO, Antman KH, editors. High Dose Cancer Chemotherapy – Pharmacology, Hematopoietins, Stem Cells. Baltimore: Williams and Wilkins, 1992.

21. Jones RB, Matthes S. Pharmacokinetics. In: Armitage JO, Antman KH, editors. High Dose Cancer Chemotherapy – Pharmacology, Hematopoietins, Stem Cells. Baltimore: Williams and Wilkins, 1992: 43–60.

22. Frei E III. Pharmacologic strategies for high dose chemotherapy. In: Armitage JO, Antman KH, editors. High Dose Cancer Chemotherapy – Pharmacology, Hematopoietins, Stem Cells. Baltimore: Williams and Wilkins, 1992: 1–13.

23. Frei E III, Cucchi CA, Rosowsky A et al. Alkylating agent resistance: in vitro studies with human cell lines. Proc Natl Acad Sci USA 1985;82:2158–62.

24. Anderson LW, Chen TL, Colvin OM et al. Cyclophosphamide and 4-hydroxycyclophosphamide/aldophosphamide kinetics in patients receiving high dose cyclophosphamide chemotherapy. Clin Cancer Res 1996;2:1481–7.

25. Stemmer SM, Cagnori PJ, Shpall EJ et al. High dose paclitaxel, cyclophosphamide, and cisplatin with autologous haematopoietic progenitor cell support: a phase I trial. J Clin Oncol 1996; 14:1463.

26. Goldberg MA, Antin JH, Guinan EC. Cyclophosphamide cardiotoxicity; analysis of dosing as a risk factor. Blood 1986;68:1114–18.

27. Tranchand B, Ploin Y-D, Minuit M-P. High dose melphalan dosage adjustment: possibility of using a test dose. Cancer Chemother Pharmacol 1989;23:95–100.

28. Groshow LB, Jones RJ, Brundrett RB. Pharmacokinetics of busulfan: correlation with veno-occlusive disease in patients undergoing

bone marrow transplantation. Cancer Chemother Pharmacol 1989;25:55–61.

29. Belani CP, Egorin MJ, Abrams JS. A novel pharmacologically based approach to dose optimisation of carboplatin when used in combination with etoposide. J Clin Oncol 1989;7:1896–902.

30. Schabel FM, Trader MW, Laster WR. Cisdichlorodiamineplatinum(II): combination chemotherapy and cross resistance studies with tumours in mice. Cancer Treat Rep 1979;63:1459–73.

31. Fleming RA, Miller AA, Stewart CF. Etoposide, an update. Clin Pharm 1989;8:274–93.

32. Santos GW, Tutschka PJ, Brookmeyer R. Marrow transplantation for acute non-lymphocytic leukaemia after treatment with busulphan and cyclophosphamide. N Engl J Med 1983;309:1347–51.

33. Ozkaynak MF, Weinberg K, Kohn D. Hepatic veno-occlusive disease post bone marrow transplantation in children conditioned with busulphan and cyclophosphamide: incidence, risk factors and clinical outcome. Bone Marrow Transplant 1991;7:467–74.

34. Buckner CD, Clift RA, Appelbaum FR. Effects of treatment regimens on post marrow transplant relapse. Semin Hematol 1991;28(suppl 4):32–6.

35. Carella AM, Santini G, Santoro A. Massive chemotherapy with non-frozen autologous bone marrow transplantation in 13 cases of refractory Hodgkin's disease. Eur J Cancer Clin Oncol 1985;21:607–13.

36. Antman KH, Rowlings PA, Vaughan WP et al. High-dose chemotherapy with autologous haematopoietic stem-cell support for breast cancer in North America. J Clin Oncol 1997;15: 1870–9.

37. Peters WP, Shpall EJ, Jones RB. High dose combination alkylating agents with bone marrow support as initial treatment for metastatic breast cancer. J Clin Oncol 1988;6:1368–76.

38. Jagganath S, Dicke KA, Armitage JO. High dose cyclophosphamide, carmustine and etoposide and autologous bone marrow transplantation for relapsed Hodgkin's disease. Ann Intern Med 1986;104:163–8.

39. Moore MR, Gordon DS, Reynolds R. Phase I trial of intravenous melphalan with high dose cyclophosphamide and etoposide followed by autologous bone marrow transplantation in patients with breast cancer or lymphoma. J Clin Oncol 1993; 12: 93 (abstract 174).

40. Kritz A, Crown JP, Motzer RJ. Beneficial impact of peripheral blood progenitor cells in patients with metastatic breast cancer treated with high dose chemotherapy plus granulocyte– macrophage colony stimulating factor. Cancer 1993;71:2515–22.

41. Spitzer TR, Cottler-Fox M, Torrisi J. Escalating doses of etoposide with cyclophosphamide and fractionated total body irradiation or busulphan as conditioning regimen for bone marrow transplantation. Bone Marrow Transplant 1989;4:559–65.

42. Przepiorka D, Dimopoulous M, Smith T. Regimen related toxicities of high dose thiotepa, busulphan and cyclophosphamide as a marrow transplant preparative regimen. Proc ASCO 1993;12:404 (abstract 1383).

43. Lotz JP, Machover D, Bellaiche A. Tandem high dose chemotherapy with VM-26, ifosfamide and carboplatin with autologous bone marrow transplantation for patients with stage IIIc–IV ovarian cancer. Proc ASCO 1993;12:257 (abstract 815).

44. Rosti G, Albertazzi L, Salvioni R. High dose chemotherapy supported with autologous bone marrow transplantation in germ cell tumours: a phase II study. Ann Oncol 1992;3:809–12.

45. Peters WP. High-dose chemotherapy and stem-cell support for primary and metastatic breast cancer. In: American Society of Clinical Oncology Full Education Book. American Society of Clinical Oncology, 1999: 139–49.

46. Appelbaum FR, Heizig GP, Ziegler JL et al. Successful engraftment of cryopreserved autologous bone marrow in patients with malignant lymphoma. Blood 1978; 52: 85–95.

47. Meloni G, De Fabritiis P, Carella AM et al. Autologous bone marrow transplantation in patients with AML in first complete remission: results of two different conditioning regimens after the same induction and consolidation therapy. Bone Marrow Transpl 1990; 5: 29–32.

48. Meloni G, De Fabritiis P, Petti MC et al. BAVC regimen and autologous bone marrow transplantation in patients with acute myelogenous leukaemia in second remission. Blood 1990; 12: 2282–5.

3

Purging, selection and minimal residual disease

Gunnar Kvalheim

CONTENTS   Introduction • Minimal residual disease in bone marrow and peripheral blood • Purging of tumour cells from bone marrow and peripheral blood progenitor cells • CD34+ cell enrichment of peripheral blood progenitor cells • Purging of tumour cells from autografts and clinical value • Minimal residual disease after high dose therapy • Conclusion

INTRODUCTION

High dose chemoradiotherapy (HDCRT) with autologous stem cell support is increasingly being used to treat selected patients who have haematological cancer as well as those with other malignancies. Previously, bone marrow has been the most frequent source of stem cell support used after high dose therapy. However, a number of studies show that peripheral blood progenitor cells (PBPC) may replace bone marrow as the major source of haemopoietic cell support in patients receiving HDCRT. The use of haemopoietic growth factors can significantly increase the number of circulating progenitor cells when administered in the recovery phase after cytotoxic treatment. Reinfusion of such cells following high dose treatment gives several advantages over the use of bone marrow: PBPC can be collected without general anaesthesia, and the use of PBPC reduces the number of days until neutrophils and platelets have reached pretransplant levels.[1–5]

In spite of these advantages, the disease-free survival of patients treated with high dose therapy has not improved significantly. Relapse of

the underlying disease still represents the major cause of death. The possible contribution of tumour cell purging to the efficacy of HDCRT with autologous stem cell transplantation is unknown, because prospective clinical studies have not been performed. However, gene-marking studies of autografted cells to trace the origin of relapse after autologous bone marrow transplantation have indicated that tumour cells remaining in the reinfused stem cell product contribute to recurrence of the disease.[6,7] This conclusion is further supported by results from studying patients with follicular lymphomas which indicate that efficient bone marrow purging improves disease-free survival.[8]

A variety of techniques have been developed for the purpose of removing tumour cells from bone marrow.[9] Monoclonal antibodies (mAbs) directed against tumour-associated antigens can be used for specific removal of the malignant cells. The mAbs can be used together with complement, coupled to toxins as immunotoxins, or in combination with iron-containing polymer beads coated with a secondary antibody. Previously, with the Clinical Stem Cell Laboratory, I have reported my experiences with purging of lymphoma cells from bone marrow employing anti-B cell or anti-T cell mAbs and magnetizeable bead, Dynabeads M-450 (Dynal A/S, Oslo, Norway).[10-14] Based on this, a purging procedure to deplete PBPCs of lymphoma cells has been developed.[15] Moreover, we have obtained data showing that the use of anti-breast cancer mAbs in combination with immunobeads efficiently removes breast cancer cells from leukapheresis products. Most solid tumour cells such as breast cancer and lymphoma cells do not express CD34 antigens. Nevertheless, positive enrichment of CD34 cells from leukapheresis products obtained from breast cancer patients has resulted in a tumour cell depletion of only 3 log.[16] Our experiences with CD34 cell enrichment employing ISOLEX 300 and immunobeads has shown a similar purging efficacy. Therefore, to eradicate tumour cells in the autografts, a combination of CD34+ cell enrichment and tumour cell purging appears to be the most efficient method currently available.

Sensitive methods developed to detect minimal residual disease before and after therapy have brought new insight into the biological behaviour of the malignant disorders treated with high dose therapy.[17-19] Remaining minimal residual disease after high dose therapy seems to predict poor prognosis. Our experience and that of others suggests that as a result of inefficient high dose conditioning regimens, patients who receive purged autografts often still have persistent minimal residual disease after treatment. Efforts must be concentrated on finding more efficient treatment regimens in autotransplantation and on the use of additional therapy (following high dose therapy) to eradicate remaining minimal residual disease.

MINIMAL RESIDUAL DISEASE IN BONE MARROW AND PERIPHERAL BLOOD

Immunocytochemistry

Sensitive immunocytochemical methods have been developed, which use tumour-associated mAbs and alkaline phosphatase anti-alkaline phosphatase (APAAP) staining techniques to detect occult micrometastatic tumour cells in blood and bone marrow.[20] In most reports, cytospins containing a total number of 0.5×10^5 to 1.0×10^5 mononuclear bone marrow cells have been tested. Recently, a new cytocentrifuge method has been developed, making it possible to test 0.5×10^6 cells on each slide. At the Norwegian Radium Hospital, we routinely perform immunocytochemical evaluation of at least four slides, giving a total number of 2×10^6 mononuclear cells from the blood or bone marrow of each patient.[4-6] The slides are incubated with the anti-cytokeratin primary antibodies AE1 and AE3 (Signet Laboratories, Dedham, MA, USA). An appropriate negative control is used. Only cells that have the antibody-binding colour-reaction morphology of epithelial cells are scored as tumour.

Polymerase chain reaction

The polymerase chain reaction (PCR) is based on an in vitro enzymatic amplification of a specific target DNA segment, resulting in a highly specific, 10^5- to 10^6-fold enrichment of the sequence of interest. Cloning the breakpoints of specific translocations makes it possible to use amplification by PCR to detect tumour cells that contain the translocation. This method has been most extensively applied to the investigation of minimal residual disease in bone marrow and blood of the t(14;18) translocation carried by lymphomas and Philadelphia chromosome-positive chronic myelogenous leukaemia.[21,22]

Use of PCR requires that the malignant cells carry a clonal somatic mutation in their genome that is absent in normal cells. Unfortunately, solid tumours such as breast cancers do not meet these requirements. In spite of this, several groups have developed reverse transcription polymerase chain reaction assays (RT-PCR) that screen for carcinoma-specific expression of mRNA in mesenchymal organs such as bone marrow and blood. The RT-PCR assay for cytokeratin-19 (CK-19) has been reported to be specific for detection of breast cancer cells in bone marrow. Recently Zippelius et al.[23] found that RT-PCR methods to detect micrometastatic epithelial cancer cells in bone marrow have a major limitation due to illegitimate transcription of tumour-associated or epithelial-specific genes in blood cells. Since seven of the eight markers used for PCR detection could be detected in a high number of bone marrow samples from normal controls, the results previously reported are questionable.

The PCR methods currently in use to detect minimal residual disease give no quantitative information about the tumour cells present in the samples tested. Procedures that include a standard added directly to the sample to be assayed, and amplified by the same primer set as the target (competitive PCR), enable an estimate to be made of the number of transcripts in blood and bone marrow samples. Recently such methodology was used to quantify RT-PCR transcripts for CK19.[24] In this study, the analysis of samples from patients without cancer enabled definition of an upper limit for the background ratio of CK19. Values above this cut-off point were regarded as positive events. Similar methods are being developed for detection of t(14;18) in B cell malignancies.[25] Real-time PCR is a new technology for quantitative PCR.[26] Its ease of operation and the reproducibility hold great promise, and at the Norwegian Radium Hospital this method is being used to assay the purging efficacy of patients with B cell lymphomas.

Clinical significance of minimal residual disease

The presence of micrometastasis in bone marrow has frequently been studied in breast cancer patients at diagnosis.[19] Depending on the mAbs used in conjunction with immunocytochemistry, the frequencies of bone marrow positive patients will differ. Since the antibodies are not tumour specific, cross-reaction with normal haemopoietic cells[27] leads to false-positive

samples. In an ongoing study at the Norwegian Radium Hospital, employing anticytokeratin mAbs AE1/AE3 or A45-B/B3 and immunocytochemistry, 26.6% of the bone marrow samples from 257 breast cancer patients were anticytokeratin positive. However, among these samples 5.4% of isotype controls stained positive, suggesting that unspecific binding of anti-CK19 mAbs to non-epithelial cells had taken place.[27] Based on this experience, the Norwegian Radium Hospital always employs morphological evaluation and negative controls when immunocytochemistry is used.

Although the immunocytochemical methods need to be standardized, this does not negate the finding by several large breast cancer studies[28,29] that detection of micrometastases in bone marrow at diagnosis is associated with increased risk of systemic relapse. At the Norwegian Radium Hospital we are currently investigating the presence of micrometastases in bone marrow and blood of patients who have operable breast cancer patients. 920 patients' samples have been evaluated.[30] Among 580 lymph node negative (LN−) breast cancers, 9.9% had CK-positive tumour cells in their bone marrow, whereas 20.6% of the 340 patients with LN+ tumours were positive. Due to the short observation time to date it remains to be seen if this study will confirm data presented by previous investigators.

In neuroblastoma and Hodgkin's disease, tumour cells can be found in 30–60% of bone marrow autografts and in 10–30% of PBPC products.[31] Previous results indicated that patients whose bone marrow and PBPC demonstrated tumour cells on immunohistochemistry have an unfavourable prognosis.[32] A possible explanation for the relatively frequent presence of tumour cells in PBPC harvests is the recent observation that stem cell mobilization with haemopoietic growth factors can induce the release of tumour cells into the bloodstream. At the Norwegian Radium Hospital, we have similar experiences in breast cancer patients. High-risk Stage II breast cancer patients were randomized to have dose escalating chemotherapy (FEC) with granulocyte colony stimulating factor (G-CSF) support or three cycles of FEC plus high dose therapy with stem cell support (protocol FBG 9401 chaired by J Bergh, Upsala, Sweden). Patients were examined by immunocytochemistry and anticytokeratin antibodies (AE1/AE3) for the presence of tumour cells in bone marrow and blood before treatment, in peripheral PBPC, and in bone marrow and blood after treatment. Of 42 patients studied, 40% presented with tumour cells in bone marrow and 7% in blood at diagnosis. In spite of tumour-reductive therapy with three cycles of chemotherapy, 17 (40%) had tumour cells in their PBPC products (Table 3.1). Among those, only two patients had tumour cells in their blood before chemotherapy.

The PCR is used in the clinic to detect micrometastatic disease in patients with lymphomas. The t(14;18) translocation, resulting in the juxtaposition of the proto-oncogene *bcl-2* with the immunoglobulin heavy-chain locus on chromosome 14, appears in approximately 85% of patients with follicular lymphomas and in 30% of high-grade diffuse non-Hodgkin's lymphomas. This technique permits the detection of one lymphoma cell among 10^5 normal cells.[21] In low-grade lymphomas bone marrow infiltration is common at diagnosis. In spite of successful tumour reduction with disappearance of enlarged lymph nodes, residual bone marrow infiltration is detected by PCR in almost all patients.[18] As in breast cancer, low-grade lymphoma cells are also mobilized into the peripheral blood with growth factors;[18] similar findings have been found in other types of cancers. Based on these observations, it can be concluded that removal of contaminating lymphoma cells from autografts used to reconstitute haemopoiesis after high dose therapy of follicular lymphomas is of potential clinical value.[21]

In addition to use of PCR methods to detect specific translocations, PCRs targeting the T cell receptor in T cell malignancies and Ig heavy chain in acute lymphoblastic leukaemia, myeloma and B cell lymphomas have recently been reported to detect residual tumour cells in bone marrow and blood with efficiency.[33] Because many of these methods for detection of minimal residual disease show persistent positive signal after therapy for several months without any sign of clinical relapse, such procedures are of limited value unless quantitative PCR is being performed.

The use of CK-19 RT-PCR to detect breast cancer cells in bone marrow has also been reported to be of clinical use.[34,35] It has been reported[35] that RT-PCR for CK19 was found in 57% of 33 LN+ patients and in 82% of 50 breast cancer patients with metastatic disease. For patients undergoing high dose therapy, the

Table 3.1 Immunocytochemical detection of epithelial tumour cells in bone marrow and blood before treatment and in mobilized peripheral blood progenitor cells (PBPC) after three cycles of chemotherapy in 42 patients: number and percentage of patients who had tumour cells among the 1×10^7 to 2×10^7 cells tested after CD45 immunomagnetic depletion

Bone marrow at diagnosis		Peripheral blood at diagnosis		PBPC after three cycles of FEC	
n	%	*n*	%	*n*	%
17	40	3	7	17	40

presence of CK19 RT-PCR positive cells in the bone marrow prior to treatment was a bad prognostic factor.

PURGING OF TUMOUR CELLS FROM BONE MARROW AND PERIPHERAL BLOOD PROGENITOR CELLS

Different procedures to purge tumour cells from autografts such as chemotherapy and mAbs either with complement or as immunotoxins or immunomagnetic beads have been extensively tested in the clinic.[9] Currently the most frequently used procedure used is based on mAbs and paramagnetic beads.

At the Norwegian Radium Hospital we developed an efficient indirect immunomagnetic purging procedure to deplete lymphoma cells from bone marrow, employing anti-B cell or anti-T cell mAbs and magnetizeable beads, Dynabeads M-450 sheep-anti-mouse (Dynal A/S, Oslo, Norway).[10–14] A mononuclear cell preparation of harvested marrow is incubated with saturated amounts of a mixture of the mAbs binding the B cell antigens CD19, CD20, CD22, CD23 and CD37, or the T cell antigens CD2, CD3, CD5 and CD7. Excess antibody is removed by washing and the beads are then added and incubated. The bead/cell rosettes formed and excess beads are removed using our own purging device or the MAX-SEP cell separator (Baxter Biotech, Irvine, California, USA). After a second cycle of purging, the cell suspension is concentrated and frozen.

Of 83 patients with non-Hodgkin's lymphomas treated with fractionated total body irradiation, high dose cyclophosphamide and immunomagnetic purged bone marrow, the median number of days to recover granulocytes ($>0.5 \times 10^9/l$) was 24 (range 11–117) and platelets ($>20 \times 10^9/l$) 24 (range 8–566).[14] Purging with immunomagnetic beads was found to be 10–100 times more efficient than targeted cell lysis with complement activating antibodies and rabbit complement[36] and up to a 5 log depletion of tumour cells was achieved when PCR was used to detect residual lym-

phoma cells after purging.[37] The same purging procedure was also successfully used to purge tumour cells from PBPC.[15] However, since the number of cells in a PBPC graft is 10 times the number found in bone marrow grafts, a large number of expensive beads are needed. Because of this, a negative depletion of tumour cells has gradually been substituted by CD34+ cell enrichment.

CD34+ CELL ENRICHMENT OF PERIPHERAL BLOOD PROGENITOR CELLS

Autografts consisting of isolated CD34+ progenitor cells from PBPC appear to give a similar reconstitution of haemopoiesis after high dose therapy to that given by unmanipulated PBPC.[15,16] Because most solid tumour cells do not express the CD34 antigen the isolated cells should not contain malignant cells. However, previous studies show that CD34 enrichment gives only a 2–4 log tumour cell depletion of breast cancer cells.[16] Given that the purity of CD34 cells obtained in these studies varies from 50% to 85%, one explanation for the modest purging effect could be that the malignant cells contaminate the CD34− fraction of the selected cells. Employing the Isolex 300i device, at the Norwegian Radium Hospital, we tested the purging efficacy of CD34+ cell enrichment in 32 patients with breast cancer. In spite of a median of 99.4% purity of CD34+ cells, immunocytochemical examination of isolated cells from individual breast cancer patients confirmed that only 3 log tumour cell depletion was obtained.[38] Similar findings have been reported by others using different devices.[16]

In lymphoma patients, B cells were present among the isolated cells even when a purity of 99.7% CD34 cells was achieved. Transformed non-Hodgkin's lymphoma patients who are candidates for high dose therapy frequently contain residual disease in their stem cell products. We therefore tested whether CD34+ cell enrichment plus B cell purging was able to deplete lymphoma cells from the PBPC grafts. In three individual clinical scaled experiments, fresh *bcl-2* negative PBPC products from lymphoma patients were spiked with 0.5% Karpas cells. By the use of the Isolex 300i, version 2.0, CD34+ cell enrichment plus purging with anti-CD19 and anti-CD20 antibodies and immunobeads were performed simultaneously. Enriched CD34+ cells from three individual experiments gave a purity of CD34+ cells of 99.6%, 99.7% and 99.5%, and the yield of CD34+ cells was 52%, 70% and 38%, respectively. Because added Karpas cells contained the *bcl-2* rearrangement, real-time PCR using a consensus Jh reverse primer and a *bcl-2* forward primer and probe was employed to measure purging efficacy. In two experiments the numbers of *bcl-2* rearranged positive cells were calculated to be 8×10^7 and 4.8×10^7 cells in PBPC before purging. After CD34+ cell enrichment and B cell depletion there were 9×10^2 and 2.2×10^3 *bcl-2* rearranged cells, respectively. Five transformed non-Hodgkin's lymphoma patients were mobilized with chemotherapy (MIME) and G-CSF. After CD34+ cell enrichment and B cell depletion of PBPC the mean purity and yield of CD34+ cells obtained were 99.0 (range 98.6–99.2) and 57.3 (range 37.4–71.1). All patients given B cell purged CD34+ cells experienced fast haemopoietic engraftment. Flow cytometric measurements of B cells after purging gave either detectable cells or a low number of B cells without a monoclonal phenotype. In one patient, tumour cells contained the *bcl-2* rearrangement. By real-time PCR, the number of tumour cells was calculated to be 3.8×10^8 in PBPC before the start and 3.6×10^4 tumour cells after purging (Table 3.2). Thus our data show that the combination of CD34+ cell enrichment and B cell purging with anti-CD20 and anti-CD19 antibodies efficiently removes tumour cells with a modest loss of CD34+ cells.

PURGING OF TUMOUR CELLS FROM AUTOGRAFTS AND CLINICAL VALUE

The purging procedure should be efficient and should give a fast and sustained haemopoietic reconstitution after high dose therapy. Table 3.3 gives the Norwegian Radium Hospital's data on lymphomas autotransplanted with purged bone marrow, unmanipulated PBPC or CD34+ cells. No differences were observed in time to haemopoietic recovery, number of platelet transfusions required and number of days in the hospital among lymphoma patients given CD34 cells or non-manipulated PBPCs. However, the use of manipulated bone marrow gave a slower reconstitution. The preliminary data also indicated that progenitor cells had a reconstitution capability after CD34+ cell enrichment and B cell purging that is identical to that when CD34+ cell enrichment was used alone.

Table 3.2 Simultaneous CD34+ cell enrichment and B cell purging with anti-CD19 and anti-CD20 monoclonal antibodies of peripheral blood cell progenitor (PBPC) from transformed non-Hodgkin lymphoma patients: purging efficacy measured by real-time polymerase chain reaction (TaqMan) using a consensus Jh reverse primer and a *bcl-2* forward primer and probe

	Total no. of cells	t(14;18) copies/10^5 cells	Total no. of t(14;18) copies
PBPC	3.2×10^{10}	1200	3.8×10^8
CD34+ cells	$4.0n \times 10^8$	9	3.6×10^4

Table 3.3 Autotransplantation in patients with malignant lymphomas: time to hematopoietic recovery, number of progenitor cells infused and types of autografts used

	Bone marrow (*n* = 83 patients)	Peripheral blood progenitor cells (*n* = 50 patients)	CD34+ cells (*n* = 22 patients)
CD34+(10^6 cells/kg)	Not determined	5.7 (1.8–20.0)	5.8 (2.7–20.6)
CFU-c (10^5/kg)	6.2 (0.7–22.0)	14.1 (0.4–62.5)	12.7 (6.4–22.4)
Days neutrophils >0.5	24 (11–140)	12 (8–24)	12 (7–17)
Days platelets >20	26 (8–566)	11 (7–43)	12 (7–15)

As can be seen in Table 3.2 the combination of CD34+ cell enrichment and B cell purging assessed by real-time PCR gave 4 log tumour cell depletion of B cell lymphoma cells. This was similar to the results reported by Dreger et al.[39]

It has been shown that patients transplanted with tumour-free purged autografts have a significantly better disease-free survival compared with those who have persistent tumour cells after purging.[8,40] Because these studies had not been randomized, the Norwegian Radium Hospital initiated a prospective study in collaboration with the European Blood and Marrow Transplant Group in relapsed follicular lymphomas (CUP trial). Patients were randomized to either chemotherapy or high dose therapy plus or minus purging of B lymphoma cells. Altogether 20 centres were trained to purge the autografts uniformly with the immunomagnetic purging procedure developed in the Norwegian Radium Hospital. Over a period of 4–5 years, 140 patients entered the study and only 89 fulfilled the criteria for randomization. Twenty-four patients were treated with chemotherapy, 33 with high dose therapy and unmanipulated autografts, and 32 with purged autografts. Unfortunately, because of the small number of patients treated, no conclusions could be drawn with regard to the effect of purging.[41] We are currently testing by real-time PCR the presence of minimal residual disease in bone marrow samples taken before and after

high dose therapy, and in the infused stem cells. Hopefully this will yield further information on the efficacy of purging and any survival benefit.

To my knowledge no other randomized studies have been conducted or are being planned to address the potential clinical benefit of purging tumour cells from autografts. Because the existing data indicate that reinfusion of tumour cells contributes to relapse of the disease, I recommend purging in all lymphoma patients with a history of previous bone marrow involvement. Where possible, the Norwegian Radium Hospital always uses real-time PCR to measure the purging efficacy and the number of tumour cells infused into the patients. These data will hopefully add to our understanding of the clinical value of purging.

MINIMAL RESIDUAL DISEASE AFTER HIGH DOSE THERAPY

A persisting PCR signal in blood after high dose therapy of low-grade lymphoma does not necessarily predict relapse. However, if a PCR signal is negative and becomes positive after high dose therapy, this is an early sign of relapse.[21] In chronic myeloid leukaemia (CML) patients PCR of *BCR-ABL* transcripts is a reliable method to detect minimal residual disease.[42] Quantification of *BCR-ABL* transcripts allows measurement of changes in the PCR signal. When this method was used after bone marrow transplantation in CML, increasing signal predicted relapse several months before this was evident from morphological examination of the bone marrow.[42] This method is also being used to measure the effect of donor T cell infusions on relapsed transplanted CML patients. Hopefully, the use of real-time PCR in both leukaemias and lymphomas will further facilitate the investigation of the clinical relevance of minimal residual disease.

The sensitivity and reliability of immunocytochemical techniques used for detection of isolated epithelial cells in bone marrow are restricted by the low number of tumour cells found on each slide. In the Norwegian Radium Hospital's high-risk stage II breast cancer study the mean number of tumour cells detected per 2×10^6 cells tested was only 3. Based on these observations, the Norwegian Radium Hospital recently reported our clinical experiences with enrichment of tumour cells from large numbers of mononuclear haemopoietic cells.[43] Cells expressing CD45 antigen were removed from the samples by use of anti-CD45 conjugated Dynabeads, and the remaining cells were examined for the presence of tumour cells by immunocytochemistry, using anti-CK mAbs. When 1×10^7 to 2×10^7 mononuclear bone marrow samples ($n = 165$) or PBPC products ($n = 22$) were examined, the immunobead procedure resulted in 85% mean depletion ($\pm 1\%$ SEM, $n = 206$) of haemopoietic cells. Of the remaining cells examined for the presence of cytokeratin-expressing epithelial cells, 23.5% were positive, compared with 11.7% of the samples after standard immunocytochemistry procedure testing 2×10^6 cells. A mean 4.1-fold higher number of positive cells were detected with the CD45-depletion procedure than with the direct cytospin procedure.

Using the CD45-depletion procedure, at the Norwegian Radium Hospital we are currently testing 1×10^7 to 2×10^7 bone marrow cells and PBPC from frozen samples from individual patients before and after high dose therapy with stem cell support. Of 14 patients who experienced an early relapse after high dose therapy, 13 had circulating tumour cells either in bone marrow before treatment ($n = 9$) or in their PBPC products ($n = 4$). No difference was observed between patients given CD34+ enriched cells or PBPC as stem cell support.[24] This may indicate that early relapse is associated with circulating tumour cells that survive the high dose chemotherapy (Table 3.2).

Table 3.4 shows data from a number of patients treated with high dose therapy in whom tumour cell contamination was examined. While these are only interim data, it would appear that late relapse occurs in patients efficiently purged, indicating that this may be failure of conditioning treatment rather than failure of purging. Enrichment of tumour cells prior to detection opens up the possibility of studying a higher number of tumour cells from each sample. Furthermore, it also permits further characterization of individual tumour cells from each patient's sample.[44] By performing double staining of individual tumour cells in the bone marrow, it has been shown that metastatic cells have a heterogeneous expression of antigens such as major histocompatibility (MHC) class I antigen and antigens against different proliferation-associated molecules.[3] Downregulation of MHC class I antigens on tumour cells was observed, which in turn might lead to escape of tumour cells from lysis by cytotoxic T lymphocytes. The lack of expression of proliferation antigens on tumour cells might also indicate that many of the micrometastatic tumour cells present in the bone marrow are dormant and resistant to chemotherapy. Until now, only a small number of patients and a limited number of tumour cells from these patients have been studied. Therefore no firm conclusions can be drawn about the clinical utility of further characterization of individual tumour cells by double-staining techniques.

Recently, promising results have been reported using mAbs as therapy against solid tumours, either alone or in combination with chemotherapy.[45-47] Because immunotherapy-based strategies can work only on patients who have low tumour load and against tumour cells expressing the target antigens, phenotyping of

Table 3.4 Minimal residual disease detected from 1×10^7 to 2×10^7 mononuclear bone marrow cells employing the immunomagnetic CD45-depletion procedure. The numbers of tumour cells found in each sample before therapy and 6–12 months after therapy in six individual patients given either nine cycles of chemotherapy or three cycles of chemotherapy plus high dose with stem cell rescue are shown

Patient	Type of treatment	Diagnosis	Time after therapy (months)		Clinical status
			6	12	
I	9 × FEC	3320	15	222	Dead
II	9 × FEC	32	0	0	Alive
III	9 × FEC	30	1	1	Alive
IV	High dose	20	0	658	Dead
V	High dose	5	0	238	Dead
VI	High dose	659	33	28	Alive
VII	High dose	41	39	225	Relapse/alive

tumour cells and monitoring of in vivo tumour cell purging efficacy will become important in the near future.

CONCLUSION

Altogether, the different methods available to detect minimal residual disease are promising. Standardization programs are developing[48] and, as outlined in this chapter, monitoring minimal residual disease will give us a better understanding of the biology of the tumour cells from individual patients. Hopefully, this will also lead to an improved and specific cancer treatment.

REFERENCES

1. Gianni A, Siena S, Bregni M et al. Granulocyte–macrophage colony-stimulating factor to harvest circulating haematopoietic stem cells for autotransplantation. Lancet 1989;2: 580–4.
2. Haas R, Mohle R, Fruehauf S et al. Patients characteristics associated with successful mobilizing and autografting of peripheral blood progenitor cells (PBPC) in malignant lymphoma. Blood 1994;83:3787–94.
3. Tricot G, Jagannath S, Vesole D et al. Peripheral bloodstem cell transplantations for multiple myeloma: identification of favorable variables for rapid engraftment in 225 patients. Blood 1995;85:588–96.
4. Vose J, Armitage JO. Clinical application of hematopoietic growth factors. Blood 1995;13: 1023–35.
5. Eaves CJ. Peripheral blood stem cells reach new heights. Blood 1993;82:1957–9.
6. Brenner MK, Rill DR, Moen RC et al. Gene-marking to trace origin of relapse after autologous bone-marrow transplantation. Lancet 1993; 341:85–6.
7. Deisseroth A, Zu Z, Claxton D et al. Genetic marking shows that Ph+ cells present in autologous transplants of chronic myelogenous leukemia (CML) contribute to relapse after autologous bone marrow in CML. Blood 1994;83: 3068–76.
8. Gribben JG, Freedman AS, Neuberg D et al. Immunologic purging of marrow assessed by PCR before autologous bone marrow transplantation for B-cell lymphoma. N Engl J Med 1991;28:1525–33.

4

Leukapheresis and mobilization

Ruth Pettengell

CONTENTS Introduction • Leukapheresis • BPC-mobilizing regimens • Second-generation regimens • Summary

INTRODUCTION

Clinically useful mobilization of haemopoietic stem cells from extravascular sites into the circulation occurs when myelopoiesis is stimulated in response to administration of myelotoxic chemotherapy, or by specific cytokines or both. Haemopoietic progenitors are found within the mononuclear cell fraction of peripheral blood leukocytes and when transplanted function like bone marrow cells to reverse bone marrow aplasia. A mixture of lineage-committed progenitors, to effect early engraftment, and primitive progenitors, to effect long-term reconstitution is required in the graft for autologous haemopoietic reconstitution after myeloablative therapy. Transplantation of CD34+ cells from bone marrow or peripheral blood has demonstrated that both primitive and lineage-committed progenitor populations reside in the CD34+ fraction.[1,2] Of the cells in adult bone marrow CD34+ cells constitute 1–5%, and they constitute approximately 0.01–0.1% of normal human marrow mononuclear cells. For both autologous and allogeneic transplantation, mobilized HPC collected by apheresis have almost completely replaced bone marrow.

LEUKAPHERESIS

Any commercially available apheresis device can be used to collect blood stem cells (BSC), using machine settings designed to collect lymphocytes or low-density mononuclear cells. Automated continuous-flow blood cell separators rather than intermittent-flow devices are faster, give higher mononuclear and CD34+ cell yields[3] and have a lower extracorporeal volume. However, they need two sites of vascular access. Depending on the protocol selected, each apheresis procedure requires approximately 2.5–4.0 hours to complete, and the collections can be repeated on a daily basis until a sufficient number of cells have been harvested. Anticoagulated blood is fed continuously into a rapidly rotating bowl in which red blood cells (RBCs), leukocytes, platelets and plasma separate into layers. The mononuclear cell layer is removed and the remainder, together with a replacement fluid if appropriate, returned to the donor. The vascular access needed for efficient apheresis is often a problem for patients who have been heavily pretreated. Central venous catheters can be used, placed in either the subclavian vein or the inferior vena cava, to resolve this problem.

Bone marrow or blood progenitor cell (BPC) collected by leukapheresis can be either immediately infused into the recipient, or stored by cryopreservation for future use. The apheresis product can be directly cryopreserved without further manipulation. The method most commonly used for cryopreservation employs the addition of the cryoprotectant dimethyl sulphoxide (DMSO) to the product at a concentration of 10% by volume. The cellular concentration of the stem cell product is adjusted to 1×10^8 to 5×10^8 cells/cm^3 with autologous serum, and the mixture is cooled in a controlled rate freezer and then stored in a liquid nitrogen freezer. The alternative method uses hydroxyethyl starch and DMSO as cryoprotectants, at a final concentration of 5% by volume. The cell concentration is adjusted as above and cells are placed directly into a $-80°C$ freezer for cooling and storage without controlled-rate freezing. This second method is only suggested for short-term storage of less than 4 months. Following cryopreservation, cells are usually thawed at the bedside and immediately reinfused. The quantitation of CD34+ cells is the most important step in the quality control of peripheral blood progenitor cell (PBPC) apheresis products. The ProCOUNT kit and software for semi-automated data acquisition and analysis represents a further step toward standardization of CD34+ cell enumeration in PBPC apheresis products. However, the occurrence of software warnings is high, and analysis or data re-evaluation by experienced staff is still mandatory. Therefore, currently there is no definite advantage of the kit and software over the existing guidelines for CD34+ analysis in PBPC grafts.[4]

Timing of collection

Following chemotherapy-induced mobilization, criteria such as the initial recovery of platelet numbers and the return of a specific number of neutrophils or specific percentage of monocytes in the neutrophil fraction have been used. Alternatively, it has been shown that the early exponential increase in white blood cells and platelets after the chemotherapy-induced nadir coincides with BPC release.[5,6] None of these methods is precise in defining the optimum time of mobilization, which generally extends over 3–4 days.

It is clear that the most accurate way to determine the day for beginning leukapheresis is related to the CD34+ concentration in the peripheral blood.[7,8] It has been an ongoing challenge for laboratories to agree on a reliable and reproducible method of enumerating CD34+ progenitor cells.[9] The method adopted in most clinically active laboratories is the simple Milan/Mulhouse protocol which takes into consideration the intensity of CD34 staining of a defined population of non-granulated (low side scatter, SSC) cells and the number of leukocytes in the sample.[9]

Mononuclear cells in DNA synthesis are proliferating stem cells. Analysis of this cell fraction by flow cytometry provides reliable results and appears to be an alternative to colony forming unit–granulocyte-macrophage (CFU-GM) assay or CD34+ cell determination for BPC quantification.[10] The Sysmex SE9500 measures HPC based on lipid content, size and nuclear density. The assay is rapid (90 s) and inexpensive (US$1.35 per sample) and the sample is run on a routine clinical analyser. A high correlation ($r = 0.90$) has been seen between CD34+ cells and HPC in clinical trials.[11,12]

The value of the Sysmex SE9000 parameters [white blood cells (WBC) count, neutrophil count, and immature myeloid index (IMI)] and Sysmex R2000 reticulocyte parameters (absolute, high and medium fluorescence reticulocytes) in predicting the optimum timing of blood stem cell harvest, in comparison with peripheral blood CD34/45, has been directly compared in 64 blood stem cell harvests from 23 patients with haematological malignancies. In this study peripheral blood CD34/45 remained the most useful predictor of yield. An IMI $> 20 \times 10^6/l$ was, however, a useful surrogate for predicting a rise in peripheral blood CD34/45 from nadir and proved to be superior to WBC or neutrophil count.[13]

There is also large inter-individual variability as exemplified by the 1.0–1.5 log range of CD34+ cells yields seen in normal donors mobilized with G-CSF alone.[14] Both steady-state[15,16] and pre-leukapheresis CD34+ cell counts from peripheral blood have been shown to be useful in predicting whether stem cell mobilization will result in the collection of sufficient cells for transplantation. In a large French study of 656 transplants in patients with both haematological malignancies and solid tumours, the number of two blood volume leukaphereses required to obtain a good harvest was calculated. A single leukapheresis was sufficient if CD34+ cells were greater than $38/\mu l$, two if CD34+ cells were between 20 and $38/\mu l$ and three to four procedures if CD34+ cells were between 10 and $20/\mu l$.[17] Other groups have produced formulae to calculate yields.[18] What is clear is that significant stem cell recruitment occurs during leukapheresis.

Adequacy of the harvest

Undoubtedly, the number of HPCs reinfused following myeloablative therapy determines the time to haemopoietic recovery.[11,19,20] Further increases in transplant cell dose over an optimal number may further accelerate platelet but not neutrophil engraftment. Various centres have established threshold doses appropriate to their own patient population – HPC-mobilizing, myeloablative and post-transplant treatment regimens – but these are difficult to compare. For most purposes, enumeration of the number of CD34+ cells in apheresis products has been regarded as a reliable index of engraftment potential. Caution is required, however, because high levels of CD34+ cells do not always indicate high stem cell numbers.[21,22] Patients who expressed HLA allele A_1 or A_{24} and radiotherapy were more likely to have discordant CD34+ and CFU-GM yields.[23] Also, the evidence that long-term haemopoietic recovery may be more accurately predicted by the subpopulation of primitive progenitors transplanted suggests that the content of CD34+CD33− and long-term culture-initiating cells in cell collection samples may be more important for predicting successful engraftment, particularly in patients with poor mobilization.

For autologous and allogeneic transplantation a cell dose of 2×10^6 to 5×10^6 CD34+ cells/kg or 10^5 CFU-GM cells/kg are recommended for optimal engraftment, although there is evidence that higher doses of CD34+ ($>15 \times 10^6$/kg) may accelerate haemopoietic engraftment further.[24] Sixty per cent of patients require greater than four leukaphereses to reach optimal harvests[25] and patients who mobilize CD34+ cells at less than 0.2×10^6/kg/day on 2–3 consecutive days have a low probability of collecting 2×10^6/kg even if aphereses were continued for 5–8 days' harvests.[14,26]

The minimum number of haemopoietic progenitor cells required to effect haemopoietic reconstitution after myeloablation has not been determined but, at below 10^6 CD34+ cells/kg, neutrophil and particularly platelet recovery is delayed. Patients who fail to mobilize an adequate number of stem cells frequently require two or more attempts at mobilization, creating added risks to the patient and increased treatment and hospital costs. In one study, additional expenditure per patient receiving suboptimal CD34+ cell numbers ($<5 \times 10^6$/kg) was approximately US$4000.[27] The dose of CD34+ cells influences engraftment also in the late post-transplant period, correlating with transfusion and antibiotic requirements, fever episodes and days of hospitalization during the first year post-transplant.[28] A further concern is that if the haemopoietic stem cells have proliferated extensively prior to transplantation and few are engrafted, stem cell senescence could limit the usefulness of the graft, leading to delayed marrow failure. In normal life, peripheral leukocyte telomeres shorten by approximately 9 base pairs per year. Senescence is seen after 30–75 population doublings (Hayflick limit).[29]

There is no generally accepted mobilization procedure for patients who fail a first mobilization attempt. In general, however, integrated regimens are associated with fewer poor mobilizers and indeed some patients who have failed previous mobilization with cyclophosphamide and granulocyte colony stimulating factor (G-CSF) have been successfully re-mobilized. G-CSF alone is an effective and non-toxic alternative but yields tend to be lower.[30] Successful harvests after a second mobilization vary from 48% to 88%.[14,26]

Poor mobilization occurs in up to 30% of patients undergoing autologous BPC collection (see Table 4.1). Statistically, lower age, marrow without disease, no prior radiation, and lower numbers of prior chemotherapy regimens, were the outstanding factors correlating with larger numbers of CD34+ cells in collections.[31] A CD34+ yield reduction of 0.2×10^6/kg has been predicted for each prior cycle of chemotherapy[32] and 1.8×10^6/kg in patients exposed to large-field irradiation.[33] Some individuals with no apparent risk factors fail to increase circulating stem cell numbers to clinically useful levels regardless of the mobilization protocol used. This failure to mobilize occurs in 10% of normal donors. The Nebraska group suggests that mobilization vigour may be the result of a genetically determined or a therapeutically induced inhibitor of mobilization. Others have shown that high levels of FLT-3 ligand (>95 pg/ml) in the bone marrow or peripheral blood is a good predictor of poor mobilization.[34]

It is important to remember that successful haemopoietic engraftment depends not only on the quality of the infused cells, but also on the recipient stroma. In heavily pretreated patients, the bone marrow stroma may have been damaged by prior chemotherapy and radiotherapy, the conditioning regimen and the underlying disease. If this is the case, marrow regeneration will be jeopardized, no matter what the number or source of the haemopoietic progenitors used for transplantation.

BPC-MOBILIZING REGIMENS

A wide variety of cytokines and cytotoxics, alone and in combination, can mobilize HPC from the marrow to the peripheral blood. The optimum HPC-mobilizing regimen will depend on the proposed application. Initial protocols, which used chemotherapy alone, have now been replaced by regimens involving the use of HGF either alone or in combination with disease-specific chemotherapeutic regimens that also mobilize BPC, thereby avoiding a specific BPC-mobilization step. Many studies suggest that the combination of chemotherapy and cytokines stimulates more early HPC into the circulation than either alone, particularly in heavily pretreated patients.[30,35,36]

Cytokines

The use of cytokines alone to mobilize BPC is particularly attractive for cancer patients in remission and for normal donors for gene therapy or allogeneic transplantation. Paradoxically, lineage-specific cytokines such as G-CSF and GM-CSF are more potent stimuli to HPC mobilization than early acting factors such as interleukin-3, FLT-3/FLK-2 ligand and KIT ligand, but the combination of early- and late-acting factors gives highest yields.[37] Cytokine-induced mobilization produces an increased number of circulating stem cells in a predictable, and for KIT and FLT-3 ligand, a prolonged time period.

G-CSF

Among the different growth factors G-CSF has been most extensively used for BPC mobilization due to its predictable mobilization time course, its efficacy in cancer patients and normal donors and the low incidence of side

---

Table 4.1 Factors predicting poor mobilization

- Prior radiotherapy
- Large amount of prior chemotherapy
- High previous alkylating dose
- Previous BEAM/miniBEAM
- Low grade non-Hodgkin's lymphoma, chronic lymphoblastic leukaemia or myeloma

effects. The biological potency of glycosylated G-CSF (lenograstim) is higher than that of non-glycosylated G-CSF (filgrastim).[38] However, bioequivalent doses of filgrastim and lenograstim have a similar effect on mobilization of CD34+ cells and immature subset kinetics.[39] The clinical relevance of the greater specific activity of lenograstim is therefore limited. Allotransplantation of G-CSF-mobilized BPC has resulted in durable and complete donor chimerism, indicating that G-CSF-mobilized BPC contain all the cells required for durable lymphohaemopoiesis. Colony forming cells and LTCIC show similar mobilization kinetics.[39] After G-CSF administration, CD34+ cell counts in the peripheral blood start increasing from day 3, peak on day 5 or 6, and decrease beyond day 7 even if G-CSF is continued.[40,41] There is wide interindividual variation in mobilization potentials in response to G-CSF. Some, but not all, authors have found CD34+ yields to be adversely affected by age and the female sex.[41,42]

The dose of G-CSF is clearly important when used as a single agent. Doses of G-CSF have ranged between 2 and 24 µg/kg/day for up to 10 days, with apheresis being performed on days 5–11.[14] The European Bone Marrow Transplantation Group (EBMT) and National Marrow Donor Program (USA) recommendation is that normal donors undergoing mobilization for allogeneic BPC transplant should receive doses of 10 µg/kg/day for 5 days, with the donor undergoing BPC collections on days 5 and 6.[43,44] Following G-CSF 10 µg/kg/day, one or two leukaphereses on days 5 and 6, processing 10–20 l, will yield CD34+ cells, in most instances, at more than 2×10^6 to 3×10^6/kg (which is the threshold set at the first International Symposium on Allogeneic BSCT).[42] Mobilization with G-CSF 10 µg/kg/day is well tolerated and the duration of side effects on average is shorter than after a surgical procedure.[45] Thrombocytopenia, probably due to both leukapheresis and G-CSF administration, is observed with platelets returning to pretreatment levels within 10 days.[39] Although G-CSF has been reported to increase platelet aggregation and platelet activity in normal donors, the incidence of vascular events and the risk of thrombotic or bleeding complications has been very low.[43] Spontaneous splenic rupture during G-CSF administration has been reported.[46,47] It does not seem that G-CSF has any late adverse effects in normal donors, although longer follow-up is still needed. The total cost of G-CSF administration and two leukaphereses is reported to be comparable to the cost of bone marrow collection.[48]

Higher doses of G-CSF (24 µg/kg/day) have been reported to improve the effectiveness of BPC collection, compared with conventional doses (10 µg/kg/day).[49] Also Knudson et al.[50] found that lower doses of G-CSF (10 µg/kg/day) were not as effective a regimen as cyclophosphamide (4 g) plus G-CSF.[26] Gazitt et al., using 32 µg/kg/day of G-CSF, successfully mobilized 88% of patients (with a median of five aphereses) who had failed to mobilize with chemotherapy plus G or GM-CSF.[26] However, other authors report success in only 32% of patients, with a median of eight aphereses using high dose G-CSF for second mobilization.[51] Higher doses of G-CSF do not reduce the wide interindividual yields in PBCD34+ cells, and in normal donors the increased side effects may be unacceptable. In children the data are clearer, and there appears to be no advantage to using greater than 10 µg/kg/day.[52]

Arbona et al.[53] investigated the schedule dependency of G-CSF alone in mobilizing BPC in normal donors and found that 6 µg/kg/day of G-CSF given 12-hourly provides better CD34+ and CFU-GM yields than 10 µg/kg/day. Kroger et al.[54] confirmed these results in a uniform breast cancer patient population. Given twice-daily, 5 µg/kg G-CSF led to almost two-fold higher progenitor cell yields for CD34+, CFU-GM and mononuclear cells and resulted in significantly fewer apheresis procedures than 10 or 15 µg/kg given once-daily.[55] Twice-daily administration also resulted in an earlier mobilization peak.[55] Given the short elimination half-life of G-CSF of around 3–4 h, regardless of the route of administration, it is not surprising that once-daily dosing may be suboptimal. In addition, kinetic studies show that the highest CD34+ cell count is reached 6–12 h after G-CSF injection, with a decrease in CD34+ cell counts within 2 h.[56] Therefore the timing of the G-CSF injection in relation to apheresis is important.

In summary, despite the wide use of G-CSF for BPC mobilization, the optimal dosing and scheduling remain to be determined. Doses up to G-CSF 10 µg/kg/day show a consistent dose–response relationship with the mobilization (and collection) of CD34+ progenitor cells.[14] Whether higher doses are superior (or cost-effective) remains to be determined, and they may produce more side effects. Although there is no direct comparison of G-CSF mobilization with cyclophosphamide plus G-CSF, it is probably not as effective.[57,58] However, one study has shown that despite a six-fold higher CD34+ yield with 4000 mg/m^2 and 57% as opposed to 13% of apheresis with G-CSF alone, achieving the target CD34+ cell dose of 5×10^6/kg in one collection, the cost of chemotherapy administration, more doses of G-CSF, transfusions, and hospitalizations caused cyclophosphamide, etoposide and G-CSF to be more expensive than G-CSF alone (US$8693 versus $7326, respectively).[59] The short-term safety profile of G-CSF mobilization in normal donors is acceptable but continued safety monitoring is required.

Pegylated G-CSF

Pegylated G-CSF has shown significantly better mobilization of BPC in mice compared with G-CSF alone. In normal volunteers neutrophil numbers are sustained for between 1 and 2 weeks from a single injection and mobilization of CD34+ cells, and progenitors may occur in a more timely manner and to around the same absolute numbers as with repeated daily injections of unmodified filgrastim. Further clinical trials are awaited.[60]

Other cytokines

Lineage-specific growth factors mobilize PBPCs and accelerate haemopoietic recovery after high dose chemotherapy. Although GM-CSF is also an effective mobilization agent it is now rarely used, mostly because of its side effect profile, which is poorer than that of G-CSF. Studies in normal donors, comparing GM-CSF (at 10 µg/kg/day) and simultaneous GM-CSF and G-CSF (at 5 µg/kg/day each) have shown no advantage of the combination of CSFs over G-CSF alone to mobilize CD34+ cells. There were, however, some qualitative differences in the BPC collected after GM-CSF and G-CSF, compared with G-CSF alone.[61]

In addition to G-CSF and GM-CSF, a number of cytokines, including interleukin-1 (IL-1), IL-3, IL-7, IL-8, IL-11, c-kit ligand (stem cell factor, SCF) and thrombopoietin (TPO), have been shown to mobilize BPC in animals and humans. Daniplestim is a genetically engineered IL-3 receptor agonist that has the advantage of having the proliferative potential of human IL-3 without some of the side effects. As with IL-3, synergy is seen with G-CSF, with around 30% more CD34+ yield per kilogram than with G-CSF alone.[62]

The effect of IL-8 is quite unique: progenitor cells were mobilized maximally at 15–30 min after the administration of IL-8 and returned to pretreatment levels within 1–4 h.[63,64] Administration of antibodies to the adhesion factor VLA-4 also results in rapid mobilization (within 30 min) of progenitor cells.[65] Alone, IL-11 and SCF mobilize progenitor but not primitive stem cells, but in combination IL-11 and SCF mobilize primitive stem cells.[66]

Recombinant human thrombopoietin (rhTPO) alone stimulates modest increases in GM-CFC (maximum seven-fold) and Meg-CFC (maximum four-fold) and acts additively with chemotherapy and G-CSF to mobilize both GM-CFC and Meg-CFC (58- and 66-fold, respectively).[67] Thrombopoietin may further increase the progenitor cell content and regenerating potential of PBPC products when combined with G-CSF. In a phase I study in 29 breast cancer patients, CD34+ cell yields were substantially higher with the first apheresis following rhTPO and G-CSF versus G-CSF alone: 4.1×10^6/kg (range 1.3–17.6) versus 0.8×10^6/kg (range 0.3–4.2), with $P = 0.0003$. Sixty-one per cent of the rhTPO- and G-CSF-mobilized group versus

10% of G-CSF-mobilized patients ($P = 0.001$) required a single apheresis to reach the threshold minimum. In addition, following high dose chemotherapy and PBPC reinfusion, the rhTPO- and G-CSF-mobilized patients engrafted a day earlier and required fewer transfusions compared with G-CSF-mobilized patients.[68]

The KIT ligand is produced in bone marrow stromal cells. Alone it has little direct colony-stimulating activity but it mobilizes well in conjunction with other cytokines. The addition of SCF to G-CSF and chemotherapy results in a dose-dependent, significantly increased mobilization of BPC, with less interindividual variation in BPC yields compared with the use of chemotherapy and G-CSF alone, resulting in fewer aphereses. In addition, the combination BPC release is sustained over 5 days compared with G-CSF alone.[25,69] In one study, the yields obtained suggest that whole blood aliquots could be used to rescue patients following myeloablative therapy.[69] In particular, the addition of KIT ligand to G-CSF appears to have a role in heavily pretreated patients. In a phase II study of 92 patients, 26 heavily pretreated lymphoma patients receiving G-CSF 10 μg/kg/day, compared with 15 patients receiving in addition SCF 20 μg/kg/day, failed to achieve a CD34+ level of 1×10^6/kg by the day 5 leukapheresis.[71] In patients with multiple myeloma the addition of SCF to filgrastim after cyclophosphamide for PBPC mobilization resulted in a significant increase in CD34+ cell yield and a concomitant reduction (three-fold) in the number of leukaphereses required to collect an optimal CD34+ cell harvest of 5×10^6/kg. The median CD34+ cell yield for the SCF group in the first leukapheresis was 11.3 compared with 4.0×10^6/kg for filgrastim alone ($P = 0.003$) and for all leukaphereses (12.4×10^6 versus 8.2×10^6/kg, respectively, $P = 0.007$).[72]

The FLK-2/FLT-3 ligand synergizes with many of the same growth factors as the KIT ligand.[73] It does not activate mast cells and so has a better side effect profile than KIT ligand. It has no effect on erythropoiesis but can stimulate B, T and dendritic cells.[74,75] In mice, the number of colony forming cells (CFCs) in peripheral blood increased approximately two-, 21-, or 480-fold after administration of FLT-3 ligand, G-CSF, or the two cytokines together, respectively, for 5 days.[76,77]

Chemotherapy plus cytokine mobilization

Many but not all cytotoxic drugs stimulate HPC release. The mechanisms by which cytotoxic drugs stimulate blood progenitor release remain unknown. No relationship has yet emerged with the mode of anti-tumour action, so the effects of individual cytotoxics on mobilization are unpredictable.

The alkylating agent cyclophosphamide is the best documented and historically the most widely used drug for HPC mobilization. Although myelosuppressive, it is relatively non-toxic to early haemopoietic progenitors. This may be related to the production by primitive haemopoietic stem cells of aldehyde dehydrogenase, which inactivates the myelotoxic 4-hydroxy-cyclophosphamide metabolite. Committed haemopoietic progenitors lose the ability to produce this enzyme and hence become susceptible to cyclophosphamide cytotoxicity.[78] Both long term culture-initiating cells (LTCICs) as well as committed progenitors (CFCs, CFU) are mobilized by cyclophosphamide. The LTCICs are released simultaneously with or slightly before the clonogenic cells.[57]

An additive or synergistic effect on CFC mobilization has been seen in all studies using G- or GM-CSF following combination chemotherapy. In addition, higher numbers of progenitors, as measured by CFC and long-term culture, are mobilized by chemotherapy and G-CSF than by G-CSF alone.[57]

The optimal dose of G-CSF after chemotherapy for BPC mobilization has not been determined. However in contrast to G-CSF used alone, there appears to be no advantage to increasing the dose of G-CSF above 5 μg/kg/day or a single vial.[79] A recent study retrospectively analysed the effect of G-CSF dose on peripheral blood CD34+ cell collection from

91 patients with haematological malignancies. The administration of low dose G-CSF [median 3.6 µg/kg/day (range 2.8–4.6)] after chemotherapy appears equivalent to administration of the standard dose [6.0 µg/kg/day (range 5.5–8.1)] in achieving satisfactory PBPC collection. This approach could allow significant savings in medical cost.[80]

The scheduling of cytokines following chemotherapy, rather than the duration (or total dose), appears to be of critical importance, as it is in the use of cytokines alone (see above). When collecting BPC in the recovery phase of chemotherapy, it may not be necessary for the drug to be continually present. Following doxorubicin/etoposide, G-CSF started immediately after the myelosuppressive stimulus and given for only 5 days gave progenitor cell yields similar to those obtained after 7–9 days of G-CSF. In addition, the day of maximum progenitor cell release was similar. Conversely, starting G-CSF at the time of the chemotherapy nadir accelerated the neutrophil recovery but did not enhance progenitor cell release over that obtained with chemotherapy alone (G Mariani, personal communication). Further data are required to confirm these observations.

Cyclophosphamide and a growth factor has been the gold standard for BPC collection. However, the dose of cyclophosphamide used, growth factor type, dose and scheduling have been variable (see Table 4.1). Broadly, the doses of cyclophosphamide needed can be categorized as high dose (6–7 g/m^2), intermediate dose (3–4 g/m^2) and low dose (1.5–2 g/m^2). High dose cyclophosphamide (7 g/m^2) has been shown to be superior to intermediate dose cyclophosphamide (4 g/m^2) at BPC mobilization. Likewise, in a sequential non-randomized study of cyclophosphamide (7 g/m^2) combined with G-CSF, compared with intermediate dose cyclophosphamide plus G-CSF, patients receiving the higher dose achieved statistically higher peaks of CD34+ cells in the peripheral blood and a significantly higher number of CD34+ cells in the leukapheresis product. Furthermore, patients who failed to mobilize with lower doses of cyclophosphamide plus G-CSF improved their yield with high dose cyclophosphamide plus G-CSF.[81]

Although, from these studies, high dose cyclophosphamide appears to be more effective at BPC mobilization than intermediate or low doses, its use is associated with a longer duration of cytopenia and a high rate of non-haematological morbidity, including haemorrhagic cystitis.[82,83] In contrast, cyclophosphamide at doses of 1.5–3 g/m^2 have now been reported with low toxicity and minimal requirements for hospitalization. Using cyclophosphamide 1.5 g/m^2 combined with G-CSF, Watts et al.[33] reported that 87% of lymphoma patients achieved an adequate harvest, defined as greater than 1×10^6/kg CD34+ cells, and 50% achieved an optimal harvest (i.e. associated with rapid engraftment) of more than 3.5×10^6/kg CD34+ cells. Cyclophosphamide at this dose was well tolerated and only 5% of patients required hospitalization. Using cyclophosphamide 3 g/m^2, 60% of lymphoma patients and 73% of myeloma patients achieved a CD34+ cell target of 2.5×10^6/kg.

Etoposide is a topoisomerase-II inhibitor and an effective CFC-mobilizing drug, even in pretreated patients. It is far less frequently used than cyclophosphamide in conventional chemotherapeutic regimens and transplant preparative regimens for common malignancies. Its use in high doses is associated with minimal non-haematological toxicity and its anti-tumour activity has been well documented.[84] Like cyclophosphamide, etoposide has low extramedullary toxicity and appeared to spare haemopoietic stem cells in preclinical studies.[85] Etoposide (2 g/m^2) and G-CSF gives peak CD34+ cell yields around day 12.[86] The efficacy of cyclophosphamide mobilization may also be augmented by the addition of etoposide, and, in a study of patients with relapsed or refractory Hodgkin's disease, 28 out of 38 patients (74%) achieved greater than the target CD34+ cell dose of 2.5×10^6/kg using this combination. In breast cancer patients cyclophosphamide 2 g/m^2 plus etoposide has proved as effective a mobilization regimen as cyclophosphamide 4 g/m^2, with significantly less toxicity.

Although it is difficult to compare studies due to the different case mix, it is clear that low to intermediate dose cyclophosphamide plus G-CSF can successfully mobilize BPC from the majority of patients with minimal toxicity. This may be further enhanced by the addition of etoposide. However, a significant proportion, particularly those who have been heavily pretreated, will fail to mobilize an optimal number even though sufficient cells are collected to proceed to high dose therapy. In addition, mobilization with cyclophosphamide has the disadvantage of requiring a specific mobilization step rather than being an integral part of therapy.

SECOND-GENERATION REGIMENS

The majority of patients for whom autologous BPC will be required, whether for transplantation or cytotoxic dose intensification, are already receiving conventional chemotherapy. For these patients, it is more convenient to base regimens to mobilize BPC on routine combination chemotherapy treatments than to devise additional cycles of mobilizing chemotherapy. In addition, patients may be at high risk of relapse and have been heavily pretreated, making delays for mobilizing regimens unacceptable.

A number of cytotoxic combinations have been used to mobilize BPC (Table 4.2), based on popular therapeutic regimens. Comparisons between them are difficult because mobilization varies widely with pretreatment, disease extent and pathology, and the mobilizing chemotherapy used. Even within a single treatment centre there can be considerable variability over time.[87,88] This is not surprising given laboratory and assay variables and the high inter-patient variability in numbers of progenitors mobilized. In general, however, these regimens are associated with fewer poor mobilizers; indeed some patients who have failed previous mobilization with cyclophosphamide and G-CSF have been successfully remobilized. However, because of the substantial impact that chemotherapy regimens have on the quantity and quality of collected CD34+ cells, anticancer effects and optimal BPC yields should be evaluated for each chemotherapy schedule. In one study, the number of CD34+ cells collected per litre of processed blood was significantly higher in the cyclophosphamide (Cy) 7 g/m^2 plus G-CSF and IVE plus G-CSF group [ifosphamide (2.5 g/m^2 for 3 days), etoposide (150 mg/m^2 for 3 days), epirubicin (100 mg/m^2 on day 1)] than in the group given cyclophosphamide 4 g/m^2 plus G-CSF and G-CSF 10 μg/kg ($P \leqslant 0.005$), but those mobilized with Cy7 plus G-CSF and IVE plus G-CSF produced significantly lower early progenitors and had a reduced plating efficiency.[58]

Lymphoma

For patients with high risk or relapsed lymphoma routine, chemotherapy can provide a dual function of mobilization and anti-lymphoma therapy. Cyclophosphamide, doxorubicin, vincristine, prednisolone (CHOP) plus G-CSF mobilizes around day but is less well studied than other regimens.[89] Pettengell et al. reported that a vincristine, doxorubicin, prednisolone, etoposide, cyclophosphamide (VAPEC-B) regimen combined with G-CSF was effective in BPC mobilization in non-Hodgkin's lymphoma (NHL) and relapsed Hodgkin's disease. In addition, optimal numbers of BPC were achieved following a single apheresis and the

---

Table 4.2 Optimization of mobilization

- Patient selection/timing
- Choice of chemotherapy/mobilization regimen
- Use of higher/split doses of granulocyte colony stimulating factor
- Use of additional cytokines
- Use of optimal collection devices/protocols

chemotherapy regimen was administered on an outpatient basis.[5,35] In common with other studies, patients with Hodgkin's disease provided fewer CD34+ cells and engrafted more slowly than NHL and solid tumour patients.[86,90] This may have been related to the frequency of prior radiation therapy and the fact that almost all patients had previously received nitrogen mustard.

Watts et al.,[91] using the lymphoma salvage regimen etoposide, methylprednisolone, cytarabine, cisplatin (ESHAP), collected CD34+ cells 4.7×10^6/kg compared with 2.9×10^6/kg for a matched series of patients mobilized with low dose cyclophosphamide (1.5 g/m^2) and G-CSF.[92] In patients with NHL, ICE chemotherapy (ifosfamide, carboplatin, etoposide) is also very effective both as a cytoreduction and mobilization regimen in patients with NHL.[93] The ifosphamide, etoposide, epirubicin (IVE) regimen combined with G-CSF (G-IVE) effectively mobilizes with more than 2.5×10^6 CD34+ cells in 87% of patients, compared with 60% of patients receiving cyclophosphamide 3 g/m^2. A CD34+ cell median of 5.06×10^6/kg per leukapheresis was collected with G-IVE, compared with 1.12×10^6/kg per leukapheresis with cyclophosphamide.[94] In another study, Martinez et al.[95] used IAPVP (ifosfamide, etoposide, Ara-C and methylprednisolone) combined with G-CSF and achieved their CD34+ cell target of 3.5×10^6/kg in all 15 patients. Interestingly this regimen appeared equally effective when using a lower dose of G-CSF (50 μg/m^2).

Successful CD34+ cell yields have been described with the salvage Dexa- (carmustine, cytarabine, etoposide, melphalan) BEAM regimen giving G-CSF from day 8. However, two to six leukapheresis procedures were required,[96] and more commonly in this heavily pretreated group yields are inadequate. Furthermore, Dexa-BEAM is severely myelosuppressive, with the median time to initiation of BPC collection being 18 days and most patients requiring 2–3 weeks of hospitalization for neutropenic sepsis.[96,97] MIME (mitoxantrone, ifosfamide, methotrexate and epirubicin) plus G-CSF is also

a more effective and less toxic mobilizing regimen than dexa-BEAM with a CD34+ cell median of 3.1×10^6/kg per leukapheresis and 94% of patients achieving the target CD34+ cell dose of 2×10^6/kg.[98]

Patients with low-grade NHL present a challenge for BPC mobilization, in particular patients who have been exposed to multiple courses of oral alkylating agents, fludarabine and radiotherapy. In several series 25% of patients given cyclophosphamide plus G-CSF fail to mobilize CD34+ cells to a level of 1×10^6/kg.[99,100] In contrast, good yields have been reported with the G-IVE and HAM (high dose Ara-C and mitoxantrone) regimens. Heavily treated patients mobilized with G-IVE collected CD34+ cells at 7.36×10^6/kg compared with 2.92×10^6/kg for patients mobilized with intermediate dose cyclophosphamide.[100] Haas et al.[101] mobilized 48 patients with the HAM regimen and CD34+ cells were collected at a median of 6.9×10^6/kg in a median of two leukaphereses, with patients mobilized in first remission and those who had received less than six cycles of previous chemotherapy tending to have better results. In summary, with the possible exception of dexa-BEAM, lymphoma salvage regimens give superior mobilization to intermediate or low dose cyclophosphamide and G-CSF.

Myeloma

High dose cyclophosphamide in combination with growth factors has been used as a standard approach to BPC mobilization in myeloma, with considerable morbidity and a mortality of up to 2%.[102] Prior radiotherapy and chemotherapy with alkylating agents have a major impact on mobilization in myeloma.[103] In one series in which patients were mobilized with Cy (3 g) plus G-CSF, those who had received prior treatment with vincristine, doxorubin, dexamethasone (VAD) achieved a CD34+ cell median of 3.25×10^6/kg per leukapheresis compared with 0.39×10^6/kg/leukopheresis for patients treated with doxorubin, carmustine, cyclophosphamide, melphalan (ABCM). In multivariate analysis, favourable factors included mobilization with chemotherapy plus cytokines ($P = 0.04$) and, especially, the addition of SCF to G-CSF ($P = 0.018$) as well as the remission status of the marrow at the time of mobilization. Several authors have compared a number of different regimens for mobilization in relapsed/refractory myeloma and showed that etoposide ($200\ mg/m^2/day \times 3$) with intermediate dose Cy (4 g) plus G-CSF was the most effective regimen in this disease.[104,105] Patients receiving this schedule mobilized a median of $12.2 \times 10^6/kg$ CD34+ cells.

Mobilizing with G-CSF alone[106] reduces procedural morbidity but also BPC yields. Significantly more CD34+ yields per apheresis were obtained in patients receiving cyclophosphamide compared with patients receiving G-CSF alone (1.98×10^6 versus $1.05 \times 10^6/kg$), resulting in a higher yield of CD34+ cells (6.8×10^6 versus $4.85 \times 10^6/kg$) in the cyclophosphamide group. However, the majority of patients achieved a CD34+ cell target of $2 \times 10^6/kg$ and engraftment kinetics of the two patient groups were not significantly different. These results have been confirmed in a randomized study[107] comparing G-CSF 16 μg/kg/day alone to Cy 6 g plus G-CSF 5 μg/kg/day. The authors concluded that for the majority of myeloma patients G-CSF alone was satisfactory for mobilization and that the higher number of CD34+ cells collected with high dose cyclophosphamide was not necessary and resulted in all patients being hospitalized. Furthermore, Cy itself has little specific antimyeloma activity. Several studies of patients with myeloma have now confirmed that the addition of SCF to filgrastim after cyclophosphamide for PBPC mobilization results in a significant increase in CD34+ cell yield and a concomitant reduction in the number of leukaphereses required to collect an optimal harvest.[72,108]

Leukaemia

Unmanipulated autologous transplantation of BPC has been performed in small numbers of patients with chronic myelocytic leukaemia (CML) for many years. In CML the goal has been to mobilize Ph-negative BPC. Recent evidence suggests that normal BPC can be collected in the early phase of recovery after chemotherapy and G-CSF for patients in chronic phase. Hydroxyurea and G-CSF is a well tolerated mobilization regimen in patients with CML. In addition, significant cytogenetic response was seen.[109,110] An Italian group has used anthracycline-based chemotherapy (idarubicin, cytarabine, etoposide, ICE or daunorubicin, cytarabine).[111] The majority of patients (24 of 29) with a median of four leukaphereses successfully mobilized. The median time from the first day of chemotherapy to the first leukapheresis was 26 days (range 14–38). Thirty per cent of harvests were Ph-negative and 45% had less than 35% Ph-positive cells in the harvest. However, only 21% achieved both a successful harvest and Ph-negativity. The use of more sensitive technologies such as the PCR has revealed persistent disease in most, apparently Ph-negative cases. This is confirmed by results showing that disease relapse occurs following transplant in these cases. Interestingly, one study using RT-PCR for BCR-ABL on cytogenetically Ph-negative leukaphereses showed that, in addition to the presence of transcripts in all collections, the number of transcripts increased from the first to the fifth apheresis.[112] In summary it is possible to mobilize and collect Ph-negative enriched PBPC in unselected patients with chronic granulocytic leukaemia. Suitable material for autologous rescue can be obtained from approximately one-third of eligible, unselected young patients.

SUMMARY

Although the first demonstration of mobilization of BPC into the circulation was achieved as long ago as 1976[113] the best mobilizing regimen remains to be defined. Using currently available regimens, mobilization can be optimized with careful attention to patient selection, the timing of apheresis and the use of optimal collection devices and protocols. Chemotherapy regimens and cytokines differ in their ability to mobilize blood progenitor cells, the timing of mobilization and the cell populations released. Improved understanding of the mechanisms of BPC mobilization will lead to the design of more effective mobilizing regimens and allow development of safe and effective protocols that facilitate collection of a sufficient number of BSCs for engraftment by a small volume apheresis and ultimately without apheresis. Current cytokines and cytotoxic combinations do not appear to have reached this goal and treatment of the small minority of patients who fail current mobilization strategies remains a problem.

REFERENCES

1. Civin CI, Trischmann T, Kadan NS et al. Highly purified CD34-positive cells reconstitute hematopoiesis. J Clin Oncol 1996;14:2224–33.
2. Shpall EJ, Jones RB, Bearman SI et al. Transplantation of enriched CD34-positive autologous marrow into breast cancer patients following high-dose chemotherapy: influence of CD34-positive peripheral-blood progenitors and growth factors on engraftment. J Clin Oncol 1994;12:28–36.
3. Mehta J, Powles R, Treleaven J et al. Prospective, concurrent comparison of the Cobe Spectra and Haemonetics MCS-3P cell separators for leukapheresis after high-dose filgrastim in patients with hematologic malignancies. J Clin Apheresis 1997;12:63–7.
4. Gutensohn K, Carrero I, Krueger W et al. Semi-automated flow cytometric analysis of CD34-expressing hematopoietic cells in peripheral blood progenitor cell apheresis products. Transfusion 1999;39(11–12):1220–6.
5. Pettengell R, Testa NG, Swindell R, Crowther D, Dexter TM. Transplantation potential of hematopoietic cells released into the circulation during routine chemotherapy for non-Hodgkin's lymphoma (see comments). Blood 1993;82:2239–48.
6. Krieger MS, Schiller G, Berenson JR et al. Collection of peripheral blood progenitor cells (PBPC) based on a rising WBC and platelet count significantly increases the number of CD34+ cells. Bone Marrow Transplant 1999; 24:25–8.
7. Elliott C, Samson DM, Armitage S et al. When to harvest peripheral-blood stem cells after mobilization therapy: prediction of CD34-positive cell yield by preceding day CD34-positive concentration in peripheral blood. J Clin Oncol 1996;14:970–3.
8. Schwella N, Beyer J, Schwaner I et al. Impact of preleukapheresis cell counts on collection results and correlation of progenitor-cell dose with engraftment after high-dose chemotherapy in patients with germ cell cancer. J Clin Oncol 1996;14:1114–21.
9. Johnsen HE, Baech J, Nikolajsen K. Validation of the Nordic flow cytometry standard for CD34+ cell enumeration in blood and autografts: report from the third workshop. Nordic Stem Cell Laboratory Group. J Hematother 1999;8:15–28.
10. Legros M, Fleury J, Cure H et al. New method for stem cell quantification: applications to the management of peripheral blood stem cell transplantation. Bone Marrow Transplant 1995;15:1–8.
11. Takamatsu Y, Harada M, Teshima T et al. Relationship of infused CFU-GM and CFU-Mk mobilized by chemotherapy with or without G-CSF to platelet recovery after autologous blood stem cell transplantation (see comments). Exp Hematol 1995;23:8–13.
12. Wall DA, Oliver DA, Gale GB, Fallon RJ. Use of the hematopoietic progenitor cell (HPC) parameter of the sysmex SE9500 to monitor stem cell pheresis. Blood 1999;94(suppl 1):140a.
13. Gowans ID, Hepburn MD, Clark DM, Patterson G, Rawlinson PS, Bowen DT. The role of the Sysmex SE9000 immature myeloid index and Sysmex R2000 reticulocyte parameters in optimizing the timing of peripheral blood stem cell harvesting in patients with lymphoma and myeloma. Clin Lab Haematol 1999;21:331–6.
14. Weaver CH, Birch R, Greco FA et al. Mobilization and harvesting of peripheral blood stem cells: randomized evaluations of different doses of filgrastim. Br J Haematol 1998; 100:338–47.
15. Fruehauf S, Haas R, Conradt C et al. Peripheral

blood progenitor cell (PBPC) counts during steady-state hematopoiesis allow to estimate the yield of mobilized PBPC after filgrastim (R-metHuG-CSF)-supported cytotoxic chemotherapy. Blood 1995;85:2619–26.

16. Husson B, Ravoet C, Dehon M, Wallef G, Hougardy N, Delannoy A. Predictive value of the steady-state peripheral blood progenitor cell (PBPC) counts for the yield of PBPC collected by leukapheresis after mobilization by granulocyte colony-stimulating factor (G-CSF) alone or chemotherapy and G-CSF (letter; comment). Blood 1996;87:3526–8.

17. Atassi MC, Coffe C, Clement A et al. Predictive factors of peripheral blood stem cell collection: A French multicentre study. Blood 1999; 94 (suppl 1): 135a.

18. Donato ML, Korbling M, Gajewski JG et al. Estimation of stem cell apheresis yield by preapheresis blood CD34+ cell count. Blood 1999; 94(suppl 1):136a.

19. Bensinger WI, Weaver CH, Appelbaum FR et al. Transplantation of allogeneic peripheral blood stem cells mobilized by recombinant human granulocyte colony-stimulating factor (see comments). Blood 1995;85:1655–8.

20. Mavroudis D, Read E, Cottler-Fox M et al. CD34+ cell dose predicts survival, posttransplant morbidity, and rate of hematologic recovery after allogeneic marrow transplants for hematologic malignancies. Blood 1996;88: 3223–9.

21. Baumann I, Swindell R, Van Hoeff ME et al. Mobilisation kinetics of primitive haemopoietic cells following G-CSF with or without chemotherapy for advanced breast cancer. Ann Oncol 1996;7:1051–7.

22. Weaver A, Ryder D, Crowther D, Dexter TM, Testa NG. Increased numbers of long-term culture-initiating cells in the apheresis product of patients randomized to receive increasing doses of stem cell factor administered in combination with chemotherapy and a standard dose of granulocyte colony-stimulating factor. Blood 1996;88:3323–8.

23. Kessinger A, Lynch J, Petersen K, Sharp JG. Patterns of mobilization in autologous peripheral blood stem cell donors. Blood 1999;94(suppl 1)135a.

24. Ketterer N, Salles G, Raba M et al. High CD34(+) cell counts decrease hematologic toxicity of autologous peripheral blood progenitor

cell transplantation. Blood 1998;91:3148–55.

25. Glaspy JA, Shpall EJ, LeMaistre CF et al. Peripheral blood progenitor cell mobilization using stem cell factor in combination with filgrastim in breast cancer patients. Blood 1997; 90:2939–51.

26. Gazitt Y, Freytes CO, Callander N et al. Successful PBSC mobilization with high-dose G-CSF for patients failing a first round of mobilization. J Hematother 1999;8:173–83.

27. Glaspy J, Lu ZJ, Wheeler C et al. Economic rationale for infusing optimal numbers of CD34+ cells in peripheral blood progenitor cells (PBPCT). Blood 1997;90(suppl 1):370a.

28. Perez-Simon JA, Martin A, Caballero D et al. Clinical significance of CD34+ cell dose in long-term engraftment following autologous peripheral blood stem cell transplantation. Bone Marrow Transplant 1999;24:1279–83.

29. Hayflick LMP. The serial cultivation of human diploid cell strains. Exp Cell Res 1961;25:585–621.

30. Mohle R, Pforsich M, Fruehauf S, Witt B, Kramer A, Haas R. Filgrastim post-chemotherapy mobilizes more CD34+ cells with a different antigenic profile compared with use during steady-state hematopoiesis (Published erratum appears in Bone Marrow Transplant 1995; 15(4):655) (see comments). Bone Marrow Transplant 1994;14(5):827–32.

31. Bensinger WI, Longin K, Appelbaum F et al. Peripheral blood stem cells (PBSCs) collected after recombinant granulocyte colony stimulating factor (rhG-CSF): an analysis of factors correlating with the tempo of engraftment after transplantation (see comments). Br J Haematol 1994;87:825–31.

32. Haas R, Mohle R, Fruhauf S et al. Patient characteristics associated with successful mobilizing and autografting of peripheral blood progenitor cells in malignant lymphoma. Blood 1994;83:3787–94.

33. Watts MJ, Sullivan AM, Jamieson E et al. Progenitor-cell mobilization after low-dose cyclophosphamide and granulocyte colony-stimulating factor: an analysis of progenitor-cell quantity and quality and factors predicting for these parameters in 101 pretreated patients with malignant lymphoma. J Clin Oncol 1997; 15:535–46.

34. Gazitt Y, Liu Q. High plasma levels of flt-3 ligand (flt3-L) in the bone marrow (BM) or peripheral blood (PB) is a good predictor of a

poor mobilization of CD34+ peripheral blood stem cells in non-Hodgkin's lymphoma (NHL) patients. Blood 1999;94(suppl 1)138a.

35. Pettengell R, Morgenstern GR, Woll PJ et al. Peripheral blood progenitor cell transplantation in lymphoma and leukemia using a single apheresis. Blood 1993;82:3770–7.

36. To LB, Haylock DN, Dowse T et al. A comparative study of the phenotype and proliferative capacity of peripheral blood (PB) CD34+ cells mobilized by four different protocols and those of steady-phase PB and bone marrow CD34+ cells. Blood 1994;84:2930–9.

37. Weaver CH, Schwartzberg L, Li W, Hazelton B, West W. High-dose chemotherapy and autologous peripheral blood progenitor cell transplant for the treatment of Hodgkin's disease. Bone Marrow Transplant 1996;17:715–21.

38. Hoglund M. Glycosylated and non-glycosylated recombinant human granulocyte colony-stimulating factor (rhG-CSF) – what is the difference? Med Oncol 1998;15:229–33.

39. Teshima A, Harada M. Mobilization of peripheral blood progenitor cells for allogeneic transplantation. Cytokines Cell Mol Ther 1997;3:101–14.

40. Stroncek DF, Clay ME, Petzoldt ML et al. Treatment of normal individuals with granulocyte-colony-stimulating factor: donor experiences and the effects on peripheral blood CD34+ cell counts and on the collection of peripheral blood stem cells (see comments). Transfusion 1996;36:601–10.

41. Grigg AP, Roberts AW, Raunow H et al. Optimizing dose and scheduling of filgrastim (granulocyte colony-stimulating factor) for mobilization and collection of peripheral blood progenitor cells in normal volunteers (see comments). Blood 1995;86:4437–45.

42. Miflin G, Charley C, Stainer C, Anderson S, Hunter A, Russell N. Stem cell mobilization in normal donors for allogeneic transplantation: analysis of safety and factors affecting efficacy. Br J Haematol 1996;95:345–8.

43. Russel N, Gratwohl A, Schmitz N. The place of blood stem cells in allogeneic transplantation. Br J Haematol 1996;93:747–53.

44. Cleaver SA, Goldman JM. Use of G-CSF to mobilise PBSC in normal healthy donors – an international survey. Bone Marrow Transplant 1998;21(suppl 3): 29–31.

45. Ordemann R, Holig K, Wagner K et al.

Acceptance and feasibility of peripheral stem cell mobilisation compared to bone marrow collection from healthy unrelated donors. Bone Marrow Transplant 1998;21(suppl 3): 25–8.

46. Brown SL, Dale DC. Biology of blood and marrow transplantation. 1997;3:341–3.

47. Anderlini P, Przepiorka D, Korbling M, Champlin R. Blood stem cell procurement: donor safety issues. Bone Marrow Transplant 1998;21(suppl 3): S35–9.

48. Anderlini P, Przepiorka D, Seong D et al. Clinical toxicity and laboratory effects of granulocyte-colony-stimulating factor (filgrastim) mobilization and blood stem cell apheresis from normal donors, and analysis of charges for the procedures (see comments) (Published erratum appears in Transfusion 1997;37(1):109). Transfusion 1996;36:590–5.

49. Zeller W, Gutensohn K, Stockschlader M et al. Increase of mobilized CD34-positive peripheral blood progenitor cells in patients with Hodgkin's disease, non-Hodgkin's lymphoma, and cancer of the testis. Bone Marrow Transplant 1996;17:709–13.

50. Knudsen LM, Gaarsdal E, Jensen L, Nielsen KJ, Nikolaisen K, Johnsen HE. Improved priming for mobilization of and optimal timing for harvest of peripheral blood stem cells. J Hematother 1996;5:399–406.

51. Weaver CH, Tauer K, Zhen B et al. Second attempts at mobilization of peripheral blood stem cells in patients with initial low CD34+ cell yields. J Hematother 1998;7:241–9.

52. Kurekci AEKJ, Koehler M. Mobilization of peripheral blood progenitor cells using 16 versus 10 mg/kg/d G-CSF in children with malignancies. Ped Transplant 1998;2:160–4.

53. Arbona C, Prosper F, Benet I, Mena F, Solano C, Garcia-Conde J. Comparison between once a day vs twice a day G-CSF for mobilization of peripheral blood progenitor cells (PBPC) in normal donors for allogeneic PBPC transplantation. Bone Marrow Transplant 1998;22:39–45.

54. Kroger N, Zeller W, Hassan HT et al. Stem cell mobilization with G-CSF alone in breast cancer patients: higher progenitor cell yield by delivering divided doses (2 × 5 microg/kg) compared to a single dose (1 × 10 microg/kg). Bone Marrow Transplant 1999;23:125–9.

55. Ponisch WLS, Edel E, Haustein B et al. Mobilization of peripheral blood progenitor cells (PBPC) in normal donors for allogeneic

PBPC transplantation: comparison between once a day versus twice a day G-CSF (Filgrastime) administration. Blood 1999;137a.

56. Watts MJ, Addison I, Ings SJ et al. Optimal timing for collection of PBPC after glycosylated G-CSF administration. Bone Marrow Transplant 1998;21:365–8.

57. Sutherland HJ, Eaves CJ, Lansdorp PM, Phillips GL, Hogge DE. Kinetics of committed and primitive blood progenitor mobilization after chemotherapy and growth factor treatment and their use in autotransplants. Blood 1994;83: 3808–14.

58. Cesana C, Regazzi E, Garau D, Caramatti C, Mangoni L, Rizzoli V. Clonogenic potential and phenotypic analysis of CD34+ cells mobilized by different chemotherapy regimens. Haematologica 1999;84:771–8.

59. Akard LP, Thompson JM, Dugan MJ et al. Matched-pair analysis of hematopoietic progenitor cell mobilization using G-CSF vs. cyclophosphamide, etoposide, and G-CSF: enhanced CD34+ cell collections are not necessarily cost-effective. Biol Blood Marrow Transplant 1999;5: 379–85.

60. Molineux G, Kinstler O, Briddell B et al. A new form of Filgrastim with sustained duration in vivo and enhanced ability to mobilize PBPC in both mice and humans. Exp Hematol 1999;27: 1724–34.

61. Niedhart J. Dose intensive therapy without progenitor cell replacement, 2nd edn. Williams and Wilkins, 1995.

62. Prosper F, Vanoverbeke K, Stroncek D, Verfaillie CM. Primitive long-term culture initiating cells (LTC-ICs) in granulocyte colony-stimulating factor mobilized peripheral blood progenitor cells have similar potential for ex vivo expansion as primitive LTC-ICs in steady state bone marrow. Blood 1997;89:3991–7.

63. Laterveer L, Lindley IJ, Hamilton MS, Willemze R, Fibbe WE. Interleukin-8 induces rapid mobilization of hematopoietic stem cells with radioprotective capacity and long-term myelolymphoid repopulating ability. Blood 1995;85:2269–75.

64. Laterveer L, Lindley IJ, Heemskerk DP et al. Rapid mobilization of hematopoietic progenitor cells in rhesus monkeys by a single intravenous injection of interleukin-8. Blood 1996;87:781–8.

65. Papayannopoulou T, Nakamoto B. Peripheralization of hemopoietic progenitors in pri-

mates treated with anti-VLA 4 integrin. Proc Natl Acad Sci USA 1993;90:9324–78.

66. Mauch P, Lamont C, Neben TY, Quinto C, Goldman SJ, Witsell A. Hematopoietic stem cells in the blood after stem cell factor and interleukin-11 administration: evidence for different mechanisms of mobilization. Blood 1995;86: 4674–80.

67. Basser RL, Rasko JE, Clarke K et al. Thrombopoietic effects of pegylated recombinant human megakaryocyte growth and development factor (PEG-rHuMGDF) in patients with advanced cancer. Lancet 1996;348:1279–81.

68. Somlo G, Sniecinski I, ter Veer A et al. Recombinant human thrombopoietin in combination with granulocyte colony-stimulating factor enhances mobilization of peripheral blood progenitor cells, increases peripheral blood platelet concentration, and accelerates hematopoietic recovery following high-dose chemotherapy. Blood 1999;93:2798–806.

69. Shpall CAWS, Turner S, Yanovich RA et al. A randomised phase 3 study of PBPC mobilisation by stem cell factor (SCF, STEMGEN) and Filgratim in patients with high-risk breast cancer. Blood 1997;10(suppl 1):2627 (abstract).

70. Weaver A, Testa NG. Stem cell factor leads to reduced blood processing during apheresis or the use of whole blood aliquots to support dose-intensive chemotherapy. Bone Marrow Transplant 1998;22:33–8.

71. Stiff PMD, Bayer R, Podiak M, Kerger C. High dose G-CSF improves stem cell mobilization and collection compared to standard doses in patients with ovarian cancer which leads to a decrease in delayed platelet engraftment following stem cell transplants. Blood 1997; 90(suppl 1):2629 (abstract).

72. Facon T, Harousseau JL, Maloisel F et al. Stem cell factor in combination with filgrastim after chemotherapy improves peripheral blood progenitor cell yield and reduces apheresis requirements in multiple myeloma patients: a randomized, controlled trial. Blood 1999;94: 1218–25.

73. Rusten LS, Lyman SD, Veiby OP, Jacobsen SE. The FLT3 ligand is a direct and potent stimulator of the growth of primitive and committed human CD34+ bone marrow progenitor cells in vitro. Blood 1996;87:1317–25.

74. Jacobsen SE, Veiby OP, Myklebust J, Okkenhaug C, Lyman SD. Ability of flt3 ligand

to stimulate the in vitro growth of primitive murine hematopoietic progenitors is potently and directly inhibited by transforming growth factor-beta and tumor necrosis factor-alpha. Blood 1996;87:5016–26.

75. McKenna HJ, de Vries P, Brasel K, Lyman SD, Williams DE. Effect of flt3 ligand on the ex vivo expansion of human CD34+ hematopoietic progenitor cells. Blood 1995;86:3413–20.

76. Sudo Y, Shimazaki C, Ashihara E et al. Synergistic effect of FLT-3 ligand on the granulocyte colony-stimulating factor-induced mobilization of hematopoietic stem cells and progenitor cells into blood in mice. Blood 1997; 89:3186–91.

77. Molineux G, McCrea C, Yan XQ, Kerzic P, McNiece I. Flt-3 ligand synergizes with granulocyte colony-stimulating factor to increase neutrophil numbers and to mobilize peripheral blood stem cells with long-term repopulating potential. Blood 1997;89:3998–4004.

78. Sahovic EA, Colvin M, Hilton J, Ogawa M. Role for aldehyde dehydrogenase in survival of progenitors for murine blast cell colonies after treatment with 4-hydroperoxycyclophosphamide in vitro. Cancer Res 1988;48:1223–6.

79. Ings SJSS, Hancock B, Watts MJ et al. Results of a BNLI randomized trial of G-CSF dose after cyclophosphamide 1.5G/M2 for progenitor cell mobilization. Blood 1999;94:666 (abstract 2956).

80. Lefrere F, Belanger C, Audat F et al. The dose of granulocyte-colony-stimulating factor after chemopriming treatment does not influence apheresis yield of progenitor cells: a retrospective study of 91 cases. Transfusion 1999; 39(11–12):1207–11.

81. Lie AK, Rawling TP, Bayly JL, To LB. Progenitor cell yield in sequential blood stem cell mobilization in the same patients: insights into chemotherapy dose escalation and combination of haemopoietic growth factor and chemotherapy. Br J Haematol 1996;95:39–44.

82. Kotasek D, Shepherd KM, Sage RE et al. Factors affecting blood stem cell collections following high-dose cyclophosphamide mobilization in lymphoma, myeloma and solid tumors. Bone Marrow Transplant 1992;9:11–17.

83. Rowlings PA, Bayly JL, Rawling CM, Juttner CA, To LB. A comparison of peripheral blood stem cell mobilisation after chemotherapy with cyclophosphamide as a single agent in doses of 4 g/m² or 7 g/m² in patients with advanced cancer. Aust NZ J Med 1992;22:660–4.

84. Gianni AM, Bregni M, Siena S et al. Granulocyte–macrophage colony-stimulating factor or granulocyte colony-stimulating factor infusion makes high-dose etoposide a safe outpatient regimen that is effective in lymphoma and myeloma patients. J Clin Oncol 1992; 10:1955–62.

85. Kushner BH, Kwon JH, Gulati SC, Castro-Malaspina H. Preclinical assessment of purging with VP-16–213: key role for long-term marrow cultures. Blood 1987;69:65–71.

86. Copelan EA, Ceselski SK, Ezzone SA et al. Mobilization of peripheral-blood progenitor cells with high-dose etoposide and granulocyte colony-stimulating factor in patients with breast cancer, non-Hodgkin's lymphoma, and Hodgkin's disease. J Clin Oncol 1997;15:759–65.

87. Tarella C, Ferrero D, Bregni M et al. Peripheral blood expansion of early progenitor cells after high-dose cyclophosphamide and rhGM-CSF. Eur J Cancer 1991;27:22–7.

88. Gianni AM, Siena S, Bregni M et al. Recombinant human interleukin-3 hastens trilineage hematopoietic recovery following high-dose (7 g/m²) cyclophosphamide cancer therapy. Ann Oncol 1993;4:759–66.

89. Craig JIOSS, Parker AC, Anthony RS. The response of peripheral blood stem cells to standard chemotherapy for lymphoma. Leuk Lymphoma 1992;6:363–8.

90. McQuaker I, Haynes A, Stainer C, Byrne J, Russell N. Mobilisation of peripheral blood stem cells with IVE and G-CSF improves CD34+ cell yields and engraftment in patients with non-Hodgkin's lymphomas and Hodgkin's disease. Bone Marrow Transplant 1999;24:715–22.

91. Watts MJ, Sullivan AM et al. A comparison of ESHAP + G-CSF vs cyclophosphamide 1.5 g/m² + G-CSF for PBSC mobilisation in pretreated lymphoma patients: a matched pair analysis. Blood 1996;88(suppl 1):396 (abstract 1571).

92. Petit J, Boque C, Cancelas JA et al. Feasibility of ESHAP + G-CSF as peripheral blood hematopoietic progenitor cell mobilisation regimen in resistant and relapsed lymphoma: a single-center study of 22 patients. Leuk Lymphoma 1999;34(1–2):119–27.

93. Moskowitz CH, Bertino JR, Glassman JR et al. Ifosfamide, carboplatin, and etoposide: a highly

effective cytoreduction and peripheral-blood progenitor-cell mobilization regimen for transplant-eligible patients with non-Hodgkin's lymphoma. J Clin Oncol 1999;17:3776–85.

94. McQuaker IG, Haynes AP, Stainer C, Anderson S, Russell NH. Stem cell mobilization in resistant or relapsed lymphoma: superior yield of progenitor cells following a salvage regimen comprising ifosfamide, etoposide and epirubicin compared to intermediate-dose cyclophosphamide. Br J Haematol 1997;98: 228–33.

95. Martinez C, Mateu R, Sureda A et al. Peripheral blood stem cell mobilization following salvage chemotherapy (IAPVP-16) plus granulocyte colony-stimulating factor and autografting for non-Hodgkin's lymphoma. Transplant Proc 1995;27:2355–6.

96. Dreger P, Kloss M, Petersen B et al. Autologous progenitor cell transplantation: prior exposure to stem cell-toxic drugs determines yield and engraftment of peripheral blood progenitor cell but not of bone marrow grafts. Blood 1995;86: 3970–8.

97. Kroger N, Zeller W, Fehse N et al. Mobilizing peripheral blood stem cells with high-dose G-CSF alone is as effective as with Dexa-BEAM plus G-CSF in lymphoma patients. Br J Haematol 1998;102:1101–6.

98. Aurlien E, Holte H, Pharo A et al. Combination chemotherapy with mitoguazon, ifosfamide, MTX, etoposide (MIME) and G-CSF can efficiently mobilize PBPC in patients with Hodgkin's and non-Hodgkin's lymphoma. Bone Marrow Transplant 1998;21:873–8.

99. Perry AR, Watts MJ, Peniket AJ, Goldstone AH, Linch DC. Progenitor cell yields are frequently poor in patients with histologically indolent lymphomas especially when mobilized within 6 months of previous chemotherapy. Bone Marrow Transplant 1998;21:1201–5.

100. McQuaker IG, Haynes AP, Anderson S et al. Engraftment and molecular monitoring of CD34+ peripheral-blood stem-cell transplants for follicular lymphoma: a pilot study. J Clin Oncol 1997;15:2288–95.

101. Haas R, Moos M, Mohle R et al. High-dose therapy with peripheral blood progenitor cell transplantation in low-grade non-Hodgkin's lymphoma. Bone Marrow Transplant 1996;17: 149–55.

102. Goldschmidt H, Hegenbart U, Haas R, Hunstein W. Mobilization of peripheral blood progenitor cells with high-dose cyclophosphamide (4 or 7 g/m^2) and granulocyte colony-stimulating factor in patients with multiple myeloma. Bone Marrow Transplant 1996;17: 691–7.

103. Kroger N, Zeller W, Hassan HT et al. Successful mobilization of peripheral blood stem cells in heavily pretreated myeloma patients with G-CSF alone. Ann Hematol 1998;76:257–62.

104. Lounici ASL, Boiron JM, Fizet D et al. Factors influencing the first-day collection of peripheral blood stem cells in multiple myeloma. Blood 1999;94(suppl 1):610–11 (abstract).

105. Demirer T, Buckner CD, Gooley T et al. Factors influencing collection of peripheral blood stem cells in patients with multiple myeloma. Bone Marrow Transplant 1996;17:937–41.

106. Alegre A, Tomas JF, Martinez-Chamorro C et al. Comparison of peripheral blood progenitor cell mobilization in patients with multiple myeloma: high-dose cyclophosphamide plus GM-CSF vs G-CSF alone. Bone Marrow Transplant 1997;20:211–17.

107. Desikan KR, Barlogie B, Jagannath S et al. Comparable engraftment kinetics following peripheral-blood stem-cell infusion mobilized with granulocyte colony-stimulating factor with or without cyclophosphamide in multiple myeloma. J Clin Oncol 1998;16:1547–53.

108. Harousseau JL. Optimizing peripheral blood progenitor cell autologous transplantation in multiple myeloma. Haematologica 1999;84: 548–53.

109. Pratt G, Johnson RJ, Rawstron AC, Barnard DL, Morgan GJ, Smith GM. Autologous stem cell transplantation in chronic myeloid leukaemia using Philadelphia chromosome negative blood progenitors mobilised with hydroxyurea and G-CSF (see comments). Bone Marrow Transplant 1998;21:455–60.

110. Johnson RJ, Smith GM. Mobilisation and reinfusion of Philadelphia negative peripheral blood mononuclear cells in chronic myeloid leukaemia with hydroxyurea and G-CSF. Leuk Lymphoma 1997;27(5–6):401–15.

111. Carella AM, Simonsson B, Link H et al. Mobilization of Philadelphia-negative peripheral blood progenitor cells with chemotherapy and rhuG-CSF in chronic myelogenous leukaemia patients with a poor response to interferon-alpha. Br J Haematol 1998;101: 111–18.

112. Corsetti MT, Lerma E, Dejana A et al. Quantitative competitive reverse transcriptase-polymerase chain reaction for BCR-ABL on Philadelphia-negative leukaphereses allows the selection of low-contaminated peripheral blood progenitor cells for autografting in chronic myelogenous leukemia. Leukemia 1999;13:999–1008.

113. Richman CM, Weiner RS, Yankee RA. Increase in circulating stem cells following chemotherapy in man. Blood 1976;47:1031–9.

Part 2
High dose chemotherapy in specific diseases

5

Autologous transplantation in acute leukaemia

Joanne Ewing and Rajesh Chopra

CONTENTS Introduction • Rationale for high dose therapy in acute myeloid leukaemia • Acute myeloid leukaemia • Acute lymphoblastic leukaemia • Purging • Comparison of peripheral blood stem cells and bone marrow • Future directions and novel therapeutic approaches in acute leukaemia

INTRODUCTION

It is now over two decades since the feasibility of myeloablative therapy with stem cell rescue for acute myeloid leukaemia (AML) was demonstrated.[1,2] This approach is being used for an increasing number of patients in first and subsequent remission. This chapter provides a critical evaluation of the evidence for use of autologous bone marrow and peripheral blood transplantation in patients with acute myeloid and acute lymphoblastic leukaemia (ALL) and

discusses the rationale for the design of ongoing trials. The role of purging in autologous stem cell transplantation (ASCT) and the relative merits of peripheral blood stem cells (PBSC) as opposed to bone marrow are discussed. Finally, some of the innovative approaches to post-remission therapy in acute leukaemia are covered. The issues to be discussed are listed in Table 5.1.

RATIONALE FOR HIGH DOSE THERAPY IN ACUTE MYELOID LEUKAEMIA

The principle of administration of high dose chemotherapy in AML is to administer treatment as further dose intensification to patients in complete remission to prevent disease relapse. Dose intensification has also been employed following relapse. The development of this approach has a number of origins. Landmark studies performed by Skipper and Schabel using the early L1210 murine model of leukaemia cell kinetics had shown that for drug-responsive tumours, whilst cell growth is exponential, a definite and steep dose–response curve exists (Fig. 5.1a). This leads to a fractional log cell kill at a given dose regardless of

---

Table 5.1 Issues in autologous transplantation in AML

- Autografting versus chemotherapy
- Autografting versus allogeneic transplantation
- Risk stratification
- Timing
- Source of haemopoietic stem cells
- Purging
- Role of immunomodulatory therapy

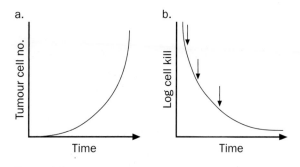

Figure 5.1
(a) Schematic representation of the Skipper–Schabel model of exponential leukaemic cell growth. (b) Schematic representation of log cell kill according to the Skipper–Schabel model – arrows represent chemotherapy courses of equal dose and interval each leading to the same fractional log cell kill. If high dose myeloablative chemotherapy is administered when the cell number is below 10^8 then residual disease will approach zero.

original cell number with the resultant exponential regression of tumour cell number.[3,4] Their theory therefore hypothesizes that by administration of a very high dose treatment at the point of minimal residual disease there will be a several log decrease in cell number resulting in complete eradication of tumour burden (Fig. 5.1b). Animal studies suggest that administration of myeloablative conditioning will achieve an 8–10 log cell kill.[5] Failure to cure would be the consequence of inadequate therapy or development of drug-resistant cells.

Norton and Simon[5] have subsequently argued that the relatively simple Skipper and Schabel model may not be relevant in the clinical setting. Human cancer does not grow exponentially in the clinical setting, and a mathematical model of tumour growth and regression based on the more complex Gompertzian theory may be more relevant (Fig. 5.2a).[6] They suggest that when a tumour is large or very small the doubling time increases due to reduced growth fraction and cell loss. Therefore at the extremes of tumour size the fractional growth rate is much slower. The response of a tumour to a given dose of

chemotherapy is proportional to the growth rate prior to treatment. Therefore, at the points of slowest growth, when the tumour cell load is either very small or very large, it is postulated that a very large treatment dose is required to achieve cure. This model is based on the same precept as the Skipper–Schabel model but takes into account the changing growth rate of tumour cells, with the conclusion that a rational approach is to use very high dose combination therapy in the setting of minimal residual disease, preferably with non-cross-resistant agents.[7] The induction–intensification strategy proposed for AML takes into account both of these models, aiming to give intensified therapy to achieve high log kill at the point of minimal residual disease when cell growth rate and therefore regression rate is low (Fig. 5.2b).

Myelotoxicity imposes a dose limitation for the use of chemotherapeutic agents and radiation therapy. The progress in the ability to

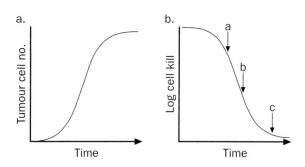

Figure 5.2
(a) Schematic representation of Gompertzian model of non-exponential tumour growth with the doubling time of the tumour increasing at the extremes of tumour size. (b) Effect of chemotherapy dose on log cell kill according to Norton–Simon model. Arrows a and b represent equal doses of chemotherapy which give rise to a cell kill which is proportional to the rate of cell growth. As the growth rate and therefore log cell kill is reduced at the point of minimal residual disease then administration of same dose consolidation courses will never achieve cure. By giving high dose myeloablative chemoradiotherapy as intensification when cell number is very small the 10^8–10^{10} log cell kill will lead to residual disease approximating to zero.

cryopreserve stem cells for transplantation was therefore a crucial breakthrough.[8] Early results from allogeneic transplantation in advanced AML demonstrated the ability of this approach to eradicate disease and, indeed, the disease-free survival (DFS) achieved in these patients was a considerable improvement on results from approaches using chemotherapy alone.[9] These studies provided the clinical rationale for the use of high dose therapy and stem cell rescue. Dicke et al. first harvested autologous marrow progenitor cells for transplant from patients in remission during the 1970s and, following myeloablative conditioning regimens, these harvested stem cells were reinfused and successfully engrafted.[2] Over the years, ASCT has become standard therapy and in 1998 approximately 1000 autologous transplant procedures for AML were undertaken in Europe (A Gratwohl, personal communication), with similar activity in the USA. One of the potential disadvantages of the use of autologous stem cells is the reinfusion of contaminating tumour blasts that are able to engraft and cause disease relapse. Attempts to avoid this hazard have been made by purging the bone marrow before reinfusion, although the clinical benefit of this approach remains unproven.

There are potential advantages to the autologous transplantation approach. The majority of patients with AML are elderly and the risk of full intensity allogeneic transplantation precludes this approach for these patients. Autologous stem cell transfer is not restricted to that minority of patients who have an HLA-matched sibling donor. Graft-versus-host disease is not a problem, in contrast to allogeneic transplantation. It is postulated that cryopreservation of the harvest actually has a beneficial tumour cell purging effect, leading to a 1 log reduction in any clonogenic AML colony forming units (CFUs).[10,11] A reduced homing potential of leukaemic blasts in comparison with the normal progenitor cells has been shown that may prevent re-establishment of disease.[12–14] There is possibly a benefit from the triggering and establishment of an autologous immune responsiveness – so-called autologous graft-versus-host disease.[15]

ACUTE MYELOID LEUKAEMIA

Benefit of intensification of post-remission therapy in acute myeloid leukaemia

Of adult patients under 60 years of age who develop acute myeloid leukaemia, around 60–80% can be expected to achieve complete remission following induction chemotherapy with a regimen combining an anthracycline with cytosine arabinoside (Ara-C). In spite of this the most common cause of treatment failure is relapse. Patients in 'morphological complete remission' may still have up to 10^{10} leukaemic cells.[16] The aim of repeated courses of intensive chemotherapy is to further reduce the tumour load and ultimately eradicate the leukaemic clone, thus achieving a cure. Clinically, there is good evidence that intensifying post-remission therapy for patients with AML gives a better DFS rate and historically the emphasis has moved from the use of prolonged low dose maintenance to shorter but more intense forms of post-remission therapy. The dose–response effect of high dose Ara-C (HDAC) in the treatment of AML is well established.[17,18] The Cancer and Leukaemia Group B (CALGB) in 1994 randomized 596 patients in complete remission to three different doses of Ara-C for four courses (3 g/m² 12-hourly for 3 days, 400 mg/m² continuous infusion for 5 days and 100 mg/m² continuous infusion for 5 days). A significant difference in DFS at 4 years was demonstrated (44%, 29% and 24%, respectively).[19] Other evidence comes from the MRC AML trials which, as they have evolved, have given greater intensity of post-remission treatment both in dose and number of courses with stepwise improvements in outcome.[20–22] The AML 10 trial indicated that those patients receiving more than four courses of treatment had a significantly reduced relapse risk.[23] This trial has raised the question of whether the optimal schedule is non-myeloablative chemotherapy alone or whether ASCT is of greater benefit.

The issue of optimal post-remission therapy in AML remains critical. Important information is now available from single-centre as well as randomized controlled trials examining autologous transplantation in first complete remission (CR1) AML.

Single-centre studies

Early single-centre studies looking at bone marrow transplantation showed that a significant survival advantage could be achieved compared to reports of best outcome from chemotherapy at the time: ASCT became accepted practice. The majority of these single-centre studies showed a durable remission rate of 45–55%.[24-33] The outcome from these trials must, however, be interpreted with great caution. The 'time-censoring' effect that inevitably occurs in this type of observational study means that during the delay to transplant some patients will relapse or die, so that those actually proceeding to transplant are already a highly selected group. Indeed, time-censoring studies have suggested that the long-term survival of patients surviving to 6 months is already around 40%.[34] There will also be referral selection bias, as those patients with a better outlook may tend to be referred to specialist centres. There is great variability in age of patients entered for transplant, with some studies including children, who seem to have a different outcome from the available treatment modalities. This makes it difficult to extrapolate these results to all patients presenting with AML, the majority of whom are over 50 years.

Variability in protocol makes broad comparisons across trials difficult. Early trials timed the stem cell collection immediately post-induction and gave a course of intensification therapy after harvest, whilst later studies used a consolidation course of HDAC prior to harvest to reduce leukaemic contamination as an in vivo purge. There are also differences in transplant conditioning regimen and in vitro purging strategy. Analysis of trial data from these early studies must take into account the continued evolution of chemotherapy regimens and comparison must always be made with best available contemporary chemotherapy protocols rather than historical comparisons. It is also pertinent to point out that refinement in transplant protocols and improvements in posttransplant care are permitting safer delivery of these intensive schedules.

Although single-centre studies were helpful in establishing the technology of stem cell transplantation they raised a number of questions that can be answered only by prospective randomized, controlled trials. The results of these trials are summarized in Table 5.2.

Prospective randomized trials comparing ASCT with chemotherapy

Adults

The first direct comparison of ASCT versus chemotherapy was reported by the EORTC/GIMEMA (European Organization for research and treatment of Cancer and Gruppo Italiano Malattie Ematologiche Maligne dell'Adulto).[35] This prospective trial entered 941 evaluable patients between 1986 and 1993. Patients were mostly under 45 years, median age 33 years. Only 66% of patients attained complete remission (CR) and were eligible for the randomization. Patients were allocated allogeneic bone marrow transplantation (ABMT) if they had a consenting HLA-matched sibling ($n = 168$). The remaining 254 were randomized to either ASCT using unpurged marrow ($n = 128$) or further chemotherapy ($n = 126$) as third course. Intermediate dose cytarabine $1 \, \text{g/m}^2$ and amsacrine were given as the second course, cytarabine $2 \, \text{g/m}^2$ 12-hourly on days 1–4, with daunorubicin $45 \, \text{mg/m}^2$ on days 5–7 as the third course in the chemotherapy arm (Fig. 5.3). Only 74% of the patients eligible for autologous transplant actually received this therapy. Analysis by intention to treat showed a 4-year DFS of 55% in the ABMT arm, and 48% in the ASCT arm, which were significantly better than 30% in the chemotherapy arm ($p = 0.05$). There was a higher relapse rate in the chemotherapy arm but many of these patients were salvaged successfully with subsequent ASCT, giving rise to a 4-year overall

Table 5.2 Results of prospective randomized studies in adults and children

Study*	Reference	Treatment	No.	Age range (years)	Disease-free survival %	P	Overall survival %	P	RR %	P	TRM (%)
EORTC/GIMEMA	35	ALLO	168		55		59		24		17
		AUTO	128		48	0.05	56	0.43	41		9
		CHEMO	126	11–59	30	0.05	46		57	<0.05	7
GOELAM	36	ALLO	67		44		53		38		22
		AUTO	67		44	NS	50	NS	44	NS	6.5
		CHEMO	61	15–50	40		55		43		3
US Intergroup	37	ALLO	120		43		46		29		21
		AUTO	111		35	NS	43	0.05	48	<0.05	14
		CHEMO	118	16–55	35		52		61		3
MRC AML10	22	ALLO	–		–		–		–		–
		AUTO	190		53‡	0.04	57‡	0.2	37	0.0007	12
		CHEMO	191	<56	39‡		45‡		58		4
BGMT 87	38	ALLO	36		66		65		18		
		AUTO	39		48	0.004	56§	NS	50		
		CHEMO	38	<15	40	NS	55§		83	0.002	
POG	39	ALLO	–		52		50		–		–
		AUTO	115		38	0.06	40	0.007	31		15
		CHEMO	117	<21	36	NS	44	NS	58	0.001	2.7
AIEOP	40	ALLO	24		51				45		0
		AUTO	35		21	0.03			78	0.03	3
		CHEMO	37	<15	27	NS			70	NS	8
CCG-2891	41	ALLO	140		70		76				
		AUTO	150		40	0.0001	45	0.09			
		CHEMO	160	<15	50	0.1	59	0.03			
MRC AML 10 Paediatric analysis	42	ALLO	61		68†		69				13
		AUTO	60		46†	0.03	70	0.2			2
		CHEMO		<15			59				4

*AIEOP, Associazione Italiana Emtologia ed Oncologia Pediatrica Cooperativa Group; BGMT 87, Bordeaux, Grenoble, Marseilles, Toulouse; CCG-2281, Children's Cancer Group; EORTC, European Organization for Research and Treatment of Cancer; GIMEMA, Gruppo Italiano Malatte Ematologiche dell'Adulto; GOELAM, Group Ouest Leucemies Aigues Myeloblastiques; MRC AML 10, Medical Research Council Acute Myeloblastic Leukaemia 10 trial; POG, Pediatric Oncology Group; RR, relapse risk; TRM, Transplant related mortality.
†ALLO, allogeneic; AUTO, autogeneic; CHEMO, chemotherapy.
‡Survival figures at 7 years.
§Survival at 3 years.

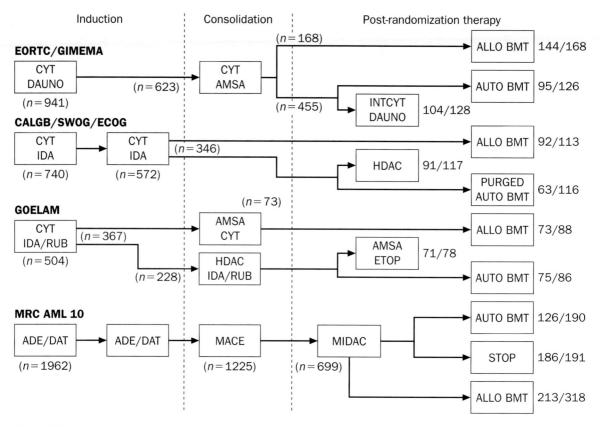

Figure 5.3
Design of prospective randomized studies of ASCT in adults. ADE, cytosine arabinoside 100 mg/m^2, daunorubicin, etoposide; ALLO, allogeneic; AMSA, amsacrine; AUTO, autologous; BMT, bone marrow transplantation; CYT, cytosine arabinoside low dose (range 100–200 mg/m^2); DAT, cytosine arabinoside 100 mg/m^2, daunorubicin, thioguanine; DAUNO, daunorubicin; ETOP, etoposide; HDAC, cytosine arabinoside high dose (3 g/m^2 for 6 days); IDA, idarubicin; MACE, cytosine arabinoside 200 mg/m^2 × 5, amsacrine, etoposide; MIDAC, cytosine arabinoside 1 g/m^2 bd for 3 days, mitozantrone; RUB, rubidazone; STOP, no further chemotherapy. Figures in parentheses represent numbers of patients at each landmark in the trial and fractions represent proportion of patients actually receiving the allocated therapy.

survival which was similar for all three groups. The time taken to treatment was a significant factor in relapse rate prior to the allotted intensification therapy. This factor demonstrates the 'time-censoring' effect and highlights the fact that even in prospective randomized studies biases may be introduced so that analysis of the data on an intention to treat basis is critical. Other problems were a suboptimal outcome in the chemotherapy arm, which may have been related to the lack of a high dose cytosine arabi-

noside (HDAC) schedule. Poor engraftment in the ASCT group was also a problem, with platelet recovery taking up to 20 weeks.

The Medical Research Council (MRC) AML 10 trial was a large collaborative trial involving over 100 centres in the United Kingdom, Republic of Ireland and New Zealand designed to examine the value of high dose therapy after four courses of consolidation treatment compared with no further chemotherapy. It addresses a rather different question to that posed by other randomized controlled trials, namely, does ASCT confer any further advantage over and above the best available intensity treatment protocol so far designed?[22] A total of 1622 patients were registered. Three hundred and eighty-one patients below 55 years were randomized after the third course of chemotherapy, representing 38% of those eligible. Of the 190 patients allocated autologous transplant only 126 received the intended therapy, and five patients in the stop arm actually received

ASCT in CR1. The reasons for this attrition include patient and physician choice as well as death or relapse before transplant could be performed. There was a suggestion of a difference when analysed by intention to treat of a DFS advantage in the autograft arm at 7 years (DFS 53% versus 39%, $P = 0.04$). When those patients surviving beyond 2 years are analysed, an overall survival advantage for ASCT can be seen in this group (Fig. 5.4). The analysis of these trials for long-term outcome will be important

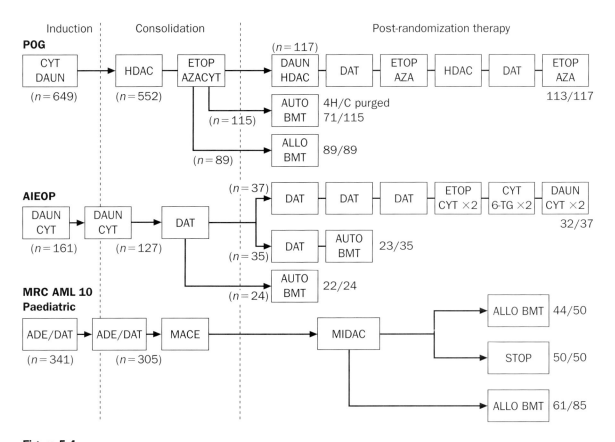

Figure 5.4

Design of prospective randomized studies of ASCT in children. ADE, cytosine arabinoside 100 mg/m², daunorubicin, etoposide; ALLO, allogeneic; AMSA, amsacrine; AUTO, autologous; AZA, azacytidine; BMT, bone marrow transplantation; CYT, cytosine arabinoside low dose (range 100–200 mg/m²); DAT, cytosine arabinoside 100 mg/m² daunorubicin, thioguanine; DAUN, daunorubicin; ETOP, etoposide; HDAC, cytosine arabinoside high dose (3 g/m² for 6 days); MACE, cytosine arabinoside 200 mg × 5, amsacrine, etoposide;. MIDAC, cytosine arabinoside 1 g/m² bd for 3 days, mitozantrone; STOP, no further chemotherapy. Figures in parentheses represent numbers of patients at each landmark in the trial and fractions represent proportion of patients actually receiving the allocated therapy.

because survival advantages may only emerge in the long term.

The US intergroup trial (ECOG/SWOG/ CALGB)[36] compared 4-hydroperoxycyclophosphamide (4-HC) purged bone marrow transplant with high dose cytarabine. As can be seen from the trial design (Fig. 5.3) a major flaw was the low dosage of treatment prior to the transplant arms of this study, with patients proceeding to autologous transplant after only two intermediate dose treatments with no high dose cytarabine consolidation prior to transplant. There were also features of the transplant protocol that may have contributed to the substantial transplant-related mortality. Busulphan was used in the conditioning regimen, leading to death from hepatic veno-occlusive disease in two patients in the ASCT and six patients in the allogeneic transplant arm. Overall mortality from the autologous transplant procedure was 14%. Four-year DFS was similar in the chemotherapy, autologous and allogeneic transplant groups (35%, 35% and 43%, respectively). There was actually an overall survival benefit demonstrated in the chemotherapy arm of this trial ($P = 0.1$). It would seem that those patients in the transplant arm suffered the disadvantages of autografting without gaining optimal beneficial effects. Salvage therapy following relapse was better in the chemotherapy group, contributing to this difference in overall rate of survival.

The GOELAM (Group Ouest Est Leucemies Aigues Myeloblastiques)[37] again showed no difference with transplantation in terms of DFS or overall survival. This group also used a second course of high dose cytarabine arabinoside (3 g/m² for eight doses) in both the chemotherapy and ASCT groups to particularly good effect, but not in the ABMT group. They were unable to show any benefit for allogeneic transplantation in this comparison.

Children

Not only does autologous transplantation have significant immediate morbidity with infection, haemorrhage, and mucositis, but there are also very significant long-term effects. Infertility,

growth and developmental effects, endocrine abnormalities, cataracts, and secondary malignancies are particularly significant for young patients. Children with acute leukaemia do well with chemotherapy alone and if they relapse respond well to salvage regimens, so any benefit which may be seen in terms of reduced relapse rate from transplantation has to be balanced with these long-term sequelae.

Both of the large randomized paediatric studies showed no survival benefit in those assigned to autograft.[39,40] The design of these trials is shown in Fig. 5.5. These trials have used multiple cycling chemotherapy blocks compared with ASCT. The largest, the Paediatric Oncology Group study (POG), randomized 232 patients under 21 years. Their 15% mortality from the autograft procedure was unusually high for this age group and no difference was seen in either DFS or overall survival. Delayed engraftment of the perfosfamide-purged marrow probably contributed to this outcome. The Italian AIEOP group found that ASCT was not superior to intensive consolidation and indeed had a relapse rate of 71% following ASCT. The ASCT was undertaken after four courses of DAT chemotherapy whereas children receiving chemotherapy had a further eight courses. This study demonstrates that even though the ASCT arm did not receive HDAC and received a nonmyeloablative conditioning regimen (BVAC), the outcome was equal to that of the additional eight courses of chemotherapy.

When 359 patients aged under 15 years registered in the MRC AML 10 trial were analysed, it was seen that ASCT or ABMT were associated with reduced relapse risk, but there was no evidence that either approach lead to better overall survival. This was mainly because of the excellent response rate to further treatment in those relapsing after chemotherapy.[42] The CCG study-2891 compared HDAC with autograft using purged marrow and actually demonstrated a benefit for intensive chemotherapy for both DFS and overall survival (Table 5.2).

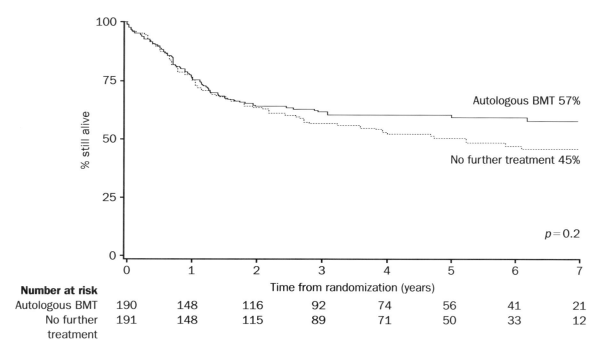

Figure 5.5
Disease-free survival in the Medical Research Council study of autologous bone marrow transplantation versus chemotherapy. Reproduced with permission from Burnett et al., Lancet 1998;351:700.

Critical analysis of prospective randomized studies

A number of general criticisms can be made of these studies. The patients undergoing randomization represent less than half of those achieving remission and therefore eligible for randomization. Of those patients randomized, many fail to receive the assigned therapy because of inter-current relapse, or patient or physician choice. A greater proportion of patients relapsing in the chemotherapy arm of these trials is successfully salvaged with autologous bone marrow transplantation. This attrition which is seen at each landmark stage in the MRC AML 10 trial is illustrated in Fig. 5.6. There were problems as seen in many studies in the randomization and delivery of assigned treatment, particularly in the ASCT arm. Analysis of the reasons for this showed that this

was due to both relapse and patient/physician choice. This will lead to an element of selection bias in the patients transplanted, making it difficult to extrapolate the data to all patients. The absence of an overall survival benefit in the majority of studies is probably related to procedural mortality of 6.5–15% and the effect of more successful salvage therapy after chemotherapy. The other factor that has been seen during the course of these trials is a sustained improvement in the outcome following chemotherapy compared with historical reports.

The varying intensity of the comparison chemotherapy arm also seems to play a critical role. The MRC AML 10 trial suggests that if the benefit of autologous transplantation is to be seen, then it is better performed after intensive consolidation therapy. The inclusion of a course of HDAC is important, whether before ASCT or

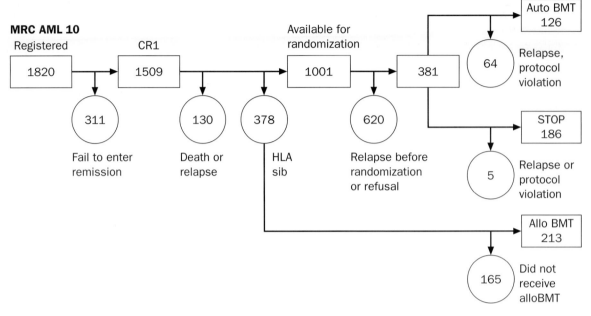

Figure 5.6
Attrition rates at each study landmark in the Medical Research Council Acute Myeloid Leukaemia 10 trial, typical of all studies. Figures in circles represent patients lost to randomization at each stage. Auto, autogeneic; Allo, allogeneic; BMT, bone marrow transplantation; CR1, first clinical remission; sib, sibling; STOP, no further chemotherapy.

before further intensification chemotherapy. The MRC trial demonstrated that when autograft is used as further consolidation compared to stopping treatment there is superior DFS and may also be a longer-term overall survival benefit. The question as to whether the function of this fifth course of therapy could be just as well served by an additional course of consolidation is to be addressed in the MRC AML 12 study.

As can be seen (Fig. 5.4), the POG and AIEOP studies looked at autografting compared with up to nine further sequential, cumulative cycles of chemotherapy. They did not report the difference in hospitalization but, given the equal outcomes, there may be benefits to undergoing one single intensive procedure rather than this extended type of chemotherapy schedule. There are few data comparing aspects of pharmacoeconomics with end points such as time spent in hospital, infection rates and antibiotic usage. If these were more widely

reported then important differences might emerge to assist decision-making. Equivalence and 'equipoise' are important factors that must be considered in randomized trial design.[41]

A number of studies (predominantly from the USA) have used 4-HC purging. The poorer engraftment associated with this manipulation may have contributed to the higher transplant-related mortality seen in the US intergroup trial and the POG study (Table 5.2).

The main conclusion that can be drawn from these results is that dose intensification, whether delivered as repeated courses of chemotherapy or as single intensive ABMT, improves DFS. Where there is a direct comparison, as in the EORTC/GIMEMA, there is a reduced relapse risk in those receiving ABMT, although this has not translated to an improvement in overall survival, due to higher procedural mortality and the better response to subsequent ABMT when relapse occurs after chemotherapy. It may well be that as the outcome from transplantation improves with better supportive care and faster marrow recovery with the use of PBSC, the improvement in relapse rates will follow into better survival.

Comparison of autologous and allogeneic bone marrow transplantation in first remission

Allogeneic transplantation has become a standard treatment. During the last two decades, outcomes from chemotherapy and ABMT have improved, so it remains important to ask whether allogeneic transplantation still has a role in first remission treatment of AML. The main disadvantages of allogeneic bone marrow transplantation are high procedure-related mortality and morbidity from chronic graft-versus-host disease. This is, however, counterbalanced by a lower relapse rate, possibly due to a graft-versus-leukaemia effect. If allogeneic transplantation can be made safer then the benefits over alternative procedures may be better defined.

No truly randomized trials are available. Most trials adopt a design whereby patients who have an HLA-matched sibling are assigned allogeneic transplantation. This design may be justified on the basis that only 25–30% of individuals in developed countries will have a sibling-matched donor. The remainder is allocated to the ABMT/chemotherapy comparison arm acting as the control. If such a design were not adopted then a far larger accrual would be necessary to attain sufficient power to detect a statistical difference.

The GOELAM, MRC and US Intergroup investigators have all assessed the role of allogeneic transplantation.[22,36,43] Relapse rate was consistently lower in all of these studies. The paediatric group analyses of the POG and CCG were able to demonstrate statistically better overall survival, but no such effect has been seen in the multicentre adult studies. In another study, the value of ABMT for DFS was confirmed in 107 patients assigned to either HLA-matched allogeneic transplant or chemotherapy (53% versus 16% DFS in the chemotherapy-alone arm) when analysed on an intention to treat basis. However, the very poor outcome of patients assigned to the chemotherapy arm is unexplained.[44] An early Dutch study randomized 117 patients to either allogeneic BMT or autografting. This study suggested that allogeneic BMT provides a better DFS than autologous BMT, although again only 59% of patients received their transplant procedure (3-year DFS: 35% autologous, 51% allogeneic bone marrow transplant, $P = 0.12$). The higher relapse rate in the autologous therapy arm was thought to be related to suboptimal cytoreductive therapy prior to harvest.[27] Mitus et al. were again able to demonstrate improved DFS in 94 patients studied.[45] In the donor/no donor analysis conducted in the MRC AML 10 trial there was no difference in overall survival although, as expected, the relapse rate was much less but the procedure-related mortality negated that effect.[43] None of these groups was able to demonstrate an overall survival advantage for allogeneic bone marrow transplantation. 'Time-censoring' effects also apply to allogeneic transplantation and, as there tends to be a longer delay to allogeneic transplant, this effect is likely to be more prominent.

Retrospective analysis of the European Group for Blood and Marrow Transplantation (EBMT) registry data 1987–1992 suggested that leukaemia-free survival was significantly better in allogeneic transplantation. Analysis of 516 allogeneic transplants and 598 autologous marrow transplants at age 3–40 years showed a significantly higher transplant-related mortality, lower relapse rates and better DFS (55% versus 42%) but no overall survival benefit.[46] Other registry-based studies, for example comparison of BGMT (Bordeaux, Grenoble, Marseilles, Toulouse) registry data, have shown allografting to be superior to autografting with lower relapse rate, higher transplant-related mortality but better overall survival.[47]

Another approach to determine when transplantation approaches are appropriate has been to seek the consensus view of a group of expert physicians by measuring a 'level of appropriateness' of therapeutic options in a range of given clinical scenarios.[48] There is a consensus view amongst physicians that allogeneic transplantation is the most effective treatment for any patient under 55 years of age with a suitable donor. Whilst there is good evidence that this results in lower rates of relapse, this has not extended to a benefit in overall survival, due to higher TRM and it has the drawback that it is only available to a small proportion of patients.

Whilst the studies comparing allogeneic transplantation consistently show a better leukaemia-free survival, the indications from several studies addressing long-term quality-of-life issues have generally shown that recipients of allogeneic transplants have more short- and long-term complications. These relate to chronic graft-versus-host disease but, in addition, there have also been demonstrated important differences in sexual function and psychosexual sequelae following allogeneic transplantation.[49,50] These important issues need to be taken into account when considering therapeutic approaches.

Transplantation in second remission and relapse

Successful salvage treatment of patients who relapse after chemotherapy has been shown to be significantly better than for those relapsing after autologous BMT.[22,30,35] Overall these patients can attain a 30% leukaemia-free survival with autografting. There is a better outcome for those with a higher duration of remission. The optimal timing of autologous transplantation is therefore debated.

A strategy to delay transplantation may be attractive, because patients potentially cured by chemotherapy need not receive transplants. No trial addresses this question, although some information may come from the MRC or GOELAM studies in which marrow was collected in CR1 in all patients so that patients relapsing after chemotherapy could be transplanted. The numbers of patients will be small:

around 110 patients relapsed following chemotherapy and only a proportion of these will enter CR2 and receive the harvest. Schiffman et al. looked at the uptake of cryopreserved autologous marrow harvested in CR1 and kept as a 'rainy day' harvest. In this study, 66% of patients relapsed and many of these received this stored marrow, but DFS was only 14%.[51]

Risk stratification

The outcome of any treatment strategy both in AML and ALL will depend on biological features of the disease independent of the treatment used. Consistent indicators of prognosis include cytogenetics and time to achieve first remission. Other prognostic factors include age, disease burden at presentation, presence of the multidrug resistance gene (MDR-1), Fab type, secondary leukaemia and leukaemia preceded by myelodysplasia (Table 5.3). Favourable karyotypes include t(8;21), inv(16) and t(15;17) whilst in contrast abnormalities of chromosome 5 or 7 or complex changes forecast a very poor outcome.[52-54] It should be possible to identify patients who are particularly likely to benefit from a particular therapeutic approach and thereby refine decisions regarding transplantation so that some patients can be saved toxic, expensive treatments. In the MRC AML10 trial the remission rates for patients assigned to the good, standard and poor risk groups were 74%, 52% and 33%, respectively, and survival from first CR 69%, 46% and 24%. Most trials to date have not taken into account cytogenetic data. Patients with poor prognostic factors seem to benefit little from intensified treatment and still have poor outcome[22] (Table 5.4). The design of the MRC AML 12 study will exclude poor risk patients defined by cytogenetics or failure to achieve <15% blasts after the second course and they will be entered into the MRC AML High Risk study to define the benefit of a number of novel strategies. Patients shown to have a particularly favourable outcome with t(15;17), t(8;21) or inv(16) who relapse following chemotherapy have a particularly good rate of CR2.

Table 5.3 Poor prognostic factors in acute myeloid leukaemia

- Adverse cytogenetic abnormalities: -5, -7, del(5q), abn(3q), complex
- Older age
- Longer time to achieve complete remission
- High white cell count at diagnosis
- Marrow blast expression of CD34
- Expression of multidrug resistance gene
- F1t3 mutation

This group is not randomized to transplant in MRC AML 12 and autograft is held in reserve for those who relapse. It would be ideal to tailor the duration of chemotherapy to the time needed to eradicate residual leukaemia cells, and the improvements in sensitivity and specificity for detecting minimal residual disease may allow the scheduling of chemotherapy to be individually determined.

Summary

In spite of considerable data, the optimal treatment of AML remains controversial and the place of autologous transplantation in the management of AML in CR1 remains to be defined.

From the available randomized controlled trials there seems to be a consistent reduction in the relapse rate, which is counterbalanced by a procedure-related mortality. Improvement in procedure-related mortality will lead to increased benefit from the autologous transplantation approach. Furthermore it may be beneficial to consolidate AML therapy with one single high dose procedure rather than to undertake multiple courses of intensive therapy. There is increasing evidence that patients themselves prefer one intensive therapeutic procedure rather than a prolonged course of therapy over months.[55] Clearly the field remains open for ongoing randomized and carefully controlled studies to examine further the role of autologous therapy and to answer some of the remaining unresolved questions.

ACUTE LYMPHOBLASTIC LEUKAEMIA

The outcome of adult ALL remains poor, with the most likely outcome being relapse and death despite 90% entering complete remission. This contrasts with the situation in children, where the majority of patients achieve a cure. Poor prognostic indices include age, cytogenetics [for example t(9;22), t(4;11)], high presenting white cell count, prolonged time to CR1, extramedullary disease at presentation and phenotype suggesting mature B lineage. The

Table 5.4 Seven-year overall survival (%) in the Medical Research Council Acute Myeloid Leukaemia 10 trial, by risk category

Risk	Autogeneic transplant	No further therapy	Overall
Good*	74	61	70
Standard	52	40	48
Poor	49	39	15

*Good risk defined by favourable cytogenetics [(t(8;21), inv(16), t(15;17)] and blasts <5% after second course.

presence of the Philadelphia chromosome has been identified as the main high risk factor, with a DFS at 2 years of around 14%.[56,57]

Results from allogeneic transplantation in first remission are no better overall than those achieved with chemotherapy[58,59] and enthusiasm over high dose therapy with autologous stem cell rescue at this stage in ALL has therefore been tempered. The major randomized study was published by Fiere et al.[60] who looked at ASCT compared with chemotherapy in first remission ALL in 191 patients. When analysed by intention to treat, the 3-year DFS rates were not significantly different (39% versus 32%). There were no differences when patients were stratified by risk factor, with a 16% survival after ASCT and 11% survival after chemotherapy in the high risk group, and 49% and 40%, respectively, in the standard risk group.[60] This group also assessed ABMT and found a survival benefit in the high risk patients but no difference in the standard risk group in the comparison with chemotherapy and ASCT.[61] Another group compared allogeneic transplantation with chemotherapy and, whilst there was no difference in overall survival or DFS when all patients were analysed on an intention to treat basis, when 96 patients with high risk ALL were examined there was better overall survival and DFS from the allograft procedure (overall 44% versus 20%, $P < 0.03$; DFS 39% versus 14%, $P = 0.01$).[62] Autologous bone marrow transplantation has been felt to be more appropriate for high risk patients in CR1 or those lacking an HLA-matched donor at relapse. The use of continuing post-remission maintenance therapy has been assessed and gave a relatively low relapse rate at 5 years of 31%, with a 5-year survival of 56%.[63]

In summary there is little evidence of a role for ASCT outside a clinical trial setting in ALL CR1 although the same arguments for use of ASCT in AML apply to ALL. The outcome of adult patients with ALL is dismal overall and particularly in those with additional risk features. Little impact has been made by chemotherapeutic approaches and novel therapies must be explored in this group of patients.

Autologous transplantation in second clinical remission

Patients who relapse following a multiagent regimen are unlikely to be cured with additional chemotherapy alone and where possible should be considered for allogeneic transplantation. A recent report from the University of Minnesota and the Dana Farber Cancer Institute of a series of consecutive ASCT and MUD transplants in both CR1 and CR2 found that when adult patients in CR2 were analysed a lower relapse risk was seen following matched unrelated donor transplant (MUD). Despite the fact that this was balanced by the higher transplant-related mortality, a statistically significant survival benefit for MUD was seen in this group.[64] Studies that attempt to make MUD transplants safer may be of benefit in high risk ALL. There is an ongoing EBMT study comparing the role of ABMT versus MUD. Outcome in recipients of HLA-matched related and unrelated bone marrow was compared to that in those receiving second ASCT. Two-year DFS was no different between the groups.[65]

PURGING

One of the prerequisites determining the success of autologous bone marrow transplantation for acute leukaemia is that reinfused stem cells should not contribute to relapse. The most common strategy, which has been adopted for in vitro purging to reduce the leukaemic contamination of the graft, has been exposure of cells in vitro to the cyclophosphamide derivatives 4-hydroperoxycyclophosphamide[66] or mafosfamide. Purging of cells using monoclonal antibodies such as CD33 or CD14/CD15 in AML and combination of B lineage or T cell immunotoxins plus 4-HC in ALL have been assessed.[67–69] Positive CD34+ stem cell selection methods employed in lymphoma and breast cancers are less relevant in leukaemia as they have been demonstrated to be stem cell disorders and many express CD34.[70] A technique based on a long-term culture technique has also been reported.[38]

Results from syngeneic transplantation, when compared with those from autologous transplant, show relapse rates of similar magnitude. This leads to the suggestion that most patients relapse post-autografting owing to an inability of the preparative conditioning regimen to ablate the tumour within the patient.[71] The degree of leukaemic contamination after purging has been compared with that prior to purging. The predictor of relapse is not the post-purge level of contamination but is related to the degree of minimal residual disease at harvest, suggesting that it is actually the patient's disease rather than reinfused cells which actually cause relapse clinically.[69,72,73] None the less there is a potential risk of infusion of occult residual leukaemic cells in the graft. Gene marking to trace the origin of disease recurrence, using a retroviral vector carrying the selectable neomycin resistance gene to mark 5% of the reinfused stem, demonstrated that in AML at relapse, some leukaemic cells did indeed carry the marker gene.[74]

There is a lack of clear clinical evidence of a benefit from purging and in practice existing techniques would seem to confer a number of disadvantages. In particular, purging may delay engraftment and this may have contributed to increased death rates in a number of randomized controlled trials.[37,39] In spite of rigorous analysis of registry data, no substantial evidence supporting marrow purging has been forthcoming.[25,28,75] Only in a selected high risk group in whom autograft was performed within 6 months, or where patients relapsed following a short remission, was any benefit seen.[28]

Appelbaum has attempted to calculate the number of patients that need to be randomized to quantify a benefit for purging. In order to undertake this he has used the following assumptions derived from the published data:

- The probability of relapse is 25% for patients in CR1 who receive syngeneic marrow and this relapse rate is equivalent to 100% effectively purged marrow.

- The probability of relapse in those receiving unpurged marrow is increased by 50% compared with those receiving syngeneic marrow.

- Marrow purging may be estimated to be effective either 50% or 100% of the time.

- Transplant-related mortality occurs in around 25% of cases whether receiving purged or unpurged marrow.

- Sample sizes are calculated based on an 80% probability of detecting a difference at the 0.05 significance level.

Using these assumptions, the number of patients required in each arm to detect an effect of purging if it is only effective 50% of the time would be 135, and if purging were 100% effective, then 31 patients would be required in each study arm.[76] Given the attrition rates seen in the MRC studies, large prospective randomized trials would be necessary and are unlikely to be forthcoming. Whether emerging targets in leukaemia cells will lend themselves to selective removal remains to be seen.

COMPARISON OF PERIPHERAL BLOOD STEM CELLS AND BONE MARROW

The first report of the use of PBSC mobilized into the peripheral blood with haemopoietic growth factors for transplantation was by Juttner et al.[77] in Australia in 1985, confirming that PBSC collected following induction regimens are capable of haemopoietic reconstitution in AML. It was believed initially that there would be reduced graft contamination due to the differences in the mobilization profile of normal cells compared with blasts. Others disagreed with this view, suggesting that the higher cell numbers infused with the PBSC may increase the dose of reinfused occult leukaemia cells.[78,79] This has never been demonstrated to be the case. Paired analysis of marrow and leukapheresis products with karyotypic markers has suggested that PBSC actually contain fewer contaminating cells.[68,73] Only one study has been reported comparing marrow with stem cell support and this showed no superiority of stem cells in terms of relapse rate.[80] The major benefit which was seen with the early A-PBSCT trials was a considerably greater speed of haemopoietic recovery, with median time to attain neutrophils $>0.5 \times 10^9/l$ being 10–15 days and platelets of $50 \times 10^9/l$ being 19 days, giving rise to benefits in procedure-related mortality, morbidity, cost and earlier discharge from hospital.[80–82] The retrospective analysis of the EBMT registry data showed that the source of stem cells does not affect relapse rate or outcome.[75]

FUTURE DIRECTIONS AND NOVEL THERAPEUTIC APPROACHES IN ACUTE LEUKAEMIA

Whilst the outcome of treatment for AML has improved substantially through the improved supportive care allowing the successful use of high doses of chemotherapeutic agents, it is unlikely that further dose escalation will have great impact on further refining these results. The dose limitations are now constrained by the organ toxicity of chemoradiotherapy rather than myelotoxicity. It is clear that a new approach is required. Developments in cellular and gene therapeutics along with better understanding of the immune system are allowing progress toward developing adoptive immunotherapy with the aim of harnessing the innate immune response to trigger cellular kill.

Autologous graft-versus-leukaemia

Allogeneic transplantation in acute leukaemia gives rise to lower relapse rates although this is often at the expense of increased transplant-related mortality. A significant component of the therapeutic effect is due to a powerful graft-versus-leukaemia effect exerted by the donor lymphocytes. The effector cells of this effect may be interleukin-2 (IL-2) responsive cytotoxic T cells. Attempts have been made to mimic this and achieve a similar benefit in autologous pro-

cedures. The stimulation of an autologous graft-versus-leukaemia effect has been attempted using interleukin-2 (IL-2) and cyclosporin following autologous transplantation.[15,83] A cytokine, IL-2, enhances lymphocyte activation and secretion of secondary cytokines (tumour necrosis factor and interferon-γ) and induces the cytotoxic endogenous LAK effector cells. Clinical phase I and II studies have been promising but the considerable toxicity has dampened the initial enthusiasm for this approach. Benyunes et al.[85] administered IL-2 after ABMT in a phase Ib study to 14 patients with AML in first relapse to induce immuno-modulatory effects.[84] Lymphokine activated killer cells (LAK) cells can lyse myeloid leukaemia cells in vitro. In spite of promising animal studies,[85] there is as yet no good clinical evidence of a benefit.[86–88]

Autologous cellular leukaemia vaccines

There is some evidence that AML cells express foreign antigens or overexpress normal cellular antigens that serve as targets for lysis. It is now possible to boost immune effector cells through gene therapy technologies. Little is known about the kinetics of leukaemia regrowth and the mechanisms by which the immune system controls residual leukaemia. Current therapeutic advances are aimed towards stimulation of the cells capable of exerting an anti-neoplastic action and this may open the way to improve management.

Autologous cellular vaccines may provide a way to harness the immune system to destroy leukaemic cells, modifying autologous cells to act as antigen-presenting cells to trigger the host immune response. It has been demonstrated that AML blasts are capable of generating an antigen-specific cytotoxic T lymphocyte (CTL) response. Acute myeloid leukaemia cells are able to escape the natural immune surveillance. One mechanism by which this occurs is the lack of key co-stimulatory molecules. The molecules B7-1 (CD80) and B7-2 (CD86), expressed on antigen-presenting cells in associ-

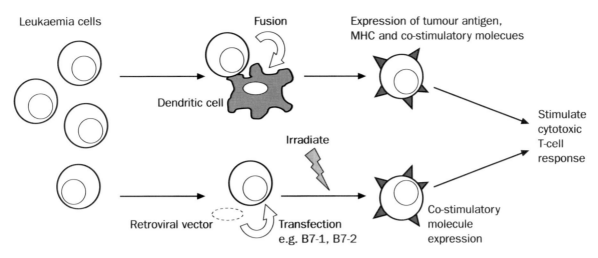

Figure 5.7
Different approaches can be taken to develop autologous cellular vaccines. The aim is to increase the antigen-presenting capacity and stimulate the host immune system to attack residual leukaemic blasts.

ation with HLA class II, provide co-stimulatory signals for T cell receptor-mediated T cell activation by binding to CD28 and CTLA-4; without these molecules engagement of the T cell receptor results in anergy or ignorance of the antigen-specific T cell, so no immune response is mounted to the tumour. Various approaches are being used to overcome this. Using a retroviral vector, B7-1 (CD80) has been introduced into murine leukaemic blasts which are then irradiated and used as a vaccine. This can stimulate an in vitro cytotoxic T cell reaction and leukaemia cell kill and protects against subsequent challenge with leukaemic cells in a murine model.[89,90] The generation of dendritic cells from AML cells in vitro using specific cytokines has been shown to be successful. These cells have been able to stimulate leukaemia-specific cytolytic activity in autologous lymphocytes[91-93] (Fig. 5.7).

Non-myeloablative conditioning regimens

Finally, substantial improvements in allogeneic transplantation protocols with better pre-emptive therapy to reduce complications may lead to a demonstrable reduction in transplant-related mortality for this group of patients. The ability to administer non-myeloablative conditioning followed by allogeneic transplant to achieve mixed chimerism harnessing the graft-versus-leukaemia effect may close the gap in transplant-related mortality in the future and may have an impact on overall survival whilst allowing this treatment option to be offered to older patients or those with coexistent morbid conditions.[94-97]

REFERENCES

1. Dicke KA, Zander A, Spitzer G et al. Autologous bone-marrow transplantation in relapsed adult acute leukaemia. Lancet 1979;1(8115):514–17.
2. Dicke KA, McCredie KB, Stevens EE, Spitzer G, Bottino JC. Autologous bone marrow transplantation in a case of acute adult leukemia. Transplant Proc 1977;9(1):193–5.
3. Skipper HE. The effects of chemotherapy on the kinetics of leukemic cell behavior. Cancer Res 1965;25(9):1544–50.
4. Skipper H, Schabel F, Wilcox W. Experimental evaluation of potential anticancer agents. XIII On the criteria and kinetics associated with 'curability'

of experimental leukaemia. Cancer Chemother Rep 1965;35:1–111.

5. Hagenbeek A, Martens ACM. Minimal residual disease in acute leukaemia. In: Jasmin C, Proctor SJ, editors. Baillières clinical haematology. London: Baillière Tindall, 1991: 609.

6. Gompertz B. On the Nature of the function expressive of the law of human mortality, and on the new mode of determining the value of life contingencies. Phil Trans R Soc Lond B 1825; 115:513–85.

7. Norton L, Simon R. Tumor size, sensitivity to therapy, and design of treatment schedules. Cancer Treat Rep 1977;61(7):1307–17.

8. Barnes DWH, Loutit JF. Radiation recovery factor and preservation by the Polge Smith Parkes technique. J Natl Cancer Inst 1955;15:1901–5.

9. Thomas E. One hundred patients with acute leukaemia. Blood 1977;49:511–33.

10. Verdonck LH, Heesben EC, van Heughton HG, Stahl GEJ, Rijksen G. The cytotoxicity of alkyl phospholipid on clonogenic leukaemia cells and on normal bone marrow progenitor cells is highly, but differentially, increased by cryopreservation. Bone Marrow Transplant 1992;9: 241–5.

11. Allieri MA, Lopez M, Douay L et al. Clonogenic leukaemic progenitor cells in acute myeloid leukaemia are highly sensitive to cryopreservation: possible purging effect for autologous bone marrow transplant. Bone Marrow Transplant 1991;7:101–5.

12. Hagenbeek AM, Martens ACM. Reinfusion of leukaemic cells with the autologous marrow graft: preclinical studies on lodging and regrowth of leukaemia. Leuk Res 1985;9:1389–95.

13. Gorin N. Collection, manipulation and freezing of haemopoietic stem cells. Clin Haematol 1986; 15(1):19–48.

14. Arlin ZF, Fried J, Clarkson BD. Therapeutic role of cell kinetics in acute leukaemia. Clin Haematol 1978;7:339–62.

15. Hess AD, Thoburn CJ. Immunobiology and immunotherapeutic implications of syngeneic/ autologous graft-versus-host disease. Immunol Rev 1997;157:111–23.

16. Campana D, Pui CH. Detection of minimal residual disease in acute leukaemia. Blood 1995; 85:1416–34.

17. Champlin R, Gajewski J, Nimer S et al. Postremission chemotherapy for adults with acute myelogenous leukaemia: improved survival with high-dose cytarabine and daunorubicin consolidation treatment. J Clin Oncol 1990; 8(7):1199–206.

18. Bishop JF, Matthews JP, Young GA et al. A randomized study of high-dose cytarabine in induction in acute myeloid leukemia (see comments). Blood 1996;87(5):1710–17.

19. Mayer RJ, Davis RB, Schiffer CA et al. Intensive postremission chemotherapy in adults with acute myeloid leukemia. Cancer and Leukemia Group B (see comments). N Engl J Med 1994; 331(14):896–903.

20. Rees J. Late intensification therapy in AML – report of the MRC AML 8 trial. Proc Am Soc Clin Oncology 1985: C621.

21. Rees JK, Gray RG, Wheatley K. Dose intensification in acute myeloid leukaemia: greater effectiveness at lower cost. Principal report of the Medical Research Council's AML9 study. MRC Leukaemia in Adults Working Party. Br J Haematol 1996;94(1):89–98.

22. Burnett AK, Goldstone AH, Stevens RM et al. Randomised comparison of addition of autologous bone-marrow transplantation to intensive chemotherapy for acute myeloid leukaemia in first remission: results of MRC AML 10 trial. UK Medical Research Council Adult and Children's Leukaemia Working Parties. Lancet 1998; 351(9104):700–8.

23. Burnett AK. Transplantation in first remission of acute myeloid leukemia (editorial; comment). N Engl J Med 1998;339(23):1698–700.

24. McMillan AK, Goldstone AH, Chopra R, Linch DC. A comparison of the outcome of ABMT in first remission acute myeloid and lymphoblastic leukemia in a single centre. Bone Marrow Transplant 1990;6(suppl 1):72.

25. Gorin NC, Aegerter P, Auvert B. Autologous bone marrow transplantation for acute leukemia in remission: an analysis of 1322 cases. Hamatol Bluttransfus 1990;33:660–6.

26. Lowenberg B, Abels J, van Bekkum DW et al. Transplantation of non-purified autologous bone marrow in patients with AML in first remission. Cancer 1984;54(12):2840–3.

27. Lowenberg B, Verdonck LJ, Dekker AW et al. Autologous bone marrow transplantation in acute myeloid leukemia in first remission: results of a Dutch prospective study. J Clin Oncol 1990;8(2):287–94.

28. Gorin NC, Labopin M, Meloni G et al. Autologous bone marrow transplantation for

acute myeloblastic leukemia in Europe: further evidence of the role of marrow purging by mafosfamide. European Co-operative Group for Bone Marrow Transplantation (EBMT). Leukemia 1991;5(10):896–904.

29. Cassileth PA, Andersen J, Lazarus HM et al. Autologous bone marrow transplant in acute myeloid leukemia in first remission. J Clin Oncol 1993;11(2):314–19.

30. Chopra R, Goldstone AH, McMillan AK et al. Successful treatment of acute myeloid leukemia beyond first remission with autologous bone marrow transplantation using busulfan/cyclophosphamide and unpurged marrow: the British autograft group experience. J Clin Oncol 1991;9(10):1840–7.

31. de Gast GC, Zwaan FE, Hagenbeek T, Verdonck LF, Lowenberg B. Autologous bone marrow transplantation in first remission AML – its relative value. Bone Marrow Transplant 1990; 6(suppl 1): 52–4.

32. Goldstone AH, Anderson CC, Linch DC et al. Autologous bone marrow transplantation following high dose chemotherapy for the treatment of adult patients with acute myeloid leukaemia. Br J Haematol 1986;64(3):529–37.

33. McMillan AK, Goldstone AH, Linch DC et al. High-dose chemotherapy and autologous bone marrow transplantation in acute myeloid leukemia. Blood 1990;76(3):480–8.

34. Gray R, Wheatley K. How to avoid bias when comparing bone marrow transplantation with chemotherapy. Bone Marrow Transplant 1991; 7(suppl 3): 9–12.

35. Zittoun RA, Mandelli F, Willemze R et al. Autologous or allogeneic bone marrow transplantation compared with intensive chemotherapy in acute myelogenous leukemia. European Organization for Research and Treatment of Cancer (EORTC) and the Gruppo Italiano Malattie Ematologiche Maligne dell'Adulto (GIMEMA) Leukemia Cooperative Groups (see comments). N Engl J Med 1995;332(4):217–23.

36. Harousseau JL, Cahn JY, Pignon B et al. Comparison of autologous bone marrow transplantation and intensive chemotherapy as postremission therapy in adult acute myeloid leukemia. The Groupe Ouest Est Leucemies Aigues Myeloblastiques (GOELAM). Blood 1997; 90(8):2978–86.

37. Cassileth PA, Harrington DP, Appelbaum FR et al. Chemotherapy compared with autologous or allogeneic bone marrow transplantation in the management of acute myeloid leukemia in first remission (see comments). N Engl J Med 1998; 339(23):1649–56.

38. Reiffers J, Stoppa AM, Attal M et al. Allogeneic vs autologous stem cell transplantation vs chemotherapy in patients with acute myeloid leukemia in first remission: the BGMT 87 study. Leukemia 1996;10(12):1874–82.

39. Ravindranath Y, Yeager AM, Chang MN et al. Autologous bone marrow transplantation versus intensive consolidation chemotherapy for acute myeloid leukemia in childhood. Pediatric Oncology Group. N Engl J Med 1996;334(22): 1428–34.

40. Amadori S, Testi AM, Arico M et al. Prospective comparative study of bone marrow transplantation and postremission chemotherapy for childhood acute myelogenous leukemia. The Associazione Italiana Ematologia ed Oncologia Pediatrica Cooperative Group. J Clin Oncol 1993; 11(6):1046–54.

41. Burnett AK, Goldstone AH, Stevens RM. Allogeneic and autologous bone marrow transplant reduce relapse risk in AML in CR1 but do not significantly improve overall survival: results of the MRC AML 10 trial. Br J Haematol 1996;93(suppl 2): 313.

42. Stevens RF, Hann IM, Wheatley K, Gray RG. Marked improvements in outcome with chemotherapy alone in paediatric acute myeloid leukemia: results of the United Kingdom Medical Research Council's 10th AML trial. MRC Childhood Leukaemia Working Party. Br J Haematol 1998;101(1):130–40.

43. Ferrant A, Doyen C, Delannoy A et al. Allogeneic or autologous bone marrow transplantation for acute non-lymphocytic leukemia in first remission. Bone Marrow Transplant 1991; 7(4):303–9.

44. Mitus AJ, Miller KB, Schenkein DP et al. Improved survival for patients with acute myelogenous leukemia (see comments). J Clin Oncol 1995;13(3):560–9.

45. Gorin NC, Labopin M, Fouillard L et al. Retrospective evaluation of autologous bone marrow transplantation vs allogeneic bone marrow transplantation from an HLA identical related donor in acute myelocytic leukemia. A study of the European Cooperative Group for Blood and Marrow Transplantation (EBMT). Bone Marrow Transplant 1996;18(1):111–17.

46. Reiffers J, Gaspard MH, Maraninchi D et al. Comparison of allogeneic or autologous bone marrow transplantation and chemotherapy in patients with acute myeloid leukaemia in first remission: a prospective controlled trial. Br J Haematol 1989;72(1):57–63.

47. Gale RP, Park RE, Dubois RW et al. Delphi-panel analysis of appropriateness of high-dose therapy and bone marrow transplants in adults with acute myelogenous leukemia in 1st remission. Leuk Res 1999;23(8):709–18.

48. Watson M, Wheatley K, Harrison GA et al. Severe adverse impact on sexual functioning and fertility of bone marrow transplantation, either allogeneic or autologous, compared with consolidation chemotherapy alone: analysis of the MRC AML 10 trial. Cancer 1999;86(7):1231–9.

49. Zittoun R, Suciu S, Watson M et al. Quality of life in patients with acute myelogenous leukaemia in prolonged first complete remission after bone marrow transplantation (allogeneic or autologous) or chemotherapy: a cross-sectional study of the EORTC-GIMEMA AML8A trial. Bone Marrow Transplant 1997;20:307–15.

50. Schiffman KCR, Clift R, Appelbaum FR et al. Consequences of cryopreserving first remission autologous marrow for use after relapse in patients with AML. Bone Marrow Transplant 1993;11:227–32.

51. Ringden O, Labopin M, Frassoni F et al. Allogeneic bone marrow transplant or second autograft in patients with acute leukemia who relapse after an autograft. Acute Leukaemia Working Party of the European Group for Blood and Marrow Transplantation (EBMT). Bone Marrow Transplant 1999;24(4):389–96.

52. Grimwade D, Walker H, Oliver F et al. The importance of diagnostic cytogenetics on outcome in AML: analysis of 1,612 patients entered into the MRC AML 10 trial. The Medical Research Council Adult and Children's Leukaemia Working Parties. Blood 1998;92(7): 2322–33.

53. Keating MJ, Smith TL, Kantarjian H et al. Cytogenetic pattern in acute myelogenous leukemia: a major reproducible determinant of outcome. Leukemia 1988;2(7):403–12.

54. Burnett AK. Karyotypically defined risk groups in acute myeloid leukaemia (comment). Leuk Res 1994;18(12):889–90.

55. Group Francais de Cytogenetique Hematologique. Cytogenetic abnormalities in adult acute lymphoblastic leukaemia: correlations with hematologic findings and outcome. A collaborative study. Blood 1996;87: 3135–42.

56. Secker-Walker L, Craig J, Hawkins J, Hoffbrand A. Philadelphia positive acute lymphoblastic leukaemia in adults: age distribution, BCR breakpoint and prognostic significance. Leukaemia 1991;5:196–9.

57. Zhang M, Hoelzer D, Horowitz M et al. Long term follow-up of adults with ALL in first remission treated with chemotherapy or bone marrow transplantation. Ann Intern Med 1995;123: 428–31.

58. Bouchiex C, David B, Sebban C et al. Immunophenotype of adult acute lymphoblastic leukaemia, clinical parameters and outcomes: an analysis of a prospective trial, including 562 tested patients (LALA87). Blood 1994;84:1603–12.

59. Fiere D, Lepage E, Sebban C et al. Adult acute lymphoblastic leukaemia: a multicentric randomised trial testing bone marrow transplantation as postremission therapy. J Clin Oncol 1993;10: 1990–2001.

60. Sebban C, Lepage E, Vernant J et al. Allogeneic bone marrow transplantation in adult acute lymphoblastic leukaemia in first complete remission: a comparative study. J Clin Oncol 1994;12: 2580–7.

61. Powles R, Mehta J, Singhal S. Autologous bone marrow or peripheral blood transplantation followed by maintenance chemotherapy for adult ALL in CR1: 50 cases from a single centre. Bone Marrow Transplant 1995;16:241–7.

62. Yeager AM, Kaizer H, Santos GW et al. Autologous bone marrow transplantation in patients with acute nonlymphocytic leukemia, using ex vivo marrow treatment with 4-hydroperoxycyclophosphamide. N Engl J Med 1986;315(3): 141–7.

63. Robertson M, Soiffer RJ, Freedman AS. Human bone marrow depleted of CD33-positive cells mediates delayed but durable reconstitution of hematopoiesis: clinical trial of MY9 monoclonal antibody-purged autografts for the treatment of acute myeloid leukaemia. Blood 1992;79:2229.

64. Voso MT, Hohaus S, Moos M et al. Autografting with CD34+ peripheral blood stem cells: retained engraftment capability and reduced tumour cell content. Br J Haematol 1999;104(2): 382–91.

65. Uckun FM, Kersey JH, Vallera DA et al. Autologous bone marrow transplantation in

high-risk remission T-lineage acute lymphoblastic leukaemia using immunotoxins plus 4-hydroperoxycyclophosphamide for purging. Blood 1990;76:1723–33.

66. Chang J, Morgenstern GR, Coutinho LH et al. The use of bone marrow cells grown up in long term culture for autologous bone marrow transplantation in acute myeloid leukaemia. An update. Bone Marrow Transplant 1989;4:4.

67. Gale R, Champlin R. How does bone marrow transplantation cure leukaemia? Lancet 1994;ii:28–30.

68. Uckun FM, Kersey JH, Haake R, Weisdorf D, Ramsay NK. Autologous bone marrow transplantation in high-risk remission B-lineage acute lymphoblastic leukaemia using a cocktail of three monoclonal antibodies (BA-1/CD24, BA-2/CD9, BA-3/CD10) plus complement and 4-HC for ex vivo marrow purging. Blood 1992;79: 1094–104.

69. Miyamoto T, Nagafuji K, Harada M, Niho Y. Significance of quantitative analysis of AML1/ETO transcripts in peripheral blood stem cells from t(8;21) acute myelogenous leukemia. Leuk Lymphoma 1997;25(1–2):69–75.

70. Brenner MK, Rill DR, Moen RC et al. Gene-marking to trace origin of relapse after autologous bone-marrow transplantation. Lancet 1993; 341(8837):85–6.

71. Appelbaum FR, Buckner CD. Overview of the Clinical relevance of autologous bone marrow transplantation. Clin Haematol 1986;15(1):1–18.

72. Juttner CA, To LB, Haylock DN, Branford A, Kimber RJ. Circulating autologous stem cells collected in very early remission from acute non-lymphoblastic leukaemia produce prompt but incomplete haemopoietic reconstitution after high dose melphalan or supralethal chemoradiotherapy. Br J Haematol 1985;61(4):739–45.

73. Sanz MA, de la Rubia J, Sanz GF et al. Busulfan plus cyclophosphamide followed by autologous blood stem-cell transplantation for patients with acute myeloblastic leukemia in first complete remission: a report from a single institution (see comments). J Clin Oncol 1993;11(9):1661–7.

74. Mehta J, Powles R, Singhal S et al. Autologous bone marrow transplantation for acute myeloid leukaemia in first remission: identification of modifiable prognostic factors. Bone Marrow Transplant 1995;16(4):499–506.

75. Korbling M, Fliedner TM, Holle R et al. Autologous blood stem cell (ABSCT) versus purged bone marrow transplantation (pABMT) in standard risk AML: influence of source and cell composition of the autograft on hemopoietic reconstitution and disease-free survival. Bone Marrow Transplant 1991;7(5):343–9.

76. To LB, Roberts MM, Haylock DN et al. Comparison of haematological recovery times and supportive care requirements of autologous recovery phase peripheral blood stem cell transplants, autologous bone marrow transplants and allogeneic bone marrow transplants. Bone Marrow Transplant 1992;9(4):277–84.

77. Henon PR, Liang H, Beck Wirth G et al. Comparison of hematopoietic and immune recovery after autologous bone marrow or blood stem cell transplants. Bone Marrow Transplant 1992;9(4):285–91.

78. Gorin NC. Autologous stem cell transplantation in acute myelocytic leukemia. Blood 1998;92(4): 1073–90.

79. Straetmans N, Herman P, Van Bockstaele DR, Michaux L, Hagemeijer A, Ferrant A. Haemopoietic defect and decreased expansion potential of bone marrow autografts from patients with acute myeloid leukaemia in first remission. Br J Haematol 1998;101(3):571–81.

80. Pendry K, Alcorn MJ, Burnett AK. Factors influencing haematological recovery in 53 patients with acute myeloid leukaemia in first remission after autologous bone marrow transplantation. Br J Haematol 1993;83(1):45–52.

81. Kasper C, Ryder WD, Durig J et al. Content of long-term culture-initiating cells, clonogenic progenitors and CD34 cells in apheresis harvests of normal donors for allogeneic transplantation, and in patients with acute myeloid leukaemia or multiple myeloma. Br J Haematol 1999;104(2): 374–81.

82. Herman P, Van Bockstaele DR, Ferrant A, Straetmans N. In vitro evaluation of the haemopoietic defect of CD34+ cells from patients with acute myeloid leukaemia in first remission. Br J Haematol 1999;106(1):142–51.

83. Yao M, Bouchet S, Harnois C et al. Quantitative and qualitative alterations of long-term culture-initiating cells in patients with acute leukaemia in complete remission. Br J Haematol 1998; 103(1):124–8.

84. Hess AD, Jones RJ, Morris LE et al. Autologous graft-versus-host disease: a new frontier in immunotherapy. Bone Marrow Transplant 1992; 10(suppl 1): 16–21.

85. Benyunes MC, Massumoto C, York A et al. Interleukin-2 with or without lymphokine-activated killer cells as consolidative immunotherapy after autologous bone marrow transplantation for acute myelogenous leukemia. Bone Marrow Transplant 1993;12(2):159–63.

86. Vourka Karussis U, Ackerstein A, Pugatsch T, Slavin S. Allogeneic cell-mediated immunotherapy for eradication of minimal residual disease: comparison of T-cell and IL-2 activated killer (LAK) cell-mediated adoptive immunotherapy in murine models. Exp Hematol 1999;27(3):461–9.

87. Benyunes MC, Higuchi C, York A et al. Immunotherapy with interleukin 2 with or without lymphokine-activated killer cells after autologous bone marrow transplantation for malignant lymphoma: a feasibility trial. Bone Marrow Transplant 1995;16(2):283–8.

88. Blaise D, Attal M, Pico JL et al. The use of a sequential high dose recombinant interleukin 2 regimen after autologous bone marrow transplantation does not improve the disease free survival of patients with acute leukemia transplanted in first complete remission. Leuk Lymphoma 1997;25(5–6):469–78.

89. Robinson N, Benyunes MC, Thompson JA et al. Interleukin-2 after autologous stem cell transplantation for hematologic malignancy: a phase I/II study. Bone Marrow Transplant 1997; 19(5): 435–42.

90. Mutis T, Schrama E, Melief CJ, Goulmy E. CD80-Transfected acute myeloid leukemia cells induce primary allogeneic T-cell responses directed at patient specific minor histocompatibility antigens and leukemia-associated antigens. Blood 1998;92(5):1677–84.

91. Mutis T, Verdijk R, Schrama E, Esendam B, Brand A, Goulmy E. Feasibility of immunotherapy of relapsed leukemia with ex vivo-generated cytotoxic T lymphocytes specific for hematopoietic system-restricted minor histocompatibility antigens. Blood 1999;93(7):2336–41.

92. Choudhury BA, Liang JC, Thomas EK et al. Dendritic cells derived in vitro from acute myelogenous leukemia cells stimulate autologous, antileukemic T-cell responses. Blood 1999;93(3): 780–6.

93. Charbonnier A, Gaugler B, Sainty D, Lafage Pochitaloff M, Olive D. Human acute myeloblastic leukemia cells differentiate in vitro into mature dendritic cells and induce the differentiation of cytotoxic T cells against autologous leukemias. Eur J Immunol 1999;29(8):2567–78.

94. Cignetti A, Bryant E, Allione B, Vitale A, Foa R, Cheever MA. CD34(+) acute myeloid and lymphoid leukemic blasts can be induced to differentiate into dendritic cells. Blood 1999;94(6): 2048–55.

95. Giralt S, Estey E, Albitar M et al. Engraftment of allogeneic hematopoietic progenitor cells with purine analog-containing chemotherapy: harnessing graft-versus-leukemia without myeloablative therapy. Blood 1997;89(12):4531–6.

96. Khouri IF, Keating M, Korbling M et al. Transplant-lite: induction of graft-versus-malignancy using fludarabine-based nonablative chemotherapy and allogeneic blood progenitor-cell transplantation as treatment for lymphoid malignancies. J Clin Oncol 1998;16(8):2817–24.

97. Slavin S, Nagler A, Naparstek E et al. Nonmyeloablative stem cell transplantation and cell therapy as an alternative to conventional bone marrow transplantation with lethal cytoreduction for the treatment of malignant and nonmalignant hematologic diseases. Blood 1998;91(3): 756–63.

6

Autografting with mobilized hematopoietic progenitor cells in chronic myeloid leukemia

Angelo Michele Carella, Enrica Lerma, Germana Beltrami and Maria Teresa Corsetti

CONTENTS Introduction • Rationale for autografting in chronic myeloid leukemia • In vitro manipulations • In vivo manipulations • Clinical results with in vivo technique employed in Genoa • Summary

INTRODUCTION

Chronic myeloid leukemia (CML) is a neoplastic disorder originating in a primitive hematopoietic stem cell.[1] The main characteristic of this mutation is the formation of a fusion gene (*bcr-abl*) with abnormal tyrosine kinase activity leading to abnormal hematopoiesis. Clinically, CML is characterized by an initial chronic phase (CP) followed by inevitable progression to an accelerated and then terminal blast phase. Allografting is currently the only curative treatment, but the majority of CML patients do not have an HLA-matched sibling donor. Unrelated donor transplants are associated with a high transplant-related mortality within the first 100 days of the procedure and can only be offered to patients under 40 years of age.

For older patients or those without compatible donors, therapy for CML includes hydroxyurea (HU), interferon-α (IFN-α) and probably tyrosine kinase inhibitors. Hydroxyurea does not modify the natural history of the disease; however, randomized studies indicate that IFN-α can induce cytogenetic remission and prolong overall survival.[2–5] Most IFN-α responders maintain molecular evidence of *bcr/abl* expression, indicating that IFN-α is unlikely to cure CML. Recently IFN-α has been combined with low dose Ara-C (LD-Ara-C), resulting in an improved cytogenetic remission rate and overall survival (OS) in comparison with IFN-α alone.[6] We have yet to evaluate whether the high cost of IFN-α (±LD-Ara-C), the incidence of side effects in 25% of patients and the low rate of long-term benefit outweigh the small increase in overall survival.

Autologous stem cell transplantation (ASCT) has been explored as an option for the treatment of these patients. In this chapter we will focus on recent advances with this procedure, particularly on in vivo manipulation techniques. Tyrosine kinase inhibitors appear to be effective therapeutically and in inducing cytogenetic remission and are currently being studied in various trials.

RATIONALE FOR AUTOGRAFTING IN CHRONIC MYELOID LEUKEMIA

There are at least two reasons for autografting in CML to improve OS. Long-term culture-initiating cells (LTC-IC) from CML patients have a poor self-maintenance capacity,[7] for reducing both normal and leukemic stem cell numbers should give normal hematopoietic stem cells a proliferative advantage. Normal hematopoietic reservoir declines with time in CML, so one should mobilize and collect Philadelphia chromosome (Ph)-negative progenitors as soon after diagnosis as possible.[8]

These observations have been confirmed after treatment with IFN-α,[4,5,9–11] intensive chemotherapy[12–15] and mobilization of Ph-negative progenitor cells after intensive chemotherapy.[16–22] Cytogenetic and other clonality studies suggest but do not prove that these cells are 'normal' hematopoietic progenitors.[23–27] In order to obtain normal progenitor cells, in vitro and in vivo approaches have been evaluated.

IN VITRO MANIPULATIONS

The Vancouver group demonstrated in a series of elegant experiments that Ph-positive cell numbers decline when put in culture, whereas previously unidentifiable Ph-negative cells emerged with preferential survival rates.[7,8,28,29] The physiological reason for this is unclear; some of the emerging Ph-negative cells show features of very primitive hematopoietic cells. On the basis of these findings, the Vancouver group devised a trial consisting of 10 days, culture of CML bone marrow and subsequent infusion into a chemotherapy-conditioned patient previously selected on the basis of the ability of his bone marrow to produce an adequate number of normal LTC-ICs in vitro. Over a 5-year period they evaluated 87 patients and selected 36 for the 10-day marrow culture, of whom 22 have been autografted. Sixteen patients remained alive up to 68 months post-autograft and five remain in complete or partial cytogenetic remission.[30] This technique is technically demanding and not feasible for most transplant units.

The Minneapolis group have shown that CD34+ DR− cells are predominantly or exclusively Ph-negative; in contrast CD34+/DR+ cells are Ph-positive. It has been recently reported that in patients in early chronic phase, CD34+DR− cells are *Bcr-Abl* mRNA negative in 80% of cases.[31] Large-scale selection with a high-speed FACS, starting with a marrow harvest of 2.0–2.5 l, results in 1×10^5 to 3×10^5/kg CD34+DR− cells. The frequencies of colony forming cells (CFC) and LTC-IC ranged from 2.6% to 8.6% and 0.187% to 0.233%, respectively. Both CD34+DR− and secondary CFC were Bcr-Abl mRNA negative. Therefore, this large-scale selection of CD34+DR− cells allows a highly purified autograft and may represent a step in the development of curative therapeutic strategies.

Other approaches include purging Ph-positive marrow cells with IFN,[32,33] incubating marrow with anti-sense oligodeoxynucleotides directed at the Bcr-Abl junctional sequences,[34,35] or the upstream sequences of MYB[36,37] CML patients. In a study conducted jointly by the Hammersmith Hospital in London and the University of Pennsylvania in Philadelphia, autologous bone marrow cells have been collected from CML patients and subjected to an in vitro purging procedure using a 24mer phosphorothioate antisense oligomer directed against codons 2–7 of the human *myb* gene.[37] Twelve patients have been recruited to this study and four have been rendered entirely or predominantly Ph-negative at the 3-month post-autograft assessment. This Ph-negativity has been transient in all cases.[36,37]

Another purging concept is to employ an agent that would preferentially protect normal progenitors from the effects of chemotherapy. MIP-1α is a candidate molecule that inhibits normal but not CML progenitors, and it may have clinical potential as a protective agent during chemotherapy or for chemotherapeutic purging of CML autografts.[38] Another novel approach involves incubation of marrow cells with ribozymes,[39–41] catalytic RNA species that can be tailored to recognize and disrupt leukemia-specific mRNA molecules.

IN VIVO MANIPULATIONS

The Genoa team has treated a large number of patients, both previously untreated and resistant to INF-α with intensive chemotherapy (idarubicin, cytosine arabinoside and etoposide – ICE or mini-ICE protocols) followed by administration of granulocyte colony stimulating factor (G-CSF).[16,17,42–44] In most cases it was possible to collect predominantly or exclusively Ph-negative myeloid progenitor cells. There is preliminary evidence that the Ph-negative progenitor cells were easier to collect in patients who had not received IFN-α.

The Swedish study adopted a different approach to in vivo purging.[45] Chronic myeloid leukemia patients were subjected to therapy of increasing intensity with the aim of achieving Ph-negativity in the bone marrow. Once Ph-negativity was achieved, patients proceeded to bone marrow harvest, which despite IFN-α treatment, was successful. A total of 194 patients have been recruited to this study; only 4% of the 118 patients who received IFN-α and hydroxyurea for 6 months became Ph-negative but increasing numbers became Ph-negative following successive cycles of chemotherapy. Overall 47 patients (18% of total) achieved Ph-negativity and 31 of these have been autografted with Ph-negative bone marrow. Of these 31 patients, 15 remained completely Ph-negative 35–65 months post-transplant. Sixty-eight percent of all patients in the study have survived at 6 years. A proportion of patients entered into the study have been allografted, which may have modified the survival data.

CLINICAL RESULTS WITH IN VIVO TECHNIQUE EMPLOYED IN GENOA

One hundred and eighty-seven patients with Ph-positive CML in different phases of the disease entered the Genoa protocol (Table 6.1). Thirty-eight patients were mobilized in blast phase, 28 patients in accelerated phase and 121 patients in chronic phase. Fifty-five patients in chronic phase were entered within a year of diagnosis and had not received IFN-α, and another 66 patients had received prior IFN-α therapy.

The treatment regimen for mobilization consisted of idarubicin 8 mg/m^2/day on days 1–5, cytosine arabinoside (Ara-C) 800 mg/m^2 by 2-h infusion on days 1–5 and etoposide 150 mg/m^2/day by 2-h infusion on days 1–3 (ICE protocol). The data from patients pretreated with IFN-α have been updated,[11] but in this chapter we will focus on patients in early-phase disease not previously treated with IFN-α (Table 6.2).

Seventeen patients received the ICE and 38 the mini-ICE protocol. In all cases G-CSF was

---

Table 6.1 The Genoa study: clinical characteristics of patients

Patients (no.)	187
Age (median, years)	47 (range, 21–62)
Phase of disease (no. of patients)	
Blastic phase (BP)	38
Accelerated phase (AP)	28
Chronic phase (CP)	66
Early CP (ECP)	55
Mobilization regimens	ICE, mini-ICE
Toxicity (>grade 2; no. of patients)	36 (22%)
Procedure-related deaths (no. of patients)	8 (5%)

Table 6.2 The Genoa study: clinical characteristics of patients in early chronic phase

Patients (no.)	55
Age (median, years)	48 (range 21–62)
White cell count at diagnosis ($\times 10^3$/l) (median)	100 (range 13–550)
Sokal index	
Low	23 (42%)
Intermediate	19 (34%)
High	13 (24%)
Time from diagnosis to mobilization (median, months)	2 (range 1–12)
Mobilization regimens (no. of patients)	
ICE	17
Mini-ICE	38

---

given at 5 µg/kg from day 8 after chemotherapy. Leukaphereses was started when the white cell count exceeded 0.8×10^9 to 1×10^9/l and CD34+ were present in the peripheral blood at >10/µl. Daily apheresis was performed until the total of CD34+ cells collected was $\geq 2 \times 10^6$/kg. All patients completed the mobilization protocol and there were no procedure-related deaths. Toxicities included alopecia, mild mucositis and diarrhea, mainly in patients treated with the ICE protocol. In five patients, grade 3 oral mucositis (World Health Organization definition) and diarrhea occurred. In contrast, patients treated with mini-ICE experienced no non-hematological toxicity. Cytogenetic analysis of collected peripheral blood progenitor cells (PBPC) showed Ph-negative cells in 33 patients (60%) and less than 34% Ph-positive cells in 11 patients (20%) (major cytogenic remission [MCyR]). Forty-four of the 55 patients (ICE, 14/17; mini-ICE, 30/38) therefore had Ph-negative or MCyR harvests (Table 6.3). In comparison, patients pretreated with IFN-α in late CP had a lower rate of complete cytogenetic remission. These results were supported by the significantly greater numbers of CD34+ cells, granulocytic macrophage colony forming units (GM-CFU) and LTC-IC in the newly diagnosed patients.

In the last 2 years minimal residual disease monitoring has been carried out in PBSC collections using a quantitative competitive (QC)

Table 6.3 Results of the Genoa study

	Cytogenetic response (% Ph-positive)	Response in peripheral blood	
		no.	%
Complete	0	33	60
Major	1–34	11	20
Minor	35–94	7	13
None	>95	4	7

Table 6.4 The Genoa study: clinical characteristics of patients autografted in early chronic phase

Age (median, years)	45 (range, 22–62)
Gender (M:F)	26:7
Previous therapy – hydroxyurea	33
Time from mobilization (median)	2 (range 1–12)
Mobilizing therapy (no. of patients)	
ICE	11
Mini-ICE	22
Cytogenetics on PBPC (no. of patients)	
Ph-negative	24
Ph-positive <34%	7
Ph-positive >34%	2
CD34+ cell dose ($\times 10^6$/kg)	4.04 (range 1.06–74.5)
CFU-GM cell dose ($\times 10^4$/kg)	19.2 (range 0.11–108.25)
High-dose therapy (no. of patients)	
IVT (Idarubicin, VP-16, TBI)	6
Busulfan	27

reverse transcriptase polymerase chain reaction (RT-PCR) for Bcr-Abl Thirty-one consecutive patients have been analyzed, 18 of them in early disease phase. This study showed that multiple stem cell collections from the same patients contained different numbers of leukemic cells and that several patients had an adequate number of progenitors for autografting in the least contaminated collection.[46] Indeed, by comparing Ph-negative collections of patients in the early phase of the disease with the correspond-

ing Ph-negative collections of another group of patients, Bcr-Abl mRNA was lower in the earlier group of patients.[46]

To date, 33 patients have been autografted (24 patients Ph-negative; seven patients MCyR; two patients Ph-positive). High dose therapy consisted of busulfan (4 mg/kg/day × 4 days) for 27 patients and a total body irradiation (TBI) containing regimen (IVT idarubicin, VP-16 and single-dose TBI) for six patients. All patients engrafted with no toxic deaths (Table 6.5). After

Table 6.5 The Genoa study: toxicity after high-dose therapy in 33 patients autografted in early chronic myeloid leukemia. Data are number of patients (percent in parentheses)

	CNS	Renal	Hepatic	Stomatitis	GI
Grade III	0	0	0	17 (52)	3 (9)
Grade II	0	1 (3)	4 (12)	7 (21)	3 (9)
Grade I	0	1 (3)	3 (9)	3 (9)	1 (3)
Total with any degree of toxicity	0	2 (6)	7 (21)	7 (21)	7 (21)

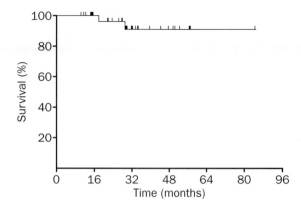

Figure 6.1
Results from the Genoa study: autografting results for chronic myeloid leukemia. Data are percentage survival after autologous stem cell transplantation early after diagnosis, with no prior interferon-α. Of 33 patients, 91% survived at >80 months.

hematopoietic recovery, all patients were treated with low dose IL-2, 2 MU daily for 5 days every 9 weeks, and IFN-α 3 MU daily for 8 weeks. After one week off therapy, the cycle was repeated a total of three times. Patients were then maintained with IFN-α alone. The median follow-up from autografting was 31 months (range 10–84 months) (Fig. 6.1). Two patients developed a blast crisis at 18 and 29 months after autografting and died of leukemia. The remaining 28 patients were in hematological remission, with 17 in complete (nine patients) or major (eight patients) cytogenetic remission, 10–56 months after autografting.

In conclusion, premobilization chemotherapy provided preferential in vivo reduction of the Ph-positive stem cell population and with G-CSF stimulated the release of primitive Ph-negative hematopoietic stem cells into the blood. A prospective randomized study comparing IFN-α ± Ara-C with autograft followed by IFN-α ± Ara-C in patients with newly diagnosed CML is ongoing (MRC/ECOG/ EBMT – CML 2000).

SUMMARY

Residual normal hematopoiesis is present at diagnosis in some patients with CML in chronic phase; leukemic cells are chemosensitive and genetic markers exist whereby leukemia cells can be identified and quantitated. We know that it is possible to mobilize 'normal' PBPC in other hematological diseases with cytogenetic markers such as Ph-positive acute lymphoblastic leukemia and myelodysplastic syndromes[47,48] and, based on the Genoa results, this approach is worth pursuing over the next few years. From a therapeutic point of view, allografting remains the treatment of choice in patients who are less than 55 years old and have an HLA-identical sibling and for younger patients with a matched unrelated donor. Normal hematopoietic reservoir declines with time in CML, so it may be desirable to mobilize and collect PBSC in order to store Ph-negative or prevalently Ph-negative stem cells as soon after diagnosis as possible, while the white cell count is controlled by HU and the search for a donor proceeds. After 6–8 months, if no donor is found, the patient can be autografted with the previously stored Ph-negative progenitors followed by IFN-α therapy. The role of tyrosine kinase inhibitors either alone or to in vivo purge patients may provide an exciting new approach to treating patients with CML.

REFERENCES

1. Federl S, Talpaz M, Estrov Z et al. The biology of chronic myeloid leukemia. N Engl J Med 1999;341:164–72.
2. Allan NC, Richards SM, Shepherd PCA. UK Medical Research Council randomized, multi-centre trial of interferon-alpha n1 for chronic myeloid leukemia: improved survival irrespective of cytogenetic response. Lancet 1995;345: 1392–7.
3. Hehlmann R, Heimpel H, Hasford H et al. Randomized comparison of interferon-alpha with busulfan and hydroxyurea in chronic myelogenous leukemia (CML). Blood 1994;84:4064–77.
4. Talpaz M, Kantarjian H, Kurzrock R et al.

Interferon-alpha produces sustained cytogenetic responses in chronic myelogenous leukemia. Ann Intern Med 1991;114:532–8.

5. ICSCML – The Italian Cooperative Study Group on Chronic Myeloid Leukemia Interferon alpha-2a as compared with conventional chemotherapy for the treatment of chronic myeloid leukemia. N Engl J Med 1994;330:820–5.

6. Guilhot F, Chastang C, Michallet M et al. Interferon-α-2b combined with cytarabine versus interferon alone in chronic myelogenous leukemia. French Chronic Myeloid Leukemia Study Group. N Engl J Med 1997;337:223–9.

7. Udomsakdi C, Eaves CJ, Swolin B et al. Rapid decline of chronic myeloid leukemic cells in long-term culture due to a defect at the leukemic stem cell level. Proc Natl Acad Sci USA 1992;89: 6192–6.

8. Udomsakdi C, Eaves CJ, Lansdorp PM et al. Phenotypic heterogeneity of primitive leukemic hematopoietic cells in patients with chronic myeloid leukemia. Blood 1992;80:2522–30.

9. Ozer H, George SL, Schiffer CA et al. Prolonged subcutaneous administration of recombinant alpha 2b interferon in patients with previously untreated Philadelphia chromosome-positive chronic-phase chronic myelogenous leukemia: effect on remission duration and survival: Cancer and Leukemia Group B study 8583. Blood 1993;82:2975–84.

10. Gordon MY, Goldman JM. Cellular and molecular mechanisms in chronic myelogenous leukaemia: biology and therapy. Br J Haematol 1996;95:10–17.

11. Carella AM, Cunningham I, Lerma E et al. Mobilization and transplantation of Philadelphia-negative peripheral blood progenitor cells early in chronic myelogenous leukemia. J Clin Oncol 1997;15:1575–82.

12. Smaller RV, Vogel J, Huguley CM Jr et al. Chronic granulocytic leukemia: cytogenetic conversion of the bone marrow with cycle-specific chemotherapy. Blood 1977;50:107–13.

13. Cunningham I, Gee T, Dowling M et al. Results of treatment of Ph-positive chronic myelogenous leukemia with an intensive treatment regimen (L-5 protocol). Blood 1979;53:375–84.

14. Sharp JC, Joyner MV, Wayne AW et al. Karyotypic conversion in Ph[1]-positive chronic myeloid leukaemia with combination chemotherapy. Lancet 1979;1:1370–2.

15. Goto T, Nishikori M, Arlin Z et al. Growth characteristics of leukemic and normal hematopoietic cells in Ph-positive chronic myelogenous leukemia and effects of intensive treatment. Blood 1982;59:793–801.

16. Carella AM, Gaozza E, Raffo MR et al. Therapy of acute phase chronic myelogenous leukemia with intensive chemotherapy, blood cell autotransplant and cyclosporine A. Leukemia 1991;5:517–21.

17. Carella AM, Podestà M, Frassoni F et al. Collection of 'normal' blood repopulating cells during early hemopoietic recovery after intensive conventional chemotherapy in chronic myelogenous leukemia. Bone Marrow Transplant 1993; 12:267–71.

18. Kantarjian HM, Talpaz M, Hester J et al. Collection of peripheral blood diploid cells from chronic myelogenous leukemia patients early in the recovery phase from myelosuppression induced by intensive chemotherapy. J Clin Oncol 1995;13:553–9.

19. Kirk JA, Reems JA, Roecklein BA et al. Benign marrow progenitors are enriched in the CD34+/HLA-DRlo population but not the CD34+/CD38lo population of chronic myeloid leukemia: an analysis using interphase fluorescence hybridization. Blood 1995;86:737–43.

20. Chalmers EA, Franklin IM, Kelsey SM et al. Treatment of chronic myeloid leukaemia in first chronic phase with idarubicin and cytarabine: mobilization of Philadelphia-negative peripheral blood stem cells. Br J Haematol 1997;96:627–34.

21. Heinzinger M, Waller CF, Rosenstiel A et al. Quality of IL-3 and G-CSF-mobilized peripheral blood stem cells in patients with early chronic phase CML. Leukemia 1998;12:333–9.

22. Fisher T, Neubauer A, Mohm J et al. Chemotherapy-induced mobilization of karyotypically normal PBSC for autografting in CML. Bone Marrow Transplant 1998;21:1029–36.

23. Lisker R, Casas L, Mutchinick O et al. Late-appearing Philadelphia chromosome in two patients with chronic myelogenous leukemia. Blood 1980;56:812–14.

24. Fialkow PJ, Martin PJ, Najfeld V et al. Evidence for a multistep pathogenesis of chronic myelogenous leukemia. Blood 1981;58:158–63.

25. Ferraris AM, Canepa L, Melani C et al. Clonal B lymphocytes lack *bcr* rearrangement in Ph-positive chronic myelogenous leukaemia. Br J Haematol 1989;73:48–50.

26. Sessarego M, Fugazza G, Frassoni F et al. Cytogenetic analysis of hemopoietic peripheral

blood cells collected by leukapheresis after intensive chemotherapy in advanced phase Philadelphia-positive chronic myelogenous leukemia. Leukemia 1992;6:715–19.

27. Raskind WH, Ferraris AM, Najfeld V et al. Further evidence for the existence of a clonal Ph-negative stage in some cases of Ph-positive chronic myelocytic leukemia. Leukemia 1993;7:1163–7.

28. Coulombel L, Kalousek DK, Eaves CJ et al. Long-term marrow culture reveals chromosomally normal hematopoietic progenitor cells in patients with Philadelphia chromosome-positive chronic myelogenous leukemia. N Engl J Med 1983;308: 1493–8.

29. Eaves C, Udomsakdi C, Cashman J et al. The biology of normal and neoplastic stem cells in CML. Leuk Lymphoma 1993;11:245–53.

30. Barnett MJ, Eaves CJ, Phillips GL et al. Autografting with cultured marrow in chronic myeloid leukemia: results of a pilot study. Blood 1994; 84:724–32.

31. Verfaillie CM, Miller WJ, Boylan K et al. Selection of benign primitive hematopoietic progenitors in chronic myelogenous leukemia on the basis of HLA-DR antigen expression. Blood 1992;79: 1003–10.

32. McGlave PB, Arthur D, Miller WJ et al. Autologous transplantation for CML using marrow treated ex vivo with recombinant human interferon gamma. Bone Marrow Transplant 1990; 6:115–20.

33. Becker M, Fabrega S, Belloc F et al. Interferon gamma is effective for BM purging in a patient with CML. Bone Marrow Transplant 1993;12: 155–8.

34. Gewirtz A. Treatment of CML with c-*myb* antisense oligodeoxynucleotides. Bone Marrow Transplant 1994;14(suppl 3): 57–61.

35. De Fabritiis P, Petti MC, Montefusco E et al. BCR-ABL antisense oligodeoxynucleotide in vitro purging and autologous bone marrow transplantation for patients with chronic myelogenous leukemia in advanced phase. Blood 1998;91:3156–62.

36. Luger SM, Ratajczak MZ, Stadtmauer EA et al. Autografting for chronic myeloid leukemia (CML) with C-MYB antisense oligodeoxynucleotide purged bone marrow: a preliminary report. Blood 1994;84(suppl 1):151 (abstract).

37. O'Brien SG, Rule SA, Ratajczak MZ et al. Autografting for CML using bone marrow purged with MYB antisense oligonucleotide. Br J Haematol 1995;89(suppl 1):12 (abstract).

38. Dunlop DJ, Wright EG, Lorimore S et al. Demonstration of stem cell inhibition and myeloprotective effects of SCI/rh MIP-1 alpha in vivo. Blood 1992;79:2221–5.

39. Kiehntopf M, Esquivel EL, Brach MA et al. Clinical applications of ribozymes. Lancet 1995;345: 1027–31.

40. Leopold LH, Shore SK, Newkirk TA et al. Multi-unit ribozyme-mediated cleavage of bcr-abl mRNA in myeloid leukemias. Blood 1995;85: 2162–70.

41. Pachuk CJ, Yoon K, Moelling K et al. Selective cleavage of bcr-abl chimeric RNAs by a ribozyme targeted to non-contiguous sequences. Nucleic Acid Res 1994;22:301–7.

42. Carella AM, Frassoni F, Melo J et al. New insights in biology and current therapeutic options for patients with chronic myelogenous leukaemia. Haematologica 1997;4:478–95.

43. Carella AM, Lerma E, Celesti L et al. Effective mobilization of Philadelphia-chromosome negative cells in chronic myelogenous leukaemia patients using a less intensive regimen. Br J Haematol 1998;100:445–8.

44. Carella AM, Lerma E, Corsetti MT et al. Autografting with Philadelphia-negative mobilized hematopoietic progenitor cells in chronic myelogenous leukemia. Blood 1999;93:1534–9.

45. Simonsson B, Oberg G, Killander A et al. Intensive treatment in order to minimize the Ph-positive clone in chronic myelogenous leukemia (CML). Bone Marrow Transplant 1994;14(suppl 3): 55–6.

46. Corsetti MT, Podestà M, Lerma E et al. Quantitative competitive reverse transcriptase-polymerase chain reaction for BCR-ABL on Philadelphia-negative leukaphereses allows the selection of low-contaminated peripheral blood progenitor cells for autografting in chronic myelogenous leukemia. Leukemia 1999;13:999–1008.

47. Carella AM, Frassoni F, Pollicardo N et al. Philadelphia-chromosome-negative peripheral blood stem cells can be mobilized in the early phase of recovery after a myelosuppressive chemotherapy in Philadelphia-chromosome-positive acute lymphoblastic leukaemia. Br J Haematol 1995;89:535–8.

48. Carella AM, Dejana A, Lerma E et al. In vivo mobilization of karyotypically normal peripheral blood progenitor cells in high-risk MDS, secondary or therapy-related acute myelogenous leukaemia. Br J Haematol 1996;95:127–30.

7

High dose chemotherapy in multiple myeloma

Jean-Luc Harousseau

CONTENTS   The role of autologous stem cell transplantation in multiple myeloma • The use of peripheral blood stem cells for autologous transplantation • Current issues in peripheral blood stem cell transplantation • Allogeneic bone marrow transplantation • Conclusion

THE ROLE OF AUTOLOGOUS STEM CELL TRANSPLANTATION IN MULTIPLE MYELOMA

In the absence of any significant improvement of conventional chemotherapy (CC) in multiple myeloma (MM), high dose chemotherapy (HDC) with autologous stem cell transplantation (ASCT) has been increasingly used in the past 15 years in this disease.

Pilot studies

After the pioneering work of McElwain et al.[1] several investigators used high dose melphalan (HDM) (140 mg/m^2 iv) without hematological support.[2–5] They demonstrated a high response rate even in refractory patients, achieving 30% clinical complete remissions (CR) in newly diagnosed patients. However, HDM induced severe myelosuppression, with a toxic death rate of approximately 10% in de novo myeloma[3,4] and >20% in pretreated patients.[2] The use of myeloid growth factors reduced the duration of neutropenia but not the risk of infection or occasional cases of protracted aplasia.[6,7] Autologous bone marrow transplantation (ABMT) reduces the hematological toxicity of

HDM[8] and allows the use of myeloablative regimens with total body irradiation (TBI)[9] or higher doses of melphalan.[10]

Both single- and multicenter studies have been published reporting the results of HDC followed by ABMT ± purging,[4,10–16] peripheral blood stem cell transplantation (PBSCT)[14,17–20] or a combination of both PBSC and bone marrow,[20,21] and CD34-selected PBSC.[22,23] Results of these studies show that autologous stem cell transplantation (ASCT) is a useful salvage therapy for primary refractory myeloma and chemosensitive relapse[24–26] but is of limited value in patients with resistant disease.[27] For patients responding to initial induction chemotherapy, ASCT is a safe (fewer than 5% toxic deaths) and effective consolidation therapy.[28] Some of the studies suggested that a CR rate of 30–50% could be achieved after ASCT in newly diagnosed myeloma patients and that this translated into prolonged remission and survival.[10,17,28] These pilot studies are difficult to analyze because patient recruitment is subject to selection bias in terms of age, performance status, renal function and response to initial chemotherapy. Historical comparisons suggest that survival of patients less than 65 years of age who respond to initial standard chemotherapy was similar to that reported in selected series of patients given early HDC.[25,29] Prospective randomized trials were needed to compare CC with HDC. In 1990, the Intergroupe Français du Myelome (IFM) initiated a trial designed to address this issue. The results of this trial were published in 1996[30] but have been recently updated, and with a median follow-up of 60 months, the new analysis confirms the published results.

The IFM 90 trial

Patients less than 65 years of age with Durie–Salmon stage II or III myeloma were eligible for the study. At the time of diagnosis, patients were randomly assigned to receive either CC or HDC. CC consisted of alternating cycles of VMCP and BVAP administered at 3-week intervals for 12 months for a total of 18 cycles. Recombinant interferon-α (IFN-α) was administered three times a week in a dose of 3 millions units/m^2 from cycle 9 until relapse. HDC was to be administered after four to six cycles of VMCP/BVAP. Patients were conditioned with HDM (140 mg/m^2) and TBI (8 Gy). IFN-α was administered at the same dosage as in the CC arm from hematological recovery until relapse. The criteria for response were as follows: CR was defined as the absence of para-

protein on serum and urine electrophoresis and ≤5% plasma cells in the marrow. Very good partial remission (VGPR) was defined as a decrease of 90% in serum paraprotein level, partial remission (PR) as a decrease of 50% in serum paraprotein level and/or a 90% decrease in urine Bence-Jones protein, and minimal response as a decrease of 25% in serum paraprotein level.

Between October 1990 and May 1993, 200 patients (100 per arm) from 33 centers were evaluated. The initial characteristics, response to initial chemotherapy and compliance to IFN treatment were comparable in both groups.

Seventy-four out of the 100 patients assigned to HDC proceeded to ABMT, with a significantly higher proportion of patients under 60 years undergoing transplantation (82% versus 58%) ($P = 0.001$). Of the 74 patients, 22 (30%) achieved CR, 16 (22%) VGPR, and 32 (43%) PR. There were two transplant-related deaths (2.7%). The probabilities of event-free survival (EFS) and overall survival (OS) 6 years after diagnosis were 29% and 58%, respectively.

The comparison of the two therapeutic modalities was made on an intention-to-treat basis, and the response rate is shown in Table 7.1. The response rate significantly improved with HDC: 38% of the patients assigned to the HDC arm had CR or VGPR, compared with 14% of patients assigned to the CC arm

---

Table 7.1 The Intergroupe Français du Myelome 90 study: response rate according to treatment

Response rate	Conventional chemotherapy ($n = 100$)	High dose therapy* ($n = 100$)	P value
Complete response	5	22	
Very good partial response	9	16	
Partial response	43	43	<0.001
Minimal response	18	7	
Progressive disease	25	12	

*Seventy-four patients did actually receive HDC.

Table 7.2 The Intergroupe Français du Myelome 90 study: parameters influencing the response

Factors	Number of patients in clinical remission or very good partial remission	P value
All patients	52/200 (26)	
Sex		0.7
Male	25/102 (24.5)	
Female	27/98 (27.6)	
Age		0.6
<60 years	34/122 (28)	
>60 years	18/78 (23)	
Durie-Salmon stage		0.08
II	18/51 (36)	
III	34/149 (23)	
M component		0.02
Immunoglobulin G	19/111 (17)	
Others	33/89 (37)	
Medullary plasmacytosis		0.5
<30	24/84 (28)	
>30	28/116 (24)	
β_2-microglobulin (mg/l)		0.05
<4	36/110 (33)	
>4	15/79 (19)	
Treatment arm		<0.001
CC	14/100 (14)	
High dose chemotherapy	38/100 (38)	

($P < 0.001$). Factors significantly associated with CR and VGPR are listed in Table 7.2.

In the CC arm, the median EFS was 18 months and median OS 42 months. The probabilities of EFS and OS 6 years after diagnosis were, respectively, 14% and 28%. In the HDC arm, the median EFS was 28 months and median OS was 57 months. The probabilities of EFS and OS 6 years after diagnosis were 25% and 43%, respectively. HDC significantly improved both the EFS ($P = 0.01$; Fig. 7.1) and the OS ($P = 0.03$; Fig. 7.2).

The only parameters influencing EFS were the serum β_2-microglobulin ($P < 0.001$) and the assigned treatment arm ($P = 0.01$) in multivariate analysis. Overall survival was related to the serum β_2-microglobulin level ($P < 0.001$). To assess the effect of treatment response on survival, the analysis focused on the 178 patients who survived more than 1 year from diagnosis. In multivariate analysis, the response to treatment was significantly related to survival ($P < 0.001$) (Fig. 7.3).

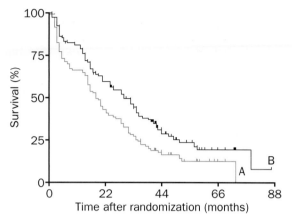

Figure 7.1
Results of the Intergroupe Français du Myelome 90 study: event-free survival according to treatment arm. Arm A: conventional chemotherapy. Arm B: autologous bone marrow transplantation.

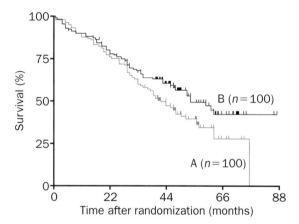

Figure 7.2
Results of the Intergroupe Français du Myelome 90 study: overall survival according to treatment arm. Arm A: conventional chemotherapy. Arm B: autologous bone marrow transplantation.

Conclusion of the IFM 90 trial

The IFM 90 trial was designed to avoid selection bias, by randomizing at diagnosis and by analyzing data on an intention-to-treat analysis.

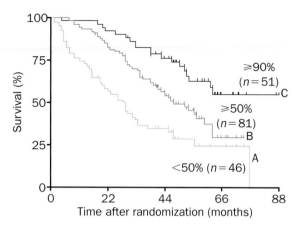

Figure 7.3
Results of the Intergroupe Français du Myelome 90 study: overall survival according to response to treatment. Arm A: minimal or no response. Arm B: partial remission. Arm C: complete remission or very good partial remission.

The study showed that HDC was significantly superior to CC in terms of response rate and 6-year EFS and OS, despite 26% of patients not completing the planned ABMT. The CC arm was a standard regimen and yielded similar results to those published,[31] so this trial demonstrates that HDC achieved a significant clinical improvement and should be offered as part of first-line therapy to younger patients.

A retrospective comparison of patients undergoing a program of double PBSCT and matched patients treated with CC according to the SWOG protocols came to a similar conclusion.[32]

THE USE OF PERIPHERAL BLOOD STEM CELLS FOR AUTOLOGOUS TRANSPLANTATION

Peripheral blood stem cells have almost completely replaced bone marrow as the source of stem cells for myeloma, because of faster hematopoietic recovery, easier accessibility and possibly lower tumor contamination. However, several issues remain regarding the use of PBSCT.

Optimizing the hematopoietic quality of the graft

In myeloma, hematopoietic progenitors were initially collected in the blood during hematopoietic recovery after moderately intensive chemotherapy such as high dose cyclophosphamide[21,33] or high dose combination chemotherapy.[17] Gianni et al. were the first to use granulocyte–macrophage colony stimulating factors (GM-CSF) after chemotherapy to increase the number of hematopoietic progenitors in stem cell harvests;[34] this was followed by other investigators who used GM-CSF or G-CSF after high dose cyclophosphamide.[21,35] Currently PBSC are collected after chemotherapeutic priming (usually high dose cyclophosphamide) plus G-CSF or GM-CSF, or G-CSF alone. In a series of 225 patients with newly diagnosed or refractory myeloma, Tricot et al. retrospectively analyzed the variables affecting PBSC mobilization and speed of engraftment.[36] They found a close correlation between the number of CD34+ cells infused and both granulocyte and platelet engraftment. Prior exposure to chemotherapy, particularly alkylating agents, significantly delayed post-transplant hematopoietic recovery. The threshold dose of CD34+ cells necessary for prompt engraftment was $\geqslant 2 \times 10^6$/kg for patients who had received chemotherapy for 24 months or less, whereas a CD34+ cell dose of $>5 \times 10^6$/kg was required for patients who had been treated for longer. Rapid platelet recovery (before day 14) was almost invariably seen (94%) when cells were infused at $>5 \times 10^6$/kg, irrespective of the duration of prior therapy. In another study of 116 patients, Marit et al. found that the number of colony forming unit–granulocyte macrophage (CFU-GM) cells infused (25×10^4/kg) was the most important predictive factor for rapid and complete hematological recovery after PBSC transplantation.[37] Previous use of alkylating agents, response to CC before the priming treatment with high dose cyclophosphamide and interval from diagnosis to priming chemotherapy were also significant factors. In a series of 103 patients treated with 7 g/m^2

cyclophosphamide plus G-CSF, Goldschmidt et al.[38] found that the duration of previous melphalan treatment was the most significant factor for predicting a poor PBSC collection and concluded that melphalan should not be given to patients prior to a PBSC harvest.

The best regimen for mobilizing an adequate PBSC harvest is unclear. High dose cyclophosphamide (up to 7 g/m^2) is extensively used and the addition of hematopoietic growth factors (GM-CSF or G-CSF) increases the PBSC yield.[21,39,40,41] Higher doses of cyclophosphamide (7 g/m^2) increase the number of PBSC harvested, compared with lower dosages ($\leqslant 4 \text{ g/m}^2$ or less),[38,42,43] and may reduce harvest contamination by malignant cells[38] and tumor cell mass.[43] The administration of high dose cyclophosphamide is associated with increased toxicity and a significant number of toxic deaths,[37,42,43] especially in pretreated patients. Stem cell collection after G-CSF alone can be considered in newly diagnosed patients, though it less effective than when it is combined with cyclophosphamide. The CD34+ cell yield achieved with G-CSF alone is usually $>2.5 \times 10^6$/kg, permitting safe and rapid hematopoietic reconstitution.[44] The main advantages of collecting PBSCs after priming with G-CSF are the reduction in toxicity and decreased expense.[45] An increased risk of mobilizing clonal myeloma cells by priming with growth factors alone has been suggested by two case reports.[46,47]

Combinations of hematopoietic growth factors could further enhance PBSC collection. Preliminary results using stem cell factor (SCF) and G-CSF are encouraging.[48,49] In heavily pretreated patients this combination allows an adequate harvest in more patients,[48] and in newly diagnosed patients target CD34+ cell yields of 5×10^6/kg are obtained, with fewer apheresis procedures.[49]

The impact of hematopoietic growth factors administered after PBSC transplantation is unclear though it appears to reduce the platelet recovery time in patients who receive low CD34+ cell numbers, but there is no discernible effect in patients who receive CD34+ cells above 5×10^6/kg.[50]

Contamination of the graft

It was hoped that PBSC harvests would be less contaminated by tumor cells than bone marrow harvests. The conflicting results obtained were partly due to different methods of detecting contamination.

Initial studies used anti-idiotypic antibodies and Southern blot analysis of immunoglobulin gene rearrangements. Several investigators showed evidence of circulating malignant precursors,[51–54] but others failed to detect immunoglobulin gene rearrangements in peripheral blood lymphocytes in the absence of circulating plasma cells.[55,56] More recent data using polymerase chain reaction (PCR) based methods confirmed that clonal cells were present in most patients with active disease. No contamination was found in remission using the low sensitivity Southern blot technique[54] but were present in reduced numbers in remission using PCR.[57] Sensitive immunofluorescence[58] and PCR-based studies have demonstrated that PBSC harvests are frequently contaminated with malignant cells.[59–63] If immunoglobulin heavy chain gene fingerprinting is used, tumor contamination is found in 44–70% of PBSC samples collected after HDC.[59–61] With allele-specific oligonucleotide PCR, tumor cells are present in almost all PBSC harvests.[61–63]

The prognostic significance of detecting malignant cells by PCR is unknown; however, Gertz et al.[64] showed that the detection of monoclonal plasma cells in harvests by immunofluorescence was associated with a shorter relapse-free survival after transplantation. In other diseases, gene marking studies have suggested that reinfused tumor cells may cause relapse,[65] although this has not been demonstrated in myeloma. Differential mobilization of myeloma cells and normal hematopoietic stem cells may be a way of reducing tumor load in autologous transplants. Gazitt et al.[66] showed that after high dose cyclophosphamide and GM-CSF priming, peak levels of myeloma cells were observed on days 5 and 6, whereas hematopoietic progenitor cell numbers peaked earlier. In contrast, Lemoli et al.[23] found concomitant mobilization of both compartments. Kiel et al.[67] found no difference in tumor load and hematopoietic stem cell yield in leukapheresis products collected on days 1 and 2.[67]

Comparison of bone marrow and peripheral blood progenitor cell autologous transplantations

Tumor cell contamination is lower in PBSC harvests than in bone marrow,[68–70] but this has not translated into an improved myeloma-free survival. A retrospective case–control study of 132 patients transplanted in 18 French centers showed that there was no difference in overall response rate, CR rate, EFS or OS;[71] however, PBSC transplantation was associated with a reduction in the median duration of neutropenia.

To answer the question of the prognostic impact of PBSC compared to bone marrow transplantation, patients in the IFM 94 trial were randomly assigned to receive PBSC or bone marrow post-treatment with HDM 140 mg/m^2 and TBI. Peripheral blood stem cells were collected with G-CSF priming after VAD therapy and growth factors were administered after transplantation. A preliminary analysis of this study shows that many patients allocated to receive bone marrow actually received PBSC because of patient or investigator preference; thus there were 145 PBSC transplantations, compared with 97 ABMT. The use of PBSC significantly reduced the mean duration of neutropenia (9.8 versus 12.2 days), thrombocytopenia (12.4 versus 23.4 days) and platelet transfusions (4.2 versus 6.6). Disease outcome measures such as response (CR and VGPR) rate, EFS and OS were not significantly different.

Graft contamination by plasma cells in ABMT is not prognostically significant.[12,13] The fact that PBSC transplantation does not prolong EFS and OS in spite of a lower tumor load in the graft could mean that relapse is also caused by persistence of clonogenic malignant cells in patients after HDC.

CURRENT ISSUES IN PERIPHERAL BLOOD STEM CELL TRANSPLANTATION

In myeloma, the current issues in PBSCT are timing, selection of patients and how to improve the results.

Timing of transplantation

Recently, JP Fermand et al. published the results of a randomized study showing no significant difference in OS between early and late PBSCT (performed as rescue treatment in case of primary resistance or at relapse).[72]

Selection of patients

Usually, PBSCT is offered to patients who are below 65 years and have a performance status 0–2 and normal renal function. The issue of age limits was emphasized in the IFM 90 trial: ASCT was performed in 82% of patients <60 years of age, versus 58% in patients aged 60–65.[30] Therefore, in the intention-to-treat analysis, ASCT was significantly superior to CC only in younger patients. The introduction of hematopoietic growth factors to transplantation practice has made PBSCT safer for older patients. Recently, the Little Rock group compared the outcome of 49 patients >65 years with 49 younger but otherwise matched patients treated with HDC.[73] The CR rate was higher in younger patients (43% versus 20%, $P = 0.02$) and the transplant-related mortality appeared to be higher in older patients (8% versus 2%). However, the EFS and OS were comparable in both groups, so the authors concluded that age was not a biologically adverse parameter for patients treated with HDC and PBSC support and should not be an exclusion criterion for transplantation. The selection criterion in this study are unknown and so the toxicity and clinical impact of the treatment in older patients remain to be determined.

Patients with renal failure are usually excluded from HDC protocols. The Little Rock group compared the outcome of 42 patients with renal failure to that of 84 pair-matched controls receiving the same treatment (melphalan 200 mg/m^2).[74] They showed that renal function improved in 50% of patients, (including dialysis-dependent patients) and that prognosis was comparable to that of the controls, concluding that renal failure should not disqualify myeloma patients from HDC.

How to improve the results of ASCT

The conditioning regimen
In the IFM 90 trial, the 6-year EFS was only 25% in the HDC arm and there was no survival curve plateau, indicating that strategies to improve outcome are needed. Achievement of CR/VGPR is significantly associated with a prolongation of survival. Therefore the aim of future studies should be to increase the CR rate by improving the conditioning regimen.

The optimal conditioning regimen for ASCT in myeloma has not been determined.[9] Since its introduction in 1987 by Barlogie et al. TBI has been used in many uncontrolled studies. The combination of TBI plus HDM 140 mg/m^2 yields CR rates ranging from 20% to 50% depending on the disease status at transplantation and criteria used to define CR. This conditioning regimen was used in the randomized IFM 90 trial and could therefore be considered standard.

The superiority of TBI-containing regimens has not been demonstrated in a prospective randomized trial. A retrospective analysis of French registry data showed no significant differences between patients treated with HDM 140 mg/m^2 plus TBI 8 Gy and patients receiving higher doses of melphalan or combinations of several alkylating agents.[25] The Royal Marsden Group reported a 70% CR rate with HDM 200 mg/m^2 in newly diagnosed patients, with minimal extramedullary toxicity.[10] The Little Rock Group also questioned the role of TBI in a population of refractory patients because HDM 200 mg/m^2 appeared superior to HDM 140 mg/m^2 plus TBI and less toxic, with 1% early deaths versus 36%.[75]

In 1995, the IFM initiated a randomized study comparing HDM 200 mg/m² and HDM 140 mg/m² plus TBI followed by PBSC autologous transplantation in patients with newly diagnosed myeloma. So far, 386 patients have been enrolled in this study. A preliminary analysis of the first 221 patients was performed (HDM 200 mg/m², 108 patients; HDM 140 mg/m² plus TBI, 113 patients). The two groups are well matched clinically, in response to initial CC and methods of PBSC collection. Currently, there is no difference in the outcome between the two groups but HDM 200 mg/m² appears less toxic and is associated with a significantly shorter median duration of neutropenia (8 versus 10 days, $P < 0.001$), reduced median number of platelet transfusions (1 versus 3, $P < 0.001$), and reduced incidence of WHO grade ≥ 3 mucositis (30% versus 52%, $P = 0.003$). If these results are confirmed by further analysis, HDM 200 mg/m² should become the standard regimen for transplantation in myeloma.

There is a clear dose–effect relationship with melphalan but the maximum tolerated dose of intravenous melphalan is unknown. In a preliminary study, Moreau et al.[76] showed that a dose of 220 mg/m² increases the area under the curve of plasma concentration without modifying other pharmacokinetic parameters. Apart from a high incidence of severe mucositis this regimen was well tolerated when supported by PBSC transplantation.

The impact of tandem transplants (IFM 94 trial)

Improved CR rates may be achieved by sequential intensive treatments. Our group explored this strategy, but the hematopoietic toxicity of the first course of HDC was excessive without PBSC support.[4] The sequential use of several courses of HDC appears to be well tolerated if PBSC with cytokine support is used.[75] Bjorkstrand et al.[77] have shown that double high-dose procedures followed by PBSC support can induce molecular remission.

The Seattle group reported the results achieved in 55 patients treated with two cycles of HDM 200 mg/m². They have shown that tandem HDM with PBPC transplants can be administered to 70% of patients under 65 years of age, resulting in an increased CR rate from 15% after cycle 1 to 55% after cycle 2.[78]

The largest experience in tandem transplantation comes from the Little Rock Group.[79] Out of 495 patients enrolled to undergo two transplants, including 315 pretreated patients, 95% completed the first course of HDM 200 mg/m² with PBSC transplantation and 73% underwent two transplants. The CR rate increased from 24% after the first transplant to 43% after two transplants. Favorable prognostic factors included a low β_2-microglobulin level, duration of prior therapy less than 12 months, sensitivity to prior standard therapy and completion of transplants within 6 months.

The impact of this aggressive strategy on EFS and OS needed further evaluation. In 1994, the IFM initiated a randomized trial (IFM 94) comparing one versus two transplants. From October 1994 to March 1997, 405 untreated patients under the age of 60 years were enrolled by 36 centers. At diagnosis they were randomized to receive either a single PBSCT (arm A = 201 patients) prepared with melphalan (140 mg/m²) plus TBI (8 Gy) or a double PBSCT (arm B = 204 patients). The first transplant was conditioned with melphalan 140 mg/m², and the second transplant with melphalan 140 mg/m² and TBI (8 Gy). Patients were initially treated with three or four cycles of the VAD regimen.

An interim analysis was performed in May 1999 on 402 eligible patients with follow-up of at least 2 years from diagnosis (median follow-up 36 months) (200 arm A, 202 arm B). In arm A, the PBSCT was performed in 83% of cases and the second HDC in 78%. On an intent-to-treat analysis there was no significant difference between arm A and arm B in terms of the CR rate (32% versus 35%), the 3-year EFS (31% versus 39%) and the 3-year OS (58% versus 66%). These results are preliminary, with a trend favoring arm B, but longer follow-up is needed before drawing any conclusions.

The source of stem cells

Contamination of the PBSC harvest by the

malignant clone remains a concern. Attempts to purge marrow with cyclophosphamide derivatives or monoclonal antibodies are possible but induce prolonged myelosuppression.[15,16,80] Selection of CD34+ progenitors appears to be a promising alternative since positive selection of CD34+ cells result in a 2.5–4.5 log depletion of plasma cells.[22,23] Several pilot studies have confirmed the feasibility of autologous transplants with CD34+ selected PBSC in myeloma.[22,23] Randomized studies comparing CD34+ selected and unselected PBSC are underway in the USA and Europe. A multicenter phase III trial comparing selected and unselected PBSC in 131 myeloma patients was recently published.[81] Successful neutrophil engraftment was achieved in all patients by day 15 and there was no significant difference between the two groups as regards platelet engraftment or survival.

Polymerase chain reaction techniques using patient-specific oligonucleotide primers show persistence of myeloma cells in CD34+ cell fractions whereas highly purified CD34+Lin− stem cells do not contain clonal myeloma cells,[63] indicating that an additional purging step may be necessary to obtain tumor-free grafts. The clinical impact of these cumbersome and expensive procedures needs to be evaluated. In a pilot study on 10 patients neutrophil and platelet engraftment was substantially delayed when compared to unmanipulated PBSC grafts.[82]

Maintenance therapy

There is no plateau in the survival curves of published series that have had adequate follow-up; therefore maintenance therapy may play a role in prolonging EFS. Several randomized studies have shown that in patients responding to CC, IFN-α maintenance prolongs remission duration by 5–12 months.[83–86] IFN-α is also used after HDC as it is theoretically more effective in patients with minimal residual disease. Only one randomized study has been published[87] that has compared IFN-α (3×10^6 IU/kg, 3 times weekly) after recovery from HDC with no further therapy. With a median follow-up of 77 months, the median PFS was significantly longer (42 versus 27 months for the control

arm), but the PFS and OS curves were no longer significantly different at the time of writing. This indicates that although IFN-α delays relapse in patients achieving CR, most patients ultimately relapse. This study involved only 85 patients, and so should be interpreted cautiously. The results of a large randomized US trial will be of interest.

Prognostic factors in patients with de novo multiple myeloma

Prognostic factors have been analyzed in two large prospective studies of patients with de novo myeloma.

In the preliminary analysis of the IFM 94 trial, univariate analysis showed that the initial β_2-microglobulin level, C-reactive protein (CRP) level, response to CC prior to ASCT and the response to ASCT were significant for OS. In multivariate analysis the initial β_2-microglobulin level was the only significant prognostic factor. In the patients who had good prognosis (β_2-microglobulin level $\leqslant 3$ mg/l) the probabilities of survival at 3 years appeared to be higher in arm B than in arm A. The patients who had poor prognosis (β_2-microglobulin >3 mg/l) appeared to have a better 3-year OS in group A.

Barlogie et al.[88] recently published the results of 'total therapy' in 231 patients with newly diagnosed MM. In multivariate analysis, superior EFS and OS were observed in the absence of unfavorable karyotypes (11q breakpoints and/or partial or complete deletion of chromosome 13) and with low β_2-microglobulin level at diagnosis ($\leqslant 4$ mg/l). Combining these factors, a subgroup of patients with a very poor prognosis was identified: those with unfavorable cytogenetics and β_2-microglobulin level >4 mg/l had a median survival of only 2.1 years, compared with 7 years for the remaining patients.

ALLOGENEIC BONE MARROW TRANSPLANTATION

Allogeneic BMT is currently performed only in patients under 50 years with an HLA identical sibling. Considering the median age of patients with MM, this strategy can only be offered to a small proportion of patients. The procedure-related death rate remains high because of high infection rate and graft-versus-host disease. A study published by the European Blood and Marrow Transplantation group has shown no advantage of allogeneic BMT compared with PBSCT.[89] Allogeneic BMT, if used early in the disease, shows encouraging results: about 33% who achieve CR after transplantation remain free of disease 6 years later.[90] Allogeneic BMT is probably the only genuinely curative therapy in myeloma because of the graft-versus-tumour effect. Recent reports of CR achieved after donor lymphocyte infusion (DLI) in patients relapsing after allogeneic BMT support the existence of a graft-versus-myeloma effect.[91,92]

Attempts to reduce the procedure-related death rate include better selection of patients, attenuated-dose conditioning regimens, T cell depletion or CD34+ cell selection. These approaches can be combined with post-transplant DLI to reduce the relapse rate.

CONCLUSION

The use of PBSC has markedly improved the feasibility and safety of autologous transplantation. It has significantly improved the EFS and OS of younger patients with myeloma. Although cure of myeloma with PBSCT remains unlikely, prolonged EFS and OS are observed in a subgroup of patients with favorable initial characteristics.[93] Recently completed and ongoing trials will clarify several issues such as the feasibility and impact of PBSCT in patients over 60 years of age, impact of tandem transplants, optimal conditioning regimen and source of stem cells. Future studies should address other issues such as the management of patients with unfavorable features or the role of innovative maintenance therapy.

REFERENCES

1. McElwain TJ, Powles RL. High dose intravenous melphalan for plasma-cell leukaemia and myeloma. Lancet 1983;2:822–4.
2. Barlogie B, Alexanian R, Smallwood L et al. Prognosis factors with high dose melphalan for refractory multiple myeloma. Blood 1988;72: 2015–19.
3. Cunningham D, Paz-Ares L, Gore ME et al. High dose melphalan for multiple myeloma: long term follow-up data. J Clin Oncol 1994;12:764–8.
4. Harousseau JL, Milpied N, Laporte JP et al. Double intensive therapy in high-risk multiple myeloma. Blood 1992;79:2827–33.
5. Lockhorst HM, Muewissen O, Verdonck LF et al. High risk multiple myeloma treated with high dose melphalan. J Clin Oncol 1992;10:47–51.
6. Barlogie B, Jagannath S, Dixon DO et al. High-dose melphalan and granulocyte–macrophage colony-stimulating factor for refractory multiple myeloma. Blood 1990;76:677–80.
7. Moreau P, Fiere D, Bezwoda WR et al. Prospective randomized placebo-controlled study of GM-CSF without stem cell transplantation after high-dose melphalan in patients with multiple myeloma. J Clin Oncol 1997;15:660–6.
8. Barlogie B, Hall R, Zander A et al. High dose melphalan with autologous bone marrow transplantation for multiple myeloma. Blood 1986;67:1298–301.
9. Barlogie B, Alexanian R, Dicke K et al. High dose chemoradiotherapy and autologous bone marrow transplantation for resistant multiple myeloma. Blood 1987;70:869–72.
10. Cunningham D, Paz-Ares L, Milan S et al. High dose melphalan and autologous bone marrow transplantation as consolidation in previously untreated myeloma. J Clin Oncol 1994;12:759–63.
11. Gore ME, Selby PS, Virer C et al. Intensive treatment of multiple myeloma and criteria for complete response. Lancet 1989;2:879–82.
12. Jagannath S, Barlogie B, Dicke K et al. Autologous bone marrow transplantation in multiple myeloma: identification of prognostic factors. Blood 1990;76:1860–6.
13. Attal M, Huguet F, Schlaifer D et al. Intensive combined therapy for previously untreated aggressive myeloma. Blood 1992;79:1130–6.
14. Dimopoulos MA, Alexanian R, Przepiorka D et al. Thiotepa, busulfan and cyclophosphamide: a new preparative regimen for autologous marrow

and blood cell transplantation in high risk multiple myeloma. Blood 1993;82:2324–8.

15. Anderson KC, Andersen J, Soiffer R et al. Monoclonal antibody-purged bone marrow transplantation therapy for multiple myeloma. Blood 1993;82:2568–76.

16. Reece DE, Barnett MJ, Connors JM et al. Treatment of multiple myeloma with intensive chemotherapy followed by autologous bone marrow transplantation using marrow purged with 4 hydroxyperoxycyclophosphamide. Bone Marrow Transplant 1993;11:139–46.

17. Fermand JP, Chevret S, Ravaud P et al. High dose chemoradiotherapy and autologous blood stem cell transplantation in multiple myeloma: results of a phase II trial involving 63 patients. Blood 1993;82:2005–9.

18. Gianni AM, Tarella C, Bregui M et al. High-dose sequential chemoradiotherapy a widely applicable regimen, confers survival benefit to patients with high-dose multiple myeloma. J Clin Oncol 1994;12:503–9.

19. Marit G, Faberes C, Pico JL et al. Autologous peripheral-blood progenitor-cell support following high-dose chemotherapy or chemoradiotherapy in patients with high-risk multiple myeloma. J Clin Oncol 1994;14:1306–13.

20. Bensinger WJ, Rowley SD, Demirer T et al. High dose therapy followed by autologous hematopoietic stem-cell infusion for patients with multiple myeloma. J Clin Oncol 1996; 14:1447–56.

21. Jagannath S, Vesole DH, Glenn L et al. Low-risk intensive therapy for multiple myeloma with combined autologous bone marrow and blood stem cell support. Blood 1992;80:1666–72.

22. Schiller G, Vescio R, Freytes C et al. Transplantation of CD34+ peripheral blood progenitor cell after high-dose chemotherapy for patients with advanced multiple myeloma. Blood 1995;86:390–7.

23. Lemoli RM, Fortuna A, Motta MR et al. Concomitant mobilization of plasma cells and hematopoietic progenitors into peripheral blood of multiple myeloma patients: positive selection and transplantation of enriched CD34+ cells to remove circulating tumor cells. Blood 1996;87: 1625–34.

24. Jagannath S, Barlogie B. Autologous bone marrow transplantation for multiple myeloma. Hematol Oncol Clin North Am 1992;6:437–49.

25. Alexanian R, Dimopoulos MA, Hester J et al. Early myeloablative therapy for multiple myeloma. Blood 1994;84:4278–82.

26. Attal M, Harousseau JL. Autologous transplantation in multiple myeloma. In: Gahrton G, Durie BGM, editors. Multiple myeloma. London: Arnold, 1996: 182–93.

27. Alexanian R, Dimopoulos M, Smith T. Limited value of myeloablative therapy for late multiple myeloma. Blood 1994;83:512–16.

28. Harousseau JL, Attal M, Divine M et al. Autologous stem cell transplantation after first remission induction treatment in multiple myeloma: a report of the French registry on autologous transplantation. Blood 1995;85: 3077–85.

29. Blade J, San Miguel JF, Montserrat F et al. Survival of multiple myeloma patients who are potential candidates for early high-dose therapy intensification/autotransplantation and who were conventionally treated. J Clin Oncol 1996; 14:2167–73.

30. Attal M, Harousseau JL, Stoppa AM et al. A prospective, randomized trial of autologous bone marrow transplantation and chemotherapy in multiple myeloma. N Engl J Med 1996; 335:91–7.

31. Gregory WM, Richards MA, Malpas JS. Combination chemotherapy versus melphalan and prednisolone in the treatment of multiple myeloma: an overview of published trials. J Clin Oncol 1992;10:334–42.

32. Barlogie B, Jagannath S, Vesole D et al. Superiority of tandem autologous transplantation over standard therapy for previously untreated multiple myeloma. Blood 1997; 89:789–93.

33. Reiffers J, Marit G, Boiron JM. Autologous blood stem cell transplantation in high risk multiple myeloma. Br J Haematol 1989;72:296.

34. Gianni AM, Sienna S, Bregni M et al. Granulocyte–macrophage colony-stimulating factor to harvest circulating haematopoietic stem cells for autotransplantation. Lancet 1989;8863: 580–4.

35. Tarella C, Boccadoro M, Omede P et al. Role of chemotherapy and GM-CSF on hemopoietic progenitor cell mobilization in multiple myeloma. Bone Marrow Transplant 1993;11:271–7.

36. Tricot G, Jagannath S, Vesole D et al. Peripheral blood stem cell transplants for multiple myeloma: identification of favorable variables for rapid engraftment in 225 patients. Blood 1996;85:588–96.

37. Marit G, Thiessard F, Faberes F et al. Factors affecting both peripheral blood progenitor cell mobilization and hematopoietic recovery following autologous blood progenitor cell transplantation in multiple myeloma patients: monocentric study. Leukemia 1998;12:1447–56.

38. Goldschmidt H, Hegenbart U, Haas R et al. Mobilization of peripheral blood progenitor cells with high-dose cyclophosphamide (4 or 7 g/m^2) and granulocyte colony stimulating factor in patients with multiple myeloma. Bone Marrow Transplant 1996;17:691–7.

39. Bensinger W, Longin K, Appelbaum F et al. Peripheral blood stem cells collected after recombinant granulocyte colony-stimulating factor: an analysis of factors correlating with the tempo of engraftment after transplantation. Br J Haematol 1994;87:825–31.

40. Martinez E, Sureda A, De Dalmases C et al. Mobilization of peripheral blood progenitor cells by cyclophosphamide and GM-CSF in multiple myeloma. Bone Marrow Transplant 1996;18:1–7.

41. Demuynck H, Delforge M, Verhoef G et al. Comparative study of peripheral progenitor cell collection in patients with multiple myeloma after single dose cyclophosphamide combined with rhGM-CSF or rhG-CSF. Br J Haematol 1995;90:384–92.

42. Kotasek D, Shepherd KM, Sage RE et al. Factors affecting blood stem cell collections following high-dose cyclophosphamide mobilization in lymphoma, myeloma and solid tumors. Bone Marrow Transplant 1992;9:11–17.

43. Goldschmidt H, Hegenbart U, Wallmeier M et al. Factors influencing collection of peripheral blood progenitor cells following high-dose cyclophosphamide and granulocyte-colony stimulating factor. Br J Haematol 1997;98:736–44.

44. Mahé B, Milpied N, Hermouet S et al. G-CSF alone mobilizes sufficient blood CD34+ cells for positive selection in newly diagnosed patients with myeloma and lymphoma. Br J Haematol 1996;92:263–8.

45. Alegre A, Tomas JF, Martinez-Chamorro C et al. Comparison of peripheral blood progenitor cell mobilization in patients with multiple myeloma: high-dose cyclophosphamide plus GM-CSF vs G-CSF alone. Bone Marrow Transplant 1997; 20:211–21.

46. Celsing F, Hast R, Stenke L, Hansson H, Pisa P. Extramedullary progression of multiple myeloma following GM-CSF treatment – grounds for caution? Eur J Haematol 1992; 49:108.

47. Vora AJ, Cheng HT, Peel J, Greaves M. Use of granulocyte colony-stimulating factor G-CSF for mobilizing peripheral blood stem cells: risk of mobilizing clonal myeloma cells in patients with bone marrow infiltration. Br J Haematol 1994; 86:180–2.

48. Tricot G, Jagannath S, Desikan KR et al. Superior mobilization of peripheral blood progenitor cell with r-met HuSCF and re-met Hu G-CSF in heavily pretreated multiple myeloma patients. Blood 1996;88(suppl 1):388 (abstract).

49. Facon T, Harousseau JL, Maloisel F et al. Stem cell factor in combination with filgrastim after chemotherapy improves peripheral blood progenitor cell yield and reduces apheresis requirements in multiple myeloma patients: a randomized controlled trial. Blood 1999;94: 1218–25.

50. Bensinger W, Appelbaum F, Rowley S et al. Factors that influence collection and engraftment of autologous peripheral blood stem cells. J Clin Oncol 1995;10:2547–55.

51. Berenson J, Wong R, Kim K, Brown N, Lichtenstein A. Evidence for peripheral blood B lymphocyte but not T lymphocyte involvement in multiple myeloma. Blood 1987;70:1550–3.

52. Chiu EKW, Ganeshaguru K, Hoffbrand AV, Mehta AB. Circulating monoclonal B lymphocytes in multiple myeloma. Br J Haematol 1989; 72:28–31.

53. Van Riet I, Heirman C, Lacor P, De Waele M, Thielemans K, Van Camp B. Detection of monoclonal B lymphocytes in bone marrow and peripheral blood of multiple myeloma patients by immunoglobulin gene rearrangement studies. Br J Haematol 1989;73:289–95.

54. Cassel A, Leibovitz N, Hornstein L et al. Evidence for the existence of circulating monoclonal B-lymphocytes in multiple myeloma patients. Exp Hematol 1990;18:1171–3.

55. Clofent G, Klein B, Commes T, Ghanem N, Lefranc M, Bataille R. No detectable malignant B cells in the peripheral blood of patients with multiple myeloma. Br J Haematol 1989;71: 357–61.

56. Billadeau D, Quam L, Thomas W et al. Detection and quantification of malignant cells in the peripheral blood of multiple myeloma patients. Blood 1992;80:1818–24.

57. Corradini P, Voena C, Omede P. Detection of cir-

culating tumor cells in multiple myeloma by a PCR-based method. Leukemia 1993;7:1879–82.

58. Witzig TE, Gertz MA, Pineda AA et al. Detection of monoclonal plasma cells in the peripheral blood stem cell harvests of patients with multiple myeloma. Br J Haematol 1995;89:640–2.

59. Bird JM, Bloxham D, Samson D et al. Molecular detection of clonally rearranged cells in peripheral blood progenitor cell harvests from multiple myeloma patients. Br J Haematol 1994;88:110–16.

60. Mariette X, Fermand JP, Brouet JL. Detection of clonal cells in peripheral blood progenitor harvests from multiple myeloma. Bone Marrow Transplant 1994;14:47–50.

61. Dreyfus F, Ribrag V, Leblond V et al. Detection of malignant B cells in peripheral stem cell collections after chemotherapy in patients with multiple myeloma. Bone Marrow Transplant 1995;15:707–11.

62. Gazitt Y, Reading CC, Hoffman R et al. Purified CD34+ Lin− thy+ stem cells do not contain clonal myeloma cells. Blood 1995;86:381–9.

63. Corradini P, Voena C, Astolfi M et al. High-dose sequential chemoradiotherapy in multiple myeloma: residual tumor cells are detectable in bone marrow and peripheral blood cell harvests and after autografting. Blood 1995;85:1596–602.

64. Gertz MA, Witzig TE, Pineda AA, Greipp PR, Kyle RA, Litzow MR. Monoclonal plasma cells in the blood stem cell harvest from patients with multiple myeloma are associated with shortened relapse-free survival after transplantation. Bone Marrow Transplant 1997;19:337–42.

65. Brenner MK, Rill DR, Moen RC et al. Gene marking to trace origin of relapse after autologous bone marrow transplantation. Lancet 1993;41: 85–6.

66. Gazitt Y, Tian E, Barlogie B et al. Differential mobilization of myeloma cells and normal hematopoietic stem cells in multiple myeloma after treatment with cyclophosphamide and granulocyte–macrophage colony-stimulating factor. Blood 1996;87:805–11.

67. Kiel K, Cremer FW, Ehrbrecht E et al. First and second apheresis in patients with multiple myeloma: no differences in tumor load and hematopoietic stem cell yield. Bone Marrow Transplant 1998;21:1109–15.

68. Fermand JP, Chevret S, Ravaud P et al. The role of autologous blood stem-cells in support of high-dose therapy for multiple myeloma. Clin North Am 1992;6:451–62.

69. Vescio RA, Han EJ, Schiller GJ et al. Quantitative comparison of multiple myeloma tumor contamination in bone marrow harvest and leukapheresis autografts. Bone Marrow Transplant 1996;18: 103–10.

70. Henry JM, Sykes PJ, Brisco MJ et al. Comparison of myeloma cell contamination of bone marrow and peripheral blood stem cell harvests. Br J Haematol 1996;92:614–19.

71. Harousseau JL, Attal M, Divine M et al. Comparison of autologous bone marrow transplantation and peripheral blood stem cell transplantation after first remission induction treatment in multiple myeloma. Bone Marrow Transplant 1995;15:963–9.

72. Fermand JP, Ravaud P, Chevret S et al. High-dose therapy and autologous peripheral blood stem cell transplantation in multiple myeloma: up-front or resume treatment? Results of a multicenter sequential randomized clinical trial. Blood 1998;92:3131–6.

73. Siegel DS, Desikan KR, Nehta J et al. Age is not a prognostic variable with autotransplants for multiple myeloma. Blood 1999;93:51–4.

74. Mehta J. (Personal Communication).

75. Vesole D, Barlogie B, Jagannath S et al. High-dose therapy for refractory multiple myeloma: improved prognosis with better supportive care and double transplants. Blood 1994;84:950–6.

76. Moreau P, Kergueris MF, Milpied N et al. A pilot study of 220 mg/m^2 melphalan followed by autologous stem cell transplantation in patients with advanced haematological malignancies: pharmacokinetics and toxicity. Br J Haematol 1996;95:527–30.

77. Bjorkstrand B, Ljungman P, Bird JM, Samson D, Gahrton G. Double high-dose chemoradiotherapy with autologous stem cell transplantation can induce molecular remission in multiple myeloma. Bone Marrow Transplant 1995;15: 367–71.

78. Weaver CH, Zhen B, Schwartzberg LS et al. Phase I-II evaluation of rapid sequence tandem high-dose melphalan with peripheral blood stem cell support in patients with multiple myeloma. Bone Marrow Transplant 1998;22:245–51.

79. Vesole D, Tricot G, Jagannath S et al. Auto-transplant in multiple myeloma: what have we learned? Blood 1996;88:838–47.

80. Gobbi M, Cavo M, Tazzari P et al. Autologous bone marrow transplantation with immuno-toxin-purged marrow for advanced multiple myeloma. Eur J Hematol 1989;51:176–81.

81. Vescio RA, Schiller G, Stewart K et al. Multicenter phase III trial to evaluate CD34+ selected versus unselected autologous peripheral blood progenitor cell transplantation in multiple myeloma. Blood 1999;93:1858–68.

82. Tricot G, Gazitt Y, Leemhuis S et al. Collection, tumor contamination, and engraftment kinetics of highly purified hematopoietic progenitor cells to support high dose therapy in multiple myeloma. Blood 1998;91:4489–95.

83. Browman G, Bergsagel DE, Sicheri D et al. Randomized trial of interferon maintenance in multiple myeloma: a study of the National Cancer Institute of Canada Trials group. J Clin Oncol 1995;13:2354–60.

84. Mandelli F, Avisati G, Amadori S et al. Maintenance therapy with recombinant interferon 2b in patients with multiple myeloma responding to conventional induction chemotherapy. N Engl J Med 1990;332:1430–4.

85. The Nordic Myeloma Study Group. Interferon α2b added to melphalan-prednisone for initial and maintenance therapy in multiple myeloma. Ann Intern Med 1996;124:212–22.

86. Westin J, Rödjer S, Turesson I et al. Interferon α2b versus no maintenance therapy during the plateau phase in multiple myeloma: a randomized study. Br J Haematol 1995;89:561–8.

87. Cunningham D, Powles R, Malpas J et al. A randomized trial of maintenance interferon following high-dose chemotherapy in multiple myeloma: long term follow-up results. Br J Haematol 1998;102:495–502.

88. Barlogie B, Jagannath S, Desikan KR et al. Total therapy with tandem transplants for newly diagnosed multiple myeloma. Blood 1999;93:55–65.

89. Björkstrand B, Ljungman P, Svensson H et al. Allogeneic bone marrow transplantation versus autologous stem cell transplantation in multiple myeloma: a retrospective case-matched study from the European Group for Blood and Marrow Transplantation. Blood 1996;88:4711–18.

90. Gahrton G, Tura S, Ljungman P et al. Prognostic factors in allogeneic bone marrow transplantation for multiple myeloma. J Clin Oncol 1995;13:1312–22.

91. Tricot G, Vesole DH, Jagannath S et al. Graft-versus-myeloma effect: proof of principle. Blood 1996;87:1196–8.

92. Verdonck L, Lokhorst H, Dekker A et al. Graft-versus-myeloma effect in two cases. Lancet 1996;347:800–1.

93. Barlogie B, Jagannath S, Naucke S et al. Long-term follow-up after high-dose therapy for high-risk multiple myeloma. Bone Marrow Transplant 1998;21:1101–7.

8

High dose chemotherapy and stem cell rescue in the treatment of low-grade non-Hodgkin's lymphoma

Elisabeth Vandenberghe

CONTENTS Epidemiology of low-grade non-Hodgkin's lymphoma • Classification of low-grade lymphomas • Conventional management and reasons for change • Peripheral blood stem cell transplantation • Purging and minimal residual disease monitoring • Adjuvant therapy • Allogeneic transplantation • Follicular lymphoma • Mantle cell lymphoma • Small lymphocytic lymphoma • Lymphoplasmacytoid lymphoma

EPIDEMIOLOGY OF LOW-GRADE NON-HODGKIN'S LYMPHOMA

Low-grade non-Hodgkin's lymphoma (LG-NHL) has an incidence of between 30 and 50 cases per million in the Western world and comprises between 23% and 46% of NHLs diagnosed. The median age of presentation is between 50 and 60 years; however, the age range is wide and patients in their 20s are occasionally diagnosed. There is a marked male predominance in some subtypes of low-grade lymphomas such as small lymphocytic lymphoma (SLL) and mantle cell lymphoma (MCL). Patients with low-grade NHLs tend to present with widespread disease and over 50% have marrow involvement at diagnosis.

Taken as a group, 50% of patients with low-grade lymphomas die of their disease within 10 years of diagnosis; however, considerable variability exists and the various subtypes of LG-NHL are associated with differing prognoses.

CLASSIFICATION OF LOW-GRADE LYMPHOMAS

The REAL classification system for lymphomas developed in 1994 (Table 8.1) is now widely used, though it is being superseded by the more comprehensive WHO classification system.[1] The low-grade lymphomas of B cell subtype are conventionally considered to include SLL, lymphoplasmacytoid lymphoma, MCL, follicle centre cell lymphoma (FCLL) and marginal zone lymphomas. The T-NHLs can behave in an indolent fashion, but are rare in the Western world, so there is little data available on the role of myeloablative chemotherapy in treating them.

The LG-NHLs may be considered to be clonal populations of B lymphocytes arrested at various points of normal B lymphoid development. They therefore possess the morphological, immunophenotypic and immunogenetic features of their normal lymphoid counterpart, and this can be useful both in the initial diagnosis

Table 8.1 The REAL classification (low-grade B lymphoid neoplasms)
B-cell chronic lymphocytic leukaemia/lymphoma
B-cell prolymphocytic leukaemia*
Lymphoplasmacytoid lymphoma
Mantle cell lymphoma
Follicle centre cell lymphoma
Marginal zone lymphoma of MALT*
Nodal marginal zone lymphoma*
Splenic marginal zone lymphoma*
Hairy cell leukaemia*
Plasmacytoma†

*No information on the role of HDC in these conditions.
†See chapter on myeloma.

of patients and for their follow-up if minimal residual disease states are achieved. Three LG-NHL are closely associated with a specific cytogenetic abnormality: the t(14;18) with upregulation of the bcl-2 oncogene is found in 80% of patients with FCCL, the t(11;14) with upregulation of cyclin D1 is found in up to 60% of patients with MCL and trisomy-12 is present in a proportion of patients with SLL.

CONVENTIONAL MANAGEMENT AND REASONS FOR CHANGE

The LG-NHLs are considered incurable with conventional treatment, which is therefore aimed at minimizing disease-related symptoms. The mainstay of treatment for most patients remains oral alkylating agents and local radiotherapy. In the last decade the adenine deaminase inhibitors such as fludarabine and chlorodeoxyadenosine have been used successfully in SLL and lymphoplasmacytoid lymphoma but have proved to be less useful in follicular lymphoma.

PERIPHERAL BLOOD STEM CELL TRANSPLANTATION

The increasing numbers of patients presenting with LG-NHL at a relatively young age and our ability to use high dose chemotherapy (HDC) with peripheral stem cell transplant (PBSCT) safely in fit patients up to the age of 65 years has led to the development of protocols exploring the safety and efficacy of this treatment in LG-NHL. There are difficulties in analysing survival data in LG-NHL, as follow-up needs to be prolonged to show a real difference between patients treated conventionally and those treated with HDC. Most of the data published to date are on highly selected patients treated at one institution or a group of collaborating institutions without randomization to a control, conventionally treated, arm. Results suggest that HDC and PBSCT may prolong survival in LG-NHL, but worryingly there appears to be no plateau in disease-free survival, suggesting that patients may not be easily cured of their disease.

PURGING AND MINIMAL RESIDUAL DISEASE MONITORING

The problem of marrow involvement and contamination of peripheral stem cell collections by clonal progenitor cells in LG-NHL is considerable. Minimal disease states can be followed up immunophenotypically; however, the most sensitive and convenient method of follow-up is by using molecular techniques such as the polymerase chain reaction (PCR). Immunoglobulin genes are invariably rearranged in low-grade lymphomas and can be used as a target for minimal residual disease (MRD) monitoring, achieving a sensitivity of 1 in 10^3 to 1 in 10^5. The rearranged bcl-2 locus (FCCL) or cyclin D1 (MCL) can also be used as a PCR target, with increased sensitivity but a lower detection rate. These techniques can be used to assess disease involvement in the marrow pre- and post-transplant, to define the number of contaminating cells in the PBSC harvest and finally to see if purging the stem cell harvest is effective at clearing clonal populations. This approach has been used by two groups treating patients with FCCL and will be discussed later.

ADJUVANT THERAPY

Patients with LG-NHL can be treated with HDC and PBSC rescue, but continuing disease either in the patient or stem cell collection remains a stumbling block in achieving long-term cure for most. Adjuvant treatments, especially if active in minimal disease states, may improve prognosis and their use has been explored particularly in FCCL. Alpha-interferon (IFN-α) has been shown to prolong remissions in conventionally treated patients with FCCL and may have a role post HDC.[2] Rituximab (MabThera) is a chimeric anti-CD20 antibody which activates complement-mediated lysis of CD20-expressing B lymphocytes and is active in about 50% of cases of relapsed FCCL and 30% of cases of relapsed MCL.[3,4]

ALLOGENEIC TRANSPLANTATION

Allogeneic bone marrow transplant is increasingly being offered to young patients with LG-NHL and though the toxic death rate is higher than in autologous procedures, the graft-versus-lymphoma effect appears to confer a considerable therapeutic advantage and possibly cure in these patients.[5,6] The development of non-myeloablative transplant protocols may be particularly useful in treating older patients with LG-NHL.[7]

The evidence supporting the use of autologous transplantation in the different sub-types of LG-NHL will be analysed and some of the current studies discussed.

FOLLICULAR LYMPHOMA

Seventy per cent of LG-NHLs are classified as FCCLs and are therefore B-NHLs with the morphological and immunophenotypic characteristics of B lymphocytes found in the germinal centre. In about 80% of cases, FCCLs are characterized by the t(14;18) (q32;q21) which leads to upregulation of the anti-apoptotic *bcl*-2 oncogene by the immunoglobulin promoter. This translocation can be detected using the PCR, providing a sensitive target for MRD detection.

Studies of PBSC in FCCL

The main questions concerning the use of HDC and PBSC rescue in FCCL are:

- does HDC confer a survival advantage in patients with FCCL?
- should HDC be used in first clinical response/partial response (CR/PR) in patients with high-risk disease, or should one wait for relapse before proceeding to HDC?
- what is the role of in vitro purging of PBSC harvests?

Large series of patients with relapsed, extensive FCCL treated with HDC and either marrow or PBSC rescue have now been reported in the literature. The Dana Farber Cancer Institute has reported the outcome of 153 patients with chemosensitive relapsed FCCL, treated with a regimen that included total body irradiation (TBI) and using purged marrow rescue. The disease-free survival (DFS) and overall survival (OS) from this series at 8 years were 42% and 66%, respectively, with a survival from diagnosis at 12 years of 69%, which contrasts favourably with a historical DFS of 2 years for relapsed FCCL treated conventionally.[8,9] St Bartholomew's Hospital, using a different antibody purging system in 64 patients, reported a DFS and OS at 4 years of 55% and 70%.[10] The University of Nebraska has reported 100 patients, with a DFS and OS of 62% and 76%, with no difference in relapse rates for those 'rescued with PBSC vs marrow or conditioned with TBI/chemotherapy vs chemotherapy only'.[11] These results are encouraging but still have to be interpreted with caution because no RCT has been carried out, the patients are frequently highly selected and longer follow-up is needed. Many other series have now been reported but are not discussed here because of small numbers or short follow-up.[12] It is generally accepted that patients who have had numerous relapses with chemoresistant disease are unlikely to benefit from HDC.

The role of HDC in newly diagnosed patients with high-risk FCCL has likewise been explored by a number of centres. Six studies are of particular interest,[11,13-17] resulting in an OS and DFS of between 64–85% and 55–70% respectively, with a median follow-up between 3–6 years. The importance of prolonged follow-up in these indolent lymphomas is emphasized by the fact that the lowest OS and PFS was found in the GOELAMS phase II study[16] comprising the series of patients with longest follow-up, although these patients were a poor risk group with a high tumour burden at presentation. Positive prognostic factors in the German study included being in clinical remission at time of mobilization and being in first (as opposed to subsequent) clinical remission.[15] The EORTC and BNLI co-operated on a randomized study looking at the role of myeloablative therapy and PBSCT in newly diagnosed low-grade lymphoma, with IFN-α maintenance in both arms, but recruitment to this study was poor and it was terminated prematurely.[2]

A further group of patients with a notoriously poor prognosis when treated conventionally are those with transformed FCCL. Three series of patients treated with HDC for transformed disease, show encouraging results. Nineteen patients treated in London had a median survival of 4.4 years, whereas the patients from the other two centres had a 5-year DFS of 36% and 46%. These results suggest a survival benefit for patients with transformed FCCL treated with HDC.[18-20]

Purging and MRD in FCCL

The problem of PBSC harvest contamination by malignant cells has been addressed in a number of studies.[13,21-23] The tumour cells can be detected by the PCR at low levels of between 1 in 10^3 to 1 in 10^5 if the immunoglobulin complementary determining region (CDR III) is used as target DNA and up to 1 in 10^5 if the rearrangement of bcl-2 is used to track the malignant clone. Amplification of the rearranged bcl-2 gene is more sensitive but may not always be detectable, whereas CDR III directed PCR is less sensitive but more reliable in MRD tracking. Two groups have shown that outcome is superior if the PBSC harvest is not contaminated by cells with a rearranged bcl-2 oncogene.[13,21,24]

Studies carried out to date to explore the efficacy of purging in reducing relapse rates have mainly used in vitro purging techniques. In vitro purging can be carried out by positive selection of the CD34-expressing stem cell fraction using columns and/or negative selection using B-lymphoid antigen-directed antibodies such as CD19 or CD20. There is no RCT showing an improvement in outcome when purging is used. The studies by Freedman et al.[21] showed an improved survival for those patients whose bcl-2 became undetectable after a negative purging system, but this may of course reflect a lower disease burden in patients whose harvest can be rendered bcl-2 negative.[21] Three studies have shown that positive CD34 selection alone or in combination with a negative selection stage can render a PBSC harvest free of detectable disease,[24-26] whereas another group using negative selection has not been able to purge effectively.[27] These differences may be due to patient selection but are more likely to reflect the use of varying MRD detection methods or purging technology. Until a prospective RCT is carried out using agreed purging technology the role of this expensive procedure will remain unclear. A case-controlled study by the European Blood and Marrow Transplant Registry (EBMT) group, comparing outcome post-transplant using purged versus unpurged bone marrow in all types of NHL, showed a similar PFS in patients with LG-NHL.[28]

Reducing the tumour load in vivo either before stem cell harvesting or after HDC and

PBSCT is another approach worth exploring. One group has shown impressive results when patients have been transplanted in CR after intensive pretransplant chemotherapy.[14] The role of the anti-CD20 antibody (rituximab) both as an in vivo purging agent prior to HDC and to eradicate residual disease after HDC is being investigated in a joint EBMT/BNLI study after pilot studies demonstrated its anti-tumour activity in over 50% of patients with relapsed FCCL.[3] Preliminary data from a series of patients given MabThera with both priming and conditioning chemotherapy showed a decrease in PCR detectable disease in the harvest, when compared to patients treated with the same regimen without MabThera. No OS and DFS data is available from this series of patients, but it demonstrates the efficacy of in vivo purging.[29] Attempts to use interleukin-2 (IL-2) to develop autologous GvH have been largely unsuccessful because of patient toxicity.

Patients who relapse after HDC frequently do so at the site of original disease, suggesting that current conditioning regimens may not eradicate the tumour. Seventeen patients with refractory FCCL were treated at the FHRC with radioimmunoconjugates using ^{131}I conjugated to the CD20 antibody, achieving high local radiotherapy doses, resulting in a high percentage of progression-free patients.[30]

Conclusion

In summary, the role and timing of high dose therapy and PBSC transplant in FCCL remains unclear but probably results in a survival advantage, especially if carried out when patients are in clinical remission before proceeding to HDC. Unfortunately there has as yet been no RCT with adequate follow-up to prove this survival advantage. The role of in vitro purging likewise remains unproven; however, the development of an in vivo method of purging using the anti-CD20 antibody may improve survival rates in future studies.

MANTLE CELL LYMPHOMA

Mantle cell lymphoma comprises between 5% and 10% of all NHLs and has characteristics of both low- and high-grade lymphoma: it is incurable with conventional therapy but has a median survival of between 2 and 5 years. The male-to-female ratio is between 4:1 and 6:1, and the median age of presentation is 60 years, albeit with a wide age range. Patients frequently present with stage IVB disease, marked splenomegaly and extranodal involvement.

Studies of PBSC in MCL

A number of groups have treated MCL patients with myeloablative chemotherapy and PBSC support with variable results. High dose chemotherapy appears to increase the remission rate significantly, but OS varies from 34% to 80% and EFS from 26% to 55% at a median time from transplant of between 18 months and 9 years.[31–36] It is noteworthy that the series with a median follow-up of only 18 months showed an EFS of 55%, probably indicating inadequate follow-up. Two interesting series[37,38] demonstrate the importance of achieving CR or good PR with first line chemotherapy followed by consolidation with HDC as part of the initial therapy plan. Another interesting series of patients who did not achieve clinical remission with anthracycline-based therapy achieved it with high dose Ara-C before proceeding to HDC, again with encouraging results.[34] Conditioning regimens include chemotherapy with or without TBI, with one study showing an improved outcome with TBI-containing conditioning.[32] Unfortunately, long-term follow-up data from these series are limited and all include unrandomized highly selected groups of patients. Fit patients under the age of 65 years with MCL are being offered myeloablative therapy with PBSC support because of their poor prognosis when treated conventionally. Survival data from most high dose procedures are submitted centrally to the

European/American BMT registries; currently a joint retrospective review is underway of patients treated in this way, which will provide some evidence for the efficacy of this approach.

Purging and MRD in MCL

The role of in vitro purging of MCLs has been explored by two groups. Neither has been able to clear the PBSC collection of clonal progenitor cells using either positive selection[35] or negative selection.[36] The role of rituximab in minimal residual disease states post-PBSCT was explored in three patients from the City of Hope series[37] and, given its proven activity in 30% of patients with relapsed MCL, will need to be investigated further.

Conclusion

A logical approach to the management of MCL is still unavailable. Given its poor prognosis with conventional treatment, it would seem reasonable to offer people HDC and PBSC support in first remission or partial remission. Cure in MCL is uncommon; however, it has been documented after allogeneic transplantation and all patients under 50 years should be considered for this form of transplantation before proceeding to an autologous procedure.[37]

SMALL LYMPHOCYTIC LYMPHOMA

Small lymphocytic lymphoma and its leukaemic counterpart chronic lymphocytic leukaemia (CLL) can be considered to be biologically the same disease. Predominantly affecting men (with a 2:1 ratio), SLL/CLL is frequently indolent and stage A disease can be associated with a survival of 10–20 years. The patients with stage B or C disease fare less well, with a median survival of 5.5 and 3.5 years, respectively. These patients with poor prognosis usually can be identified by the progressive

nature of their disease and poor response to therapy, including the adenine deaminase inhibitors. Poor prognosis in SLL/CLL is also associated with atypical morphology, unusual combinations of surface marker antigens CD38 expression and an abnormal karyotype.

Studies of PBSC in SLL

The use of PBSC transplants in CLL/SLL has already been reported by a number of groups which have reported encouraging preliminary results.[38,39] Rabinowe et al.[38] performed autologous BMTs in 15 patients with CLL, of whom five remained in clinical remission after 1 year. Khouri et al.[39] carried out autologous procedures on 11 patients with advanced disease (of whom seven had purged stem cell harvests) and achieved a molecular remission in five and morphological remission in 10; six remained in clinical remission 2–29 months after the procedure.

In the UK, the Medical Research Council is coordinating a pilot protocol in patients under the age of 60 years with stage B/C disease or rapidly progressive stage A disease, using fludarabine initially to obtain the best possible remission, followed by a cyclophosphamide/TBI-based myeloablative therapy and PBSCT with CD34 selected stem cells. Initial results demonstrate that successful mobilization is possible after fludarabine, purging with CD34 selection eliminates clonal progenitor cells in a proportion of patients, and some patients attain a molecular CR (personal communication).

CampathIH is a monoclonal antibody directed at the, and in phase II studies has been active in treating refractory disease. It may be possible in the future to explore its use in MRD states after autologous transplantation.

Conclusion

The role of HDC in SLL/CLL needs to be investigated further, preferably in the context of a RCT. Pilot studies indicate that it may be useful in younger patients with progressive disease and that current purging techniques can clear PBSC harvests of neoplastic cells.

LYMPHOPLASMACYTOID LYMPHOMA

This LG-NHL is rarely found in patients under the age of 60 years and is usually associated with an extremely indolent course, which responds to oral alkylating agents and fludarabine. Clinical presentation is frequently due to hyperviscosity secondary to an IgM paraprotein produced by the clonal lymphoplasmacytoid cells. A pilot protocol developed by the Arkansas group and used in six patients confirmed that melphalan $\pm$ TBI with PBSC rescue was a feasible, active regimen; however, no long-term episode-free survival or survival data are available yet.[40]

REFERENCES

1. Harris NL, Jaffe ES, Stein H et al. A revised European American classification of lymphoid neoplasms: a proposal from the International Lymphoma Study Group. Blood 1994;84:1361–92.
2. Hagenbeek A, Marcus R for the EORTC and BNLI. Protocol (20963): marrow ablative chemoradiotherapy and autologous stem cell transplantation followed by interferon-α maintenance treatment versus interferon-α maintenance treatment alone after a chemotherapy induced remission in patients with stages III or IV follicular non-Hodgkin's lymphoma. A prospective randomised phase III clinical trial. www.eortc.be
3. McLaughlin P, Grillo-Lopez A, Link B et al. Rituximab chimeric antiCD20 monoclonal antibody therapy for relapsed indolent lymphoma: half of patients respond to a four dose treatment program. J Clin Oncol 1998;16:2825–33.
4. Coiffier B, Haioun N, Ketterer A et al. Rituximab for the treatment of patients with relapsing or refractory aggressive lymphoma: a multicentre phase II study. Blood 1998; 92: 1927–32.
5. van Beisen K, Sobocinski K, Rowlings P et al. Allogeneic bone marrow transplantation for low grade lymphoma. Blood 1998;92:1832–6.
6. Chopra R, Goldstone AH, Pearce R et al. Autologous versus allogeneic bone marrow transplantation for low grade lymphoma. Blood 1992;10:1690–5.
7. Khouri I, Keating M, Korbling M et al. Transplant-lite: induction of graft versus malignancy using fludarabine-based non-ablative chemotherapy and allogeneic blood progenitor-cell transplantation as treatment for lymphoid malignancies. J Clin Oncol 1998;16:2817–24.
8. Gallagher CJ, Gregory G, Jones AE et al. Follicular lymphoma. Prognostic factors for response and survival. J Clin Oncol 1986;4:1470–80.
9. Friedberg JW, Freedman AS. High dose therapy and stem cell transplantation in follicular lymphoma. Ann Haematol 1999;78:203–11.
10. Rohatiner A, Johnson P, Price C et al. Myeloablative therapy with autologous bone marrow transplantation as consolidation therapy for recurrent follicular lymphoma. J Clin Oncol 1994;12:1177–84.
11. Bierman P, Vose J, Anderson J et al. High dose therapy with autologous hematopoietic rescue for follicular low-grade non-Hodgkin's lymphoma. J Clin Oncol 1997;15:445–50.
12. Bastion Y, Brice P, Haioun C et al. Intensive therapy with peripheral blood progenitor cell support in 60 patients with poor prognosis follicular lymphoma. Blood 1998;86:3257–62.
13. Freedman A, Gribben J, Neuberg D et al. High dose therapy and autologous bone marrow transplantation in patients with follicular lymphoma during first remission. Blood 1996;88:2780–6.
14. Fouillard L, Laporte J, Labopin M et al. Autologous stem cell transplantation for non-Hodgkin's lymphoma: the role for graft purging and radiotherapy post transplantation – results of a retrospective analysis of 120 patients grafted in a single institution. J Clin Oncol 1998;16:2803–16.
15. Voso MT, Martin S, Abdallah A. High dose therapy and autologous blood stem cell transplantation in patients with follicular lymphoma. Bone Marrow Transplant 1999;23(suppl 3):5.
16. Colombat PH, Cornillet P, Deconinck E et al. Value of autologous stem cell transplantation with purged bone marrow as first line therapy for follicular lymphoma with high tumour burden: a Goelams phase II study. Bone Marrow Transplant 2000;26:971–7.
17. Horning SJ, Negrin RS, Hoppe RT et al. High dose therapy and autologous bone marrow

transplantation for follicular lymphoma in first or partial remission: results of a phase II clinical trial. Blood 2001;97:404–9.

18. Foran J, Apostolides J, Pappamichael D et al. High dose therapy with autologous haematopoietic support in patients with transformed follicular lymphoma: a study of 27 patients from a single centre. Ann Oncol 1998;9:865–9.

19. Friedberg J, Neuberg D, Gribben J et al. Autologous bone marrow transplantation following histologic transformation of indolent B cell non-Hodgkin's lymphoma. Blood 1998;92:727a.

20. Chen C, Crump M, Tsang R et al. Auto-transplants for histologically transformed follicular non-Hodgkin's lymphoma. Br J Haematol 2001;113:202–8.

21. Freedman AS, Ritz J, Neuberg D et al. Autologous bone marrow transplantation in 69 patients with a history of low grade B-cell non-Hodgkin's lymphoma. Blood 1991;77:2524–9.

22. Colombat Ph, Cornillet C, Foussard JS et al. Value of autologous stem cell transplantation with purged stem cells as first line therapy of follicular lymphoma with high tumour burden. Bone Marrow Transplant 1999;23 (suppl 1):514.

23. McQuaker I, Haynes A, Anderson S et al. Engraftment and molecular monitoring of CD34+ peripheral blood stem cell transplants for follicular lymphoma: a pilot study. J Clin Oncol 1997;15:2288–95.

24. Tarella C, Corradini P, Astolfi M et al. Negative immunomagnetic ex vivo purging combined with high dose chemotherapy with peripheral blood progenitor cell autograft in follicular lymphoma patients: evidence for long term clinical and molecular remissions. Leukaemia 1999;13:1456–62.

25. Dreger P, Viehmann K, von Neuhoff N et al. Autografting of highly purified peripheral blood progenitor cells following myeloablative therapy in patients with lymphoma: a prospective study of the long term effects on tumour eradication, reconstitution of haematopoiesis and immune recovery. Bone Marrow Transplant 1999;24:153–61.

26. Voso MT, Hohaus S, Moos M et al. Autografting with CD34+ve peripheral blood cells: retained engraftment capability and reduced tumour cell content. Br J Haematol 1999;104:382–91.

27. Pappa VI, Wilkes S, Salam A et al. Use of the polymerase chain reaction and direct sequencing analysis to detect cells with the t(14;18) in autologous bone marrow from patients with follicular lymphoma before and after in vitro purging. Bone Marrow Transplant 1998;2:553–8.

28. William C, Goldstone AH, Pearce R et al. Purging of bone marrow in autologous bone marrow transplantation for non-Hodgkin's lymphoma: a case matched comparison with unpurged cases by the European Blood and Bone Marrow Transplantation Lymphoma Registry. J Clin Oncol 1996;14:2454–64.

29. Voso MT, Pantel G, Weis M et al. In vivo depletion of B cells using a combination of high dose cytosine arabinoside/mitaxantrone and rituximab for autografting in patients with non-Hodgkin's lymphoma. Br J Haematol 2000;109:729–35.

30. Liu S, Eary J, Petersdorf S et al. Follow-up of relapsed B-cell lymphoma patients treated with Iodine 131 labelled anti-CD20 antibody and autologous stem cell rescue. J Clin Oncol 1998;16:3270–8.

31. Conde E, Bosch F, Arranz R. Autologous stem cell transplantation (ASCT) for mantle cell lymphoma. The experience of the GEL/TAMO Spanish cooperative group. Bone Marrow Transplant 1999;23(suppl 1):515.

32. Milpied N, Gaillard F, Moreau P et al. High-dose therapy with stem cell transplantation for mantle cell lymphoma: results and prognostic factors, a single center experience. Bone Marrow Transplant 1998;22:645–50.

33. Blay JY, Sebban C, Surbiguet C et al. High-dose chemotherapy with hematopoietic stem cell transplantation in patients with mantle cell or diffuse centrocytic non-Hodgkin's lymphomas: a single center experience on 18 patients. Bone Marrow Transplant 1998;21:51–4.

34. Kroger N, Hoffknecht M, Dreger P et al. Long-term disease-free survival of patients with advanced mantle-cell lymphoma following high-dose chemotherapy. Bone Marrow Transplant 1998;21:55–7.

35. Ketterer N, Salles G, Espinouse D et al. Intensive therapy with peripheral stem cell transplantation in 16 patients with mantle cell lymphoma. Ann Oncol 1997;8:701–4.

36. Haas R, Brittinger G, Meusers P. Myeloablative therapy with blood stem cell transplantation is effective in mantle cell lymphoma. Leukemia 1996;1:1975–9.

37. Khouri IF, Romaguera J, Kantarijian H et al.

Hyper-CVAD and high dose methotrexate/cytarabine followed by stem cell transplantation: an active regimen for aggressive mantle-cell lymphoma. J Clin Oncol 1998;16:3803–9.

38. Dreger P, Martin S, Kuse A et al. The impact of autologous stem cell transplantation on the prognosis of mantle cell lymphoma: a joint analysis of two prospective studies with 46 patients. Haem J 2000;1:87–94.

39. Suzan F, Belanger C, Ribrag V et al. Preliminary report of a strategy assessing a CHOP-regimen and high dose Ara-C (DHAP) followed by high-dose chemotherapy with autologous peripheral blood stem cell transplantation (APBSCT) for mantle cell lymphoma (MCL). Blood 1998;92 (suppl 1):1916.

40. Geisler CH, Andersen NS, Elonen et al. Nordic Mantle Cell Lymphoma (MCL) Protocol: preliminary results of primary purged autologous peripheral blood-stem-cell transplantation. Bone Marrow Transplant 1999;23(suppl 1):520.

41. Andersen NS, Donovan JW, Borus JS et al. Failure of immunologic purging in mantle cell lymphoma assessed by polymerase chain reaction detection of minimal residual disease. Blood 1997;90:4212–21.

42. Corradini P, Ladetto M, Astolfi M et al. Clinical and molecular remission after allogeneic blood cell transplantation in a patient with mantle-cell lymphoma. Br J Haematol 1996;94:376–8.

43. Rabinowe S et al. Autologous and allogeneic bone marrow transplantation for poor prognosis patients with B-cell chronic lymphocytic leukaemia. Blood 1993;82:1366–76.

44. Khouri I, Keating M, Vriesendorp H et al. Autologous and allogeneic bone marrow transplantation for chronic lymphocytic leukaemia, preliminary results. J Clin Oncol 1994;12:748–58.

45. Desikan R, Dhodapkar M, Siegel D et al. High dose therapy with autologous peripheral blood stem cell support for Waldenstrom's macroglobulinaemia: a pilot study. Blood 1998;(suppl 1): no. 2721.

9

High dose chemotherapy and stem cell transplantation in Hodgkin's disease

John W Sweetenham

INTRODUCTION

High dose chemotherapy (HDC) and autologous stem cell transplantation (ASCT) is a widely applied treatment in adult patients with Hodgkin's disease, most commonly used in those with relapsed or refractory disease. Despite its widespread use, however, its role in the treatment of patients with Hodgkin's disease remains unclear. This is mainly a reflection of the fact that, to date, only two randomized trials comparing HDC and ASCT with conventional chemotherapy have been reported. Current clinical practice has been influenced largely by phase II studies from single centres, and registry-derived data.

The use of allogeneic bone marrow transplantation in Hodgkin's disease has also been reported, although its use has been limited by donor availability and by very marked regimen-related toxicity. However, some activity has been reported, and interest in this approach has been revived by early reports of the use of 'mini-transplantation' strategies in lymphoma.

BACKGROUND

Management policies for patients with Hodgkin's disease have changed substantially in the last decade. In early-stage disease, the use of extended field radiotherapy is declining, and being replaced by a 'risk-adapted' approach. Although the standard treatment for 'good risk' early-stage disease is with sub-total nodal radiotherapy, an increasing number of patients are now receiving 'adjuvant' chemotherapy, with more limited radiotherapy fields. Most patients who have 'poor risk' early-stage disease now receive combination chemotherapy, supplemented by involved field radiotherapy.[1,2]

In advanced-stage disease, anthracycline-containing combination chemotherapy regimens have replaced alkylating agent based therapy as standard.[3] These regimens have been shown to produce higher disease-free and overall survival rates, and to have a lower potential for long-term toxicity, such as secondary leukaemia and impaired reproductive function. Novel, dose-intensive regimens such as

Stanford V and BEACOPP are now being assessed in randomized trials in comparison with standard chemotherapy.[4,5] The identification of prognostic factors for patients with advanced Hodgkin's disease has recently been described,[6] and novel strategies are being developed for those patients with 'poor risk' advanced disease. Potential applications of HDC are therefore changing. Improvements in supportive care of patients undergoing HDC, particularly the development of peripheral blood progenitor cell transplantation, have widened its applicability. This has led to its use relatively early in the course of the disease, including as a component of first-line therapy in some patients. However, the potential long-term toxicities of HDC and the increasing likelihood of tumour control with 'conventional dose' chemotherapy may limit the use of stem cell transplantation for this disease in the future.

At present, HDC and ASCT is used mostly for patients with relapsed or refractory disease after failure of 'conventional dose' chemotherapy.

HIGH DOSE CHEMOTHERAPY AND AUTOLOGOUS STEM CELL TRANSPLANTATION

For relapsed disease

The use of 'conventional dose' salvage therapy in patients who relapse after treatment with combination chemotherapy produces high remission rates. In a series from the National Cancer Institute in the USA, in patients relapsing after MOPP (mustine, vincristine, procarbazine, prednisone) chemotherapy, retreatment with MOPP produced second complete remission rates of around 50%, with a median second remission duration of 21 months.[7] The most important prognostic factor for achievement of second remission was the duration of the initial remission. In those patients with an initial remission of less than 12 months, only 29% achieved a second complete remission with

MOPP. In contrast, the second remission rate in those with an initial remission of greater than 12 months was 93%. Despite this high remission rate in the 'favourable' group, only 17% were alive and free of disease at 20 years.

Non-cross-resistant regimens have also been widely used as second-line therapy for patients with relapsed disease. Encouraging results have been reported in single-centre studies using this approach. For example, in studies from Milan, 5-year progression-free survival (PFS) has been reported in 51% of patients treated with further conventional chemotherapy following relapse more than 12 months after treatment with MOPP, ABVD (doxorubicin, bleomycin, vinblastine, dacarbazine), or alternating MOPP/ABVD.[8] Various second-line regimens were used, including MOPP, ABVD or CEP (lomustine, etoposide, prednimustine).

These results have not been reproduced in multicentre studies. In a randomized study conducted by the Cancer and Leukaemia Group B (CALGB), patients receiving ABVD as first-line therapy were treated with MOPP at relapse, with a 5-year failure-free survival rate of only 31%.[3] The outcome for patients who received MOPP as initial therapy, and ABVD at relapse was worse, with only 15% failure free at 5 years.

Results of the use of HDC and ASCT in this setting have apparently been superior. For example, Chopra et al.[9] have reported a 5-year freedom from progression rate of 47% in a series of 52 patients receiving HDC and ASCT at first relapse after combination chemotherapy.[9] Comparable results were reported from Vancouver in 58 patients receiving HDC and ASCT in first relapse, in whom the 5-year freedom from progression was 61%.[10] Similar results have also been reported from other single centres.[11,12] In a study from Stanford University, the outcome for 60 patients with relapsed or refractory disease treated with HDC and ASCT was compared with a matched group of historical controls who received conventional dose salvage therapy.[13] Four-year event-free survival (EFS) and freedom from progression (FFP) were higher in the group treated with HDC and ASCT (Fig. 9.1), although no overall survival difference was observed. For the group of patients who relapsed after an initial remission of less than 1 year, an overall survival advantage was observed for patients receiving HDC (Fig. 9.2). A large registry-based study from the European Group for Blood and Marrow Transplantation (EBMT) reported a 45% EFS at 5 years in 139 patients with Hodgkin's disease treated with HDC and ASCT in first relapse after chemotherapy (Fig. 9.3).[14]

The results of two randomized trials comparing high dose with conventional dose salvage therapy have now been reported. In a small randomized trial conducted by the British National Lymphoma Investigation (BNLI), 40 patients with Hodgkin's disease in first or subsequent relapse were randomized to receive HDC with BEAM (carmustine, etoposide, cytosine arabinoside, melphalan) and autologous bone marrow transplantation (ABMT) or conventional dose therapy, using the same drugs at lower dose ('mini-BEAM').[15] There was a significant difference in EFS for patients receiving

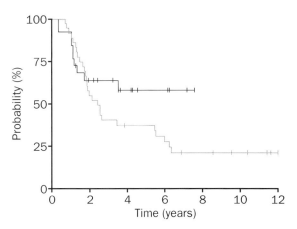

Fig. 9.2

Overall survival for patients with relapsed Hodgkin's disease and an initial remission duration of less than 12 months treated with high dose therapy and autologous stem cell transplantation (solid line) or conventional dose salvage therapy (broken line). Reproduced with permission from Yuen et al., Blood 1997;89:814–22.[13]

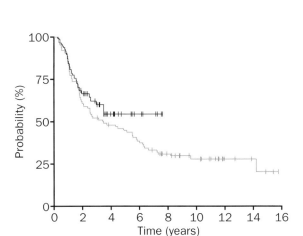

Fig. 9.1

Overall survival in Hodgkin's disease patients with relapsed or refractory disease treated with high dose therapy and autologous stem cell transplantation (solid line) or conventional dose salvage chemotherapy (broken line). Reproduced with permission from Yuen et al., Blood 1997;89:814–22.[13]

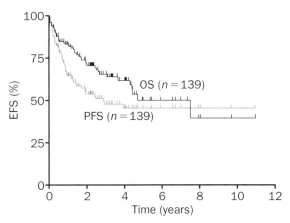

Fig. 9.3

Event-free survival (EFS), as overall (OS) and progression-free survival (PFS), for patients receiving high dose therapy and autologous stem cell transplantation following first relapse after chemotherapy. Reproduced with permission from Sweetenham et al., Bone Marrow Transplant 1997;20:745–52.[14]

BEAM compared with mini-BEAM (3-year EFS = 53% for BEAM versus 10% for mini-BEAM, $P = 0.025$), although there was no overall survival difference. The overall survival in this study is, however, difficult to interpret, since some patients who relapsed after mini-BEAM 'crossed over' to receive BEAM and ASCT and were subsequently progression free.

The German Hodgkin's Disease Study Group and the EBMT have recently completed a randomized study with a similar design.[16] One hundred and sixty-one patients with relapsed Hodgkin's disease were entered. All were initially treated with two cycles of dexa-BEAM (dexamethasone, BEAM). Responding patients were then treated according to randomized arm, either with two further courses of dexa-BEAM, or BEAM and ASCT. One hundred and thirty-nine patients were evaluable. With a median follow-up of 34 months, there was a significant improvement in time to treatment failure (TTF) for patients receiving BEAM and ASCT compared with those receiving further dexa-BEAM. However, there was no difference in overall survival. As with the BNLI study, this is partly due to the ability of HDC and ASCT to salvage patients who relapsed after receiving conventional dose therapy.

Prognostic factors

The selection of appropriate patients for HDC and ASCT at relapse remains uncertain. Analysis of prognostic factors in previous studies has produced conflicting results. Several studies have shown that the response of the disease to conventional dose chemotherapy given immediately prior to the HDC (disease status) is predictive of long-term outcome. These studies show superior survival for patients undergoing ASCT having achieved a further complete remission (CR) to chemotherapy, compared with those whose disease has responded but who have not achieved a CR ('responsive relapse').[9,12,14] The group who fail to respond to conventional dose salvage ('resistant relapse') have the worst outcome (Fig. 9.4). However, this observation is not consistent in all published series, and long-term disease-free

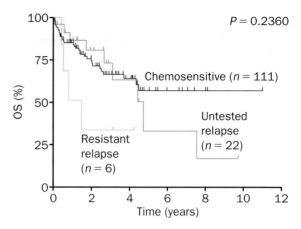

Fig. 9.4

Overall survival (OS) for patients with Hodgkin's disease treated with high dose therapy and autologous stem cell transplantation in first relapse following chemotherapy, according to disease status at time of transplantation. Reproduced with permission from Sweetenham et al., Bone Marrow Transplant 1997;20:745–52.[14]

survival (DFS) is observed in up to 30% of patients classified as having chemoresistant disease at relapse.

The initial remission duration has been identified as a predictive factor for survival in some series,[9,10] although studies from Nebraska[12] and from the EBMT[14] have failed to confirm this. Factors such as disease bulk at the time of ASCT, and the presence of B symptoms or extranodal disease have also been shown to be predictive in some series. Early treatment-related mortality has been between 0% and 10% in most published reports.

Summary

Although only two small randomized trials have been reported, there is general acceptance that HDC and ASCT should be considered as 'standard therapy' for patients whose disease has relapsed after two prior combination chemotherapy regimens such as MOPP and ABVD, and many centres proceed to HDC following relapse after only one of these regimens. With the increasing use of seven- or eight-drug combination chemotherapy regimens as first-line therapy, the use of HDC at first relapse is also regarded as standard, especially if the initial remission duration is less than 12 months. Although the benefit of HDC and ASCT at first relapse in patients with an initial remission of greater than 1–2 months is less clear, the long-term results of conventional dose second-line regimens are poor, and there is evidence to suggest that survival after HDC and ASCT may be superior.

For patients who fail to enter remission after induction therapy

Patients who do not enter remission after first-line combination chemotherapy have a poor outlook. In a study from Milan, 41% of patients who failed to respond to alternating MOPP/ABVD and were then treated with the CEP regimen achieved a complete response, but only 12% were alive at 5 years, and all of these had active disease.[17] Similar results were reported from the National Cancer Institute in the USA,[7] with a 16-month median overall survival (OS), and from Stanford University, where the 4-year OS for patients with primary refractory Hodgkin's disease was only 38%, with a corresponding 4-year PFS of 19%.[13]

Several retrospective studies have reported encouraging results in patients treated with HDC and ASCT after failure to enter remission. In a series from London, 46 patients with primary refractory Hodgkin's disease were treated with BEAM and ABMT.[9] The 5-year PFS for this group was 33%. Comparable results have been observed in Milan using high dose sequential therapy with ASCT.[18] The group from Stanford University have reported a 4-year PFS of 52% and OS of 44% in patients with primary refractory disease receiving HDC and ASCT. These results were significantly better than those for a matched population of historical controls who received conventional dose second-line therapy.[13,19]

The Autologous Blood and Marrow Transplant Registry of North America (ABMTR) has recently reported a series of 122 patients with Hodgkin's disease who underwent HDC and ASCT having failed to achieve remission after induction chemotherapy.[20] Definition of induction failure in this series was restricted to patients who had obvious disease progression after induction therapy, or who had biopsy-proven persistent disease in residual radiographic abnormalities. The 3-year actuarial PFS and OS in this series were 38% and 50%, respectively. The EBMT has reported comparable results in 175 patients with Hodgkin's disease failing to enter remission after one or two induction chemotherapy regimens.[21] This series included patients with disease progression, and those with either stable or minimally responsive disease following initial chemotherapy. The 5-year actuarial PFS and OS were 36% and 32%, respectively (Fig. 9.5).

Although the results of HDC and ASCT appear superior, all of these results must be interpreted cautiously. In addition to the potential selection bias inherent in retrospective analyses, the definition of induction failure is inconsistent in these studies. Assessment of response in Hodgkin's disease is problematic,

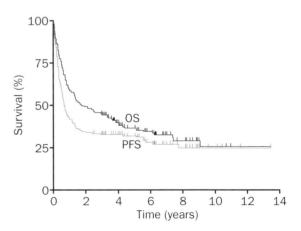

Fig. 9.5
Overall (OS) and progression-free survival (PFS) for patients with Hodgkin's disease receiving high dose therapy and autologous stem cell transplantation after failure of induction therapy. Reproduced with permission from Sweetenham et al., J Clin Oncol 1999;17:3101–9.[21]

particularly in patients with bulky mediastinal disease at presentation, where residual masses are common after chemotherapy.[22,23] These masses may contain active disease but may represent fibrotic masses with no active disease. Previous studies have demonstrated that the presence of a residual mass in the mediastinum after chemotherapy is associated with a higher relapse rate than in patients with no residual mass. However, between 60% and 70% of patients with residual masses remain progression free. Therefore, the failure to achieve a clinical and/or radiological remission after chemotherapy does not always imply the persistence of active Hodgkin's disease. The group of patients who have stable or only minimally responsive disease after chemotherapy may therefore be distinct from those who have obvious disease progression.

Only two of the published series have attempted to address this issue. In the ABMTR series, only patients with definite disease progression or those with tissue confirmation of disease in residual masses were included. In the EBMT series, there was no difference in outcome for patients who had obvious disease progression after first-line therapy, compared with those who had stable, or minimally responsive disease (Fig. 9.6).

Early treatment-related mortality has been relatively high in these patients, with most studies reporting rates between 10% and 20%.

Prognostic factors
As with relapsed disease, the optimal selection of patients with refractory disease for HDC and ASCT is unclear. Previous studies have identified various factors which have predictive value, including disease bulk at the time of ASCT, performance status, presence of B symptoms, bone marrow involvement, stage, extranodal disease, relapse within a previously irradiated field, elevated serum lactate dehydrogenase (LDH), and extent of prior therapy.[9–13,18,19,24–27] However, identification of these factors has been inconsistent, reflecting the small patient numbers in most series, and their retrospective nature.

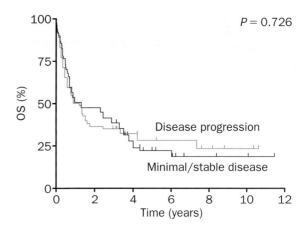

Fig. 9.6
Overall survival (OS) for patients with Hodgkin's disease receiving high dose therapy and autologous stem cell transplantation after failure of induction therapy according to response to prior chemotherapy. Reproduced with permission from Sweetenham et al., J Clin Oncol 1999;17:3101–9.[21]

Summary
The quality of evidence for the use of HDC and ASCT in refractory Hodgkin's disease is poor and is based entirely on retrospective studies. These suggest that it may be superior to conventional dose therapy, producing long-term DFS in about 30% of patients. For patients with disease progression after induction chemotherapy, the use of HDC and ASCT is generally regarded as standard, although it is associated with a relatively high treatment-related mortality. For patients with minimally responsive or stable disease after induction chemotherapy, the effect of HDC and ASCT is less clear, although the EBMT series suggest that it may improve outcome compared with conventional dose therapy. However, confirmation of this requires prospective, randomized studies for comparison with conventional dose salvage. Such studies will require precise criteria for the assessment of residual masses, using imaging techniques such as gallium scintigraphy and positron emission tomography (PET), which may provide information on the viability of disease within residual masses.[28,29]

HIGH DOSE CHEMOTHERAPY AND AUTOLOGOUS STEM CELL TRANSPLANTATION AS A COMPONENT OF FIRST-LINE THERAPY FOR PATIENTS WITH 'POOR RISK' HODGKIN'S DISEASE

In view of the apparent activity of HDC and ASCT for relapsed and refractory Hodgkin's disease, it has also been used as a component of first-line therapy in patients with 'poor risk' disease. In most reports, HDC has been given to consolidate complete remission in patients thought to be at high risk of subsequent relapse. These retrospective studies have observed long-term DFS of 70–90%.[30–33] However, interpretation of these data is difficult because of their retrospective nature and the variable definition of poor risk disease.

A prospective, randomized trial comparing conventional dose chemotherapy using ABVD with HDC and ASCT is in progress, but the definition of 'poor risk' in the eligibility for this trial is controversial.[34] The International Prognostic Factors Project on Advanced Hodgkin's Disease has recently described reproducible clinical prognostic factors at presentation for patients with advanced Hodgkin's disease,[35] but these were not available when the present randomized study was initiated.

Nevertheless, irrespective of the results of this trial, the role of HDC and ASCT as a component of first-line therapy is doubtful. The projected long-term DFS for the poorest risk group in the International Prognostic Factors Project was approximately 40%. Emerging reports of the long-term toxicity of HDC (see below) have identified major effects on reproductive function in both sexes, as well as a risk of secondary malignancy.

In view of the effectiveness of HDC and ASCT as a salvage therapy, poor risk patients should probably receive conventional dose, anthracycline-based induction therapy, reserving HDC and ASCT for patients with relapsed or refractory disease. This approach will mean that 40% of patients with poor risk disease will not be exposed to the potential short- and long-term toxicity of HDC, and the overall survival for the entire cohort of patients is unlikely to be compromised.

TRANSPLANT-RELATED ISSUES

Source of stem cells

Peripheral blood stem cells have almost completely replaced bone marrow as the preferred source of autologous stem cell support for patients with Hodgkin's disease. A single, case-matched study from the EBMT showed an apparently higher relapse rate for patients receiving peripheral blood stem cells compared with bone marrow, but this has not been confirmed.[36]

High dose regimen

The most widely used high dose regimens for patients with Hodgkin's disease have been BEAM, CBV (cyclophosphamide, carmustine, etoposide) and high dose cyclophosphamide with total body irradiation (TBI). Although no randomized comparisons of these regimens have been performed, there is no evidence to suggest that any specific regimen has superior activity. In the EBMT studies, no difference in survival was noted for patients receiving chemotherapy only compared with TBI-based regimens.[14,21] However, the use of TBI-based regimens is limited by the fact that many patients have received prior mediastinal radiotherapy.

Pre-transplant 'debulking' chemotherapy
Although conventional dose salvage therapy is usually given prior to HDC in patients with relapsed/refractory disease, its effect on outcome is unknown. The potential advantages of pre-transplant therapy are:

- to 'test' disease sensitivity and
- to 'debulk' disease prior to HDC.

Since disease sensitivity at ASCT has been shown to be a predictive factor for subsequent PFS and OS, this may provide useful prognostic information. However, since long-term DFS is well documented in patients who have chemoresistant disease, it is difficult to exclude patients from HDC on the basis of their response to conventional dose salvage.

Disease bulk at the time of ASCT has been shown to be predictive of long-term outcome in some series. However, since it is closely related to disease sensitivity, its predictive value is often lost in multivariate analysis. The long-term value of 'debulking' chemotherapy prior to high dose therapy is therefore unclear. In some studies, a proportion of patients have proceeded to HDC and ASCT without prior therapy, in 'untested' relapse.[9,14] These patients have been shown to have long-term outcomes similar to those receiving prior chemotherapy. However, many of the patients in untested relapse had non-bulky disease at the time of ASCT, and may represent a more favourable subgroup.

Although there is no clear evidence for its value, most centres give initial conventional dose salvage. This is often necessary for logistic reasons, since admission for HDC may have to be planned some weeks in advance. In addition, this therapy may be used to mobilize peripheral blood stem cells. However, there is no evidence that prolonged conventional dose treatment, or the achievement of complete remission prior to HDC and ASCT, has any impact on long-term DFS.

Long-term complications

Frequently reported late complications of HDC and ASCT for Hodgkin's disease include chronic lung damage and infection. Male infertility is almost invariable. Female fertility is very rare, although it has been reported. Induction of early ovarian failure, with the premature onset of the menopause, is common. Second malignancies, including myelodysplastic syndrome and acute myeloid leukaemia, have been reported, with a variable incidence between 5% and 25%.[37–39] However, second malignancies, and impaired reproductive func-

tion are well-recognized complications of the standard treatment regimens in Hodgkin's disease that were in regular use until 5–10 years ago. The relative contribution of initial chemotherapy and HDC to the risk of second malignancy is therefore unclear.

ALLOGENEIC STEM CELL TRANSPLANTATION

The use of allogeneic bone marrow transplantation (BMT) for Hodgkin's disease has been described in several small series[40–43] and, more recently, in two large registry studies. It is associated with a high treatment-related mortality, although relapse rates in surviving patients appear to be lower than after autologous transplantation, implying the existence of a graft-versus-lymphoma effect.

One hundred consecutive patients with relapsed or refractory Hodgkin's disease receiving allogeneic BMT, and registered with the International Bone Marrow Transplant Registry (IBMTR), were reported by Gajewski et al.[44] The 3-year DFS and OS rates were 15% and 21%, respectively. The treatment-related mortality in this group of poor risk, heavily pretreated patients was high, and although the relapse rate in surviving patients was low, the potential survival benefit of this lower relapse rate was offset by the high treatment-related toxicity. In a study from the EBMT, 45 patients receiving allogeneic BMT for relapsed/refractory Hodgkin's disease were matched for most major prognostic factors with a group receiving autologous stem cells.[45] No difference in OS or PFS was observed. The long-term OS and PFS for patients undergoing allogeneic BMT were 25% and 15%, respectively, compared with corresponding values of 37% and 24% for ASCT. As with the IBMTR study, the toxic death rate was very high (48% at 4 years) for patients receiving allogeneic BMT.

In view of its high toxicity, and donor availability, allogeneic transplantation is not considered as a routine procedure in Hodgkin's disease. However, the observation of an apparent graft-versus-lymphoma effect provides a rationale for further investigation of its role. Current studies are exploring several strategies which may reduce the treatment-related toxicity, including the use of allogeneic peripheral blood stem cells, the use of conditioning regimens with reduced toxicity in the allogeneic setting (including BEAM) and the use of non-myeloablative conditioning ('mini-transplantation').

CONCLUSIONS

High dose chemotherapy and ASCT now has an established role in the treatment of relapsed and refractory Hodgkin's disease, despite the relative lack of evidence from large-scale randomized trials. Current indications for its use are summarized in Table 9.1. Encouraging early results from trials of new multi-drug brief-

Table 9.1 Present indications for high dose therapy and stem cell transplantation in Hodgkin's disease

Indication	Current use	Level of evidence	Comments
Second or subsequent relapse after chemotherapy	Established	2 randomized trials; both show superior event-free survival on high dose arm	No survival benefit in either trial, but may be due to 'crossover' design (see text)
First relapse after chemotherapy	Standard	Phase II single-institution and registry-based retrospective studies	Modern use of 7 or 8 drug regimens as initial therapy suggests that this should be standard approach irrespective of initial remission duration
Failure of induction therapy	Standard	Phase II single-institution and registry-based retrospective studies	Definition of induction failure influences results; prospective study required
First-line therapy of 'poor risk' disease	Experimental	Phase II trial in progress	Definition of poor risk is controversial; probably has no role in view of potential long-term toxicity and activity of HDC at relapse
Allogeneic transplantation	Experimental	Registry-based and single-institution retrospective studies	High early toxicity; graft-versus-lymphoma effect demonstrated
'Mini-allografting'	Experimental	No studies at present	–

duration chemotherapy regimens suggest that the use of HDC may decline in the future. However, new approaches to therapy are still required, particularly for patients with primary refractory disease. In this context, non-myeloablative therapy, using allogeneic peripheral blood progenitor cells is currently under investigation.

REFERENCES

1. Carde P, Hagenbeek A, Hayat M et al. Clinical staging versus laparotomy and combined modality with MOPP versus ABVD in early stage Hodgkin's disease: The H6 twin randomized trials from the European Organisation for Research and Treatment of Cancer Lymphoma Cooperative Group. J Clin Oncol 1993;11:2258–72.

2. Horning SJ, Hoppe RT, Mason J et al. Stanford–Kaiser Permanente G1 study for clinical stage I to IIA Hodgkin's disease: subtotal lymphoid irradiation versus vinblastine, methotrexate and bleomycin chemotherapy and regional irradiation. J Clin Oncol 1997;15: 1736–44.

3. Canellos GP, Anderson JR, Propert KJ et al. Chemotherapy of advanced Hodgkin's disease with MOPP, ABVD, or MOPP alternating with ABVD. N Engl J Med 1992;327:1478–84.

4. Bartlett NL, Rosenberg SA, Hoppe RT et al. Brief chemotherapy, Stanford V, and adjuvant radiotherapy for bulky or advanced-stage Hodgkin's disease: a preliminary report. J Clin Oncol 1995; 13:1080–8.

5. Diehl V, Franklin J, Hasenclever D et al. BEACOPP, a new dose-escalated and accelerated regimen, is at least as effective as COPP/ABVD in patients with advanced-stage Hodgkin's lymphoma: Interim report from a trial of the German Hodgkin's Lymphoma Study Group. J Clin Oncol 1998;16:3810–21.

6. Hasenclever D, Diehl V. A prognostic score for advanced Hodgkin's disease. N Engl J Med 1998; 339:1506–14.

7. Longo DL, Duffey PL, Young RC et al. Conventional-dose salvage combination chemotherapy in patients relapsing with Hodgkin's disease after combination chemotherapy: the low probability for cure. J Clin Oncol 1992;10:210–18.

8. Bonfante V, Santoro A, Divizzi L et al. Outcome of patients with Hodgkin's disease relapsing after alternating MOPP/ABVD. Proc ASCO 1993;12:364 (abstract).

9. Chopra R, McMillan AK, Linch DC et al. The place of high dose BEAM therapy and autologous bone marrow transplantation in poor-risk Hodgkin's disease. A single center 8-year study of 155 patients. Bone Marrow Transplant 1993; 81:1137–45.

10. Reece DE, Phillips GL. Intensive therapy and autologous stem cell transplantation for Hodgkin's disease in first relapse after combination chemotherapy. Leuk Lymphoma 1996;21: 245–52.

11. Nademanee A, O'Donnell MR, Snyder DS et al. High-dose chemotherapy with or without total body irradiation followed by autologous bone marrow and/or peripheral blood stem cell transplantation for patients with relapsed and refractory Hodgkin's disease: results in 85 patients with analysis of prognostic factors. Blood 1995;85:1381–90.

12. Bierman PJ, Anderson JR, Freeman MB et al. High-dose chemotherapy followed by autologous hematopoietic rescue for Hodgkin's disease patients following first relapse after chemotherapy. Ann Oncol 1996;7:151–6.

13. Yuen AR, Rosenberg SA, Hoppe RT et al. Comparison between conventional salvage therapy and high-dose therapy with autografting for recurrent or refractory Hodgkin's disease. Blood 1997;89:814–22.

14. Sweetenham JW, Taghipour G, Milligan D et al. High-dose therapy and autologous stem cell rescue for patients with Hodgkin's disease in first relapse after chemotherapy: results from the EBMT. Bone Marrow Transplant 1997;20:745–52.

15. Linch DC, Winfield D, Goldstone AH et al. Dose intensification with autologous bone marrow transplantation in relapsed and resistant Hodgkin's disease: results of a BNLI randomised trial. Lancet 1993;341:1051–4.

16. Schmitz N, Sextro M, Pfistner D et al. High-dose therapy (HDT) followed by hematopoietic stem cell transplantation (HSCT) for relapsed chemosensitive Hodgkin's disease (HD): final results of a randomized GHSG and EBMT trial. Proc ASCO 1999;18:2 (abstract).

17. Santoro A, Viviani S, Valagussa P et al. CCNU, etoposide and prednisone (CEP) in refractory Hodgkin's disease. Semin Hematol 1986;13 (suppl 1):23–6.

18. Gianni AM, Siena S, Bregni M et al. High-dose sequential chemoradiotherapy with peripheral blood progenitor cell support for relapsed or refractory Hodgkin's disease – a 6-year update. Ann Oncol 1993;4:889–95.

19. Horning SJ, Chao NJ, Negrin RS et al. High-dose therapy and autologous hematopoietic progenitor cell transplantation for recurrent or refractory Hodgkin's disease: analysis of the Stanford University results and prognostic indices. Blood 1997;89:801–13.

20. Lazarus HM, Rowlings PA, Zhang M-J et al. Autotransplants for Hodgkin's disease in patients never achieving remission: a report from the Autologous Blood and Marrow Transplant Registry. J Clin Oncol 1999;17:534–45.

21. Sweetenham JW, Carella AM, Taghipour G et al. High dose therapy and autologous stem cell transplantation for adult patients with Hodgkin's disease who fail to enter remission after induction chemotherapy: results in 175 patients reported to the EBMT. J Clin Oncol 1999;17:3101–9.

22. Jochelson M, Mauch P, Balikian J et al. The significance of the residual mediastinal mass in treated Hodgkin's disease. J Clin Oncol 1995; 13:637–40.

23. Radford JA, Cowan RA, Flanagan M et al. The significance of residual mediastinal abnormality on the chest radiograph following treatment for Hodgkin's disease. J Clin Oncol 1988;6:940–6.

24. Yahalom J, Gulati SC, Toia M et al. Accelerated, hyperfractionated total-lymphoid irradiation, high-dose chemotherapy, and autologous bone marrow transplantation for refractory and relapsing patients with Hodgkin's disease. J Clin Oncol 1993;11:1062–70.

25. Ribrag V, Nasr F, Bouhris JH et al. VIP (etoposide, ifosfamide and cisplatinum) as a salvage intensification program in relapsed or refractory Hodgkin's disease. Bone Marrow Transplant 1998;21:969–74.

26. Lancet JE, Rapoport AP, Brasacchio R et al. Autotransplantation for relapsed or refractory Hodgkin's disease: long-term follow up and analysis of prognostic factors. Bone Marrow Transplant 1998;22:265–71.

27. Josting A, Katay I, Rueffer U et al. Favorable outcome of patients with relapsed or refractory Hodgkin's disease treated with high-dose chemotherapy and stem cell transplantation at the time of maximal response to conventional salvage therapy (Dexa-BEAM). Ann Oncol 1998; 9:289–95.

28. Salloum E, Schwab Brandt D, Caride VJ et al. Gallium scans in the management of patients with Hodgkin's disease: A study of 101 patients. J Clin Oncol 1997;15:518–27.

29. Bangerter M, Moog F, Buchmann I et al. Whole-body 2-[^{18}F]-fluoro-2-deoxy-D-glucose positron emission tomography (FDG-PET) for accurate staging of Hodgkin's disease. Ann Oncol 1998; 9:1117–22.

30. Carella AM, Prencipe E, Pungolino E et al. Twelve years experience with high-dose therapy and autologous stem cell transplantation for high-risk Hodgkin's disease patients in first remission after MOPP/ABVD chemotherapy. Leuk Lymphoma 1996;21:63–72.

31. Moreau P, Milpied N, Mechinaud-Lacroix F et al. Early intensive therapy with autotransplantation for high-risk Hodgkin's disease. Leuk Lymphoma 1993;12:51–7.

32. Bradley SJ, Pearce R, Taghipour G et al. First remission autologous bone marrow transplantation for Hodgkin's disease: Preliminary EBMT data. Leuk Lymphoma 1995;15(suppl 1):51.

33. Nademanee A, Molina A, Stein A et al. High-dose therapy and autologous stem cell transplantation (AHSCT) as consolidation therapy during first complete remission (CR) or partial remission (PR) in patients with unfavorable prognosis and advanced stage Hodgkin's disease (HD). Blood 1997;90(suppl 1):114 (abstract).

34. Federico M, Clo V, Carella AM. Preliminary analysis of clinical characteristics of patients enrolled in the HD01 protocol: a randomised trial of high-dose therapy and autologous stem cell transplantation versus conventional therapy for patients with advanced Hodgkin's disease responding to first line therapy. Leuk Lymphoma 1995;15(suppl 1):63.

35. Hasenclever D, Diehl V. A prognostic score for advanced Hodgkin's disease. N Engl Med 1998; 339:1506–14.

36. Majolino I, Pearce R, Taghipour G et al. Peripheral-blood stem-cell transplantation versus autologous bone marrow transplantation in Hodgkin's and non-Hodgkin's lymphomas: a new matched analysis of the European Group for Blood and Marrow Transplantation registry data. J Clin Oncol 1997;15:509–17.

37. Traweek ST, Slovak ML, Nademanee A et al. Clonal karyotypic hematopoietic cell abnormali-

ties occurring after autologous bone marrow transplantation for Hodgkin's disease. Blood 1994;84:957–63.

38. Darrington DL, Vose JM, Anderson JR et al. Incidence and characterization of secondary myelodysplastic syndrome and acute myelogenous leukemia following high-dose chemoradiotherapy and autologous stem-cell transplantation for lymphoid malignancies. J Clin Oncol 1994;12:2527–34.

39. Miller JS, Arthur DC, Litz CE et al. Myelodysplastic syndrome after autologous bone marrow transplantation: an additional late complication of curative cancer therapy. Blood 1994;83:3780–6.

40. Jones RJ, Ambinder RF, Piantadosi S et al. Evidence of a graft versus lymphoma effect associated with allogeneic bone marrow transplantation. Blood 1991;77:649–53.

41. Appelbaum FR, Sullivan KM, Thomas ED et al. Allogeneic bone marrow transplantation in the treatment of MOPP resistant Hodgkin's disease. J Clin Oncol 1985;3:1490–4.

42. Phillips GL, Reece DE, Barnett MJ et al. Allogeneic bone marrow transplantation for refractory Hodgkin's disease. J Clin Oncol 1989; 7:1039–45.

43. Phillips GL, Herzig RH, Lazarus HM et al. High-dose chemotherapy, fractionated total body irradiation and allogeneic marrow transplantation for malignant lymphoma. J Clin Oncol 1986;4: 480–8.

44. Gajewski JL, Phillips GL, Sobocinski KA et al. Bone marrow transplantation from HLA-identical siblings in advanced Hodgkin's disease. J Clin Oncol 1996;14:1291–6.

45. Milpied N, Fielding AK, Pierce RM et al. Allogeneic bone marrow transplant is not better than autologous transplant for patients with relapsed Hodgkin's disease. J Clin Oncol 1996;14:1291–6.

10

High dose chemotherapy in aggressive lymphomas

Bertrand Coiffier and Gilles Salles

CONTENTS   Introduction • High dose chemotherapy in relapsing patients • High dose chemotherapy in refractory patients • High dose chemotherapy as part of the first-line treatment • High dose chemotherapy in patients with partial response at the end of the first treatment • High dose chemotherapy in patients with non-DLCL aggressive lymphomas • Open questions regarding the optimal HDC modalities in lymphoma patients • Future directions for autologous transplantation in lymphoma patients

INTRODUCTION

Aggressive lymphomas comprise several entities in the World Health Organization lymphoma classification:[1-3] diffuse large B cell lymphoma (DLCL), peripheral T cell lymphoma (PTCL), anaplastic large cell lymphoma (ALCL), Burkitt's lymphoma and lymphoblastic lymphoma. Often, mantle cell lymphoma is added to this list because of its refractoriness to the different treatments, even if its initial presentation more often looks like an indolent lymphoma. Each of these entities has different clinical characteristics and a specific pattern of outcome[4] but they also have similarities, particularly in terms of the different therapeutic approaches that have been proposed.[5] A large proportion of patients with these lymphomas may be cured by the initial treatment; how many depends on the entity, the presence of adverse prognostic factors at diagnosis [as defined in the International Prognostic Index (IPI)],[6,7] and the age of the patients or the presence of active concomitant diseases.

High-dose chemotherapy (HDC) with autolo-gous haemopoietic stem cell support has been used in aggressive lymphomas for 20 years[8] and it has become apparent that in relapses some patients may benefit from HDC.[9] However, for relapsing patients survival benefit was not demonstrated in a randomized trial until 1995.[10] Since such benefit was demonstrated, physicians have tried to include HDC in each phase of the treatment of lymphoma; however, its therapeutic advantage for all but the sensitive relapsing patients is still under debate.[11] Even though HDC is now recognized as the standard therapy for some patients, many questions remain to be answered. High dose chemotherapy may be used in lymphoma patients as part of the first-line treatment, in patients who have a partial response after first-line treatment, in relapsing patients or in refractory patients.

The first trials of HDC were done with bone marrow cells, but peripheral blood stem cells are now used and have greater effectiveness: haematological recuperation is quicker with peripheral blood stem cells, with fewer infectious complications.[12,13] The registry data from the European Group for Blood and Marrow

Transplantation (EBMT) indicate that about 3000 autologous transplants were performed in patients with lymphoproliferative disorders in European countries during the year 1998 and lymphoma represented the major indication for HDC, before breast cancer, Hodgkin's disease and myeloma.[14] Moreover, more than 90% of patients received haemopoietic stem cells with a peripheral blood origin.

Most of the data presented in the present chapter are derived from clinical trials using autologous bone marrow stem cells, because there are only a few published studies that have used peripheral blood stem cells. Most studies refer to 'aggressive lymphomas', and very few to specific entities. Thus, the data will be presented for the treatment of aggressive lymphomas in general, and specific points concerning each specific disease entity will be presented at the end of the chapter. General data for haemopoietic stem cell (HSC) harvest, the selection of HSC, or complications of the HDC are described in other chapters and will not be described here.

HIGH DOSE CHEMOTHERAPY IN RELAPSING PATIENTS

High dose chemotherapy supported with haemopoietic stem cell transplantation was initially used in relapsing or refractory patients, and the first compilation of 100 cases clearly indicated that patients with a chemosensitive relapse were the most likely to benefit from HDC.[9] Several non-randomized studies further indicated that about 20–40% of relapsing patients with intermediate or high-grade lymphoma experienced prolonged remission after HDC.[15–18] In a retrospective analysis of 244 patients failing the LNH-84 regimen, the administration of HDC appeared as an independent factor for survival (relative risk 0.59; 95% confidence interval 0.37–0.91) in responding patients aged below 60 years.[18] However, the Parma study is the only randomized trial performed in relapsing aggressive lymphoma patients to assess the role of HDC.[10] From 1987

until 1994, 215 lymphoma patients received two courses of salvage chemotherapy consisting of dexamethasone, high dose cytarabine and cis-platinum (DHAP) and the 109 responding patients were then randomized to receive either HDC with autologous bone marrow cell transplantation or four more courses of DHAP. A higher rate of complete response was observed in patients treated with HDC (78% versus 41%) and overall survival and disease-free survival were significantly higher in these patients (Table 10.1). It should be noted that only patients who achieved complete response (CR) clinical remission with first therapy and without bone marrow involvement were included in the study, and that only half of the patients responded to the DHAP salvage therapy and were therefore randomized. In these selected, favourable patients, the Parma trial clearly established that HDC was the best available treatment. Because of these results and the results of non-randomized studies that showed the same benefit for patients treated with HDC, the International Consensus Conference on High-Dose Therapy with Hematopoietic Stem Cell Transplantation in Aggressive Non-Hodgkin's Lymphomas, held in Lyon in April 1998, considered HDC to be the standard treatment for relapsing patients under 65 years with aggressive lymphoma.[11]

Several studies have addressed the prognostic influence of different parameters at diagnosis or at time of relapse (Table 10.2).[9,16,18,19] One of the pre-eminent prognostic factors was the delay between the first-line induction therapy and the relapse: patients relapsing within 1 year of the initiation of their first treatment were unlikely to respond to salvage therapy and then to HDC, while patients relapsing more than 1 year after their first treatment could gain a substantial benefit from HDC.[24] Other factors identified were the disease status at time of HDC (CR versus partial response versus stable or refractory disease), the number of previous lines of treatment (first-line versus second-line versus subsequent lines), the presence of a large tumour, lactic dehydrogenase (LDH) above normal level, and performance status at time of

Table 10.1 Results of the PARMA randomized trial in relapsing aggressive lymphomas[10,80]

	High-dose chemotherapy plus autotransplant (%)	DHAP (%)	p value
5-year event-free survival	46	12	0.0001
5-year overall survival	53	32	0.038
8-year event-free survival	36	11	<0.002
8-year overall survival	47	27	0.042

Table 10.2 Prognostic factors for aggressive lymphoma patients undergoing stem cell transplantation; only studies including at least 100 patients are presented

Author	No. of patients	Prognostic parameters
Philip et al. (1987)[9]	100	Chemosensitivity, remission at time of HDC
Petersen et al. (1990)[17]	101	Disease history, performance status
Vose et al. (1993)[20]	158	Chemosensitivity, tumour mass, number of previous treatments, LDH level
Conde et al. (1974)[21]	104	Performance status, remission at time of HDC
Mills et al. (1995)[22]	107	Chemosensitivity, tumour mass, number of previous lines of treatment
Majolino et al. (1997)[23]	1915	Chemosensitivity, number of previous lines of treatment
Blay et al. (1998)[19]	109	International Prognostic Index at time of relapse

relapse (Table 10.2). The results of the PARMA study also showed that relapsing patients with one or more adverse factors of the IPI were more likely to benefit from transplantation than those without any adverse prognostic factor at relapse.[19]

A 1997 randomized study addressed the optimal schedule of dose intensification supported with autologous peripheral stem cells in relapsing patients. The LNH-RP93 trial[25] included 66 patients with relapsing or refractory aggressive lymphoma who received a first course of salvage chemotherapy followed by peripheral blood stem cell harvest. Patients without progression were then randomized between immediate HDC with the ICE regimen (ifosfamide, carboplatin and etoposide) or the administration of two additional courses of intensive chemotherapy before HDC. Despite a higher toxicity and the occurrence of some progressions during this intensive chemotherapy, the progression-free survival and overall survival were significantly higher in patients who received additional courses of salvage chemotherapy. Therefore, these preliminary results support the concept that a maximum response to salvage therapy should be obtained before proceeding to HDC or that HDC is associated with the best results when it is used at a time of minimal persisting tumour. It is not indicated for untested relapsing patients.

Taken together, these data indicate that the standard treatment for patients with aggressive lymphoma who relapse after complete remission should be intensive salvage therapy until the best achievable response, followed by HDC and autologous transplant.[11] There has been no randomized study that addresses the therapeutic value of HDC in patients who have bone marrow involvement or specific lymphomas. Nevertheless, if these patients respond to the salvage therapy they may also benefit from HDC, as shown in phase II studies. After HDC, 50% of patients experienced a new progression, and some additional therapy may be worthwhile. Trials are underway with modulators of the immune system but their role remains to be demonstrated.

HIGH DOSE CHEMOTHERAPY IN REFRACTORY PATIENTS

Refractoriness to therapy has several definitions but the best one is progression during treatment or during the 6 months after its completion. In this situation, very few patients may be salvaged by any therapy. However, if 10–15% of these patients responded to another type of chemotherapy, HDC may prolong this response in half of them. Patients in relapse and who did not respond to the first salvage regimen are unlikely to respond to a subsequent salvage regimen, but the rare patient who responds may also benefit from HDC.[26] Thus, HDC may be recommended only for a small subset of these patients. However, a recent registry data analysis suggested that some primary refractory patients with aggressive lymphoma might be assisted by HDC supported by autologous transplant.[27] Prospective studies are needed to better identify which refractory patients may benefit from HDC.

HIGH DOSE CHEMOTHERAPY AS PART OF THE FIRST-LINE TREATMENT

Because of the efficacy of HDC in relapsing patients who responded to salvage therapy, several groups have included HDC with autologous transplant as a part of the first-line therapy for patients with poorer outcome. Three different strategies have been explored:

- HDC in patients achieving a complete response after a full course of conventional chemotherapy;
- HDC following abbreviated standard induction therapy;
- high dose induction at the outset.[11]

The first two approaches were usually restricted to patients identified for their poor outcome, using different criteria. Many studies were initiated before the description of the International Prognostic Index,[6] which can predict the outcome of subgroups based on five simple criteria: age, stage, LDH level, performance status and the number of extranodal sites. Therefore, it remains difficult to make an accurate comparison of the patients included in these studies.

In patients achieving a complete response after full course conventional chemotherapy

The LNH87-2 clinical trial, by the Groupe d'Etudes des Lymphomes de l'Adulte (GELA, France), compared HDC using the CBV regimen (cyclophosphamide 6000 mg/m^2, carmustine 300 mg/m^2 and etoposide 1000 mg/m^2), supported by bone marrow stem cells, with outpatient consolidation chemotherapy in patients who achieved a complete remission after a high dose cyclophosphamide, doxorubicin, vincristine, prednisolone (CHOP) induction regimen (ACVB or doxorubicin 75 mg/m^2 day 1, cyclophosphamide 1200 mg/m^2 day 1, vindesine 3 mg/m^2 days 1 and 5, bleomycin 15 mg/m^2 days 1 and 5, and prednisone 60 mg/m^2 days 1–5).[28,29] A total of 541 patients were randomized and the updated results showed no significant difference between the two treatment arms when considering the whole population included in the trial.[26] However, when the poor-prognosis patients, defined by high–intermediate or high risk in the IPI, were considered, the 8-year progression-free survival and overall survival were significantly higher in patients who received transplanted cells (Table 10.3). In the final analysis of the trial, with a median follow-up of 8 years, the benefit observed in the group of poor risk patients treated with HDC increased in terms of disease-free survival and became statistically significant for overall survival, compared with the previous analyses.[30]

In another recently published study, patients were randomized at study entry to receive standard induction therapy (12-week VACOP-B regimen with etoposide, doxorubicin, cyclophosphamide, vincristine, prednisone, and bleomycin) or the same regimen followed by HDC.[31] Patients who were randomized to receive standard therapy and achieve a CR were simply followed; patients who obtained a partial response, no response or relapse underwent conventional salvage therapy with the DHAP regimen. Patients randomized to standard induction therapy and HDC were restaged following induction therapy; patients with complete or partial response and non-responders proceeded to HDC with the BEAM regimen (carmustine, etoposide, cytarabine, melphalan). Sixty patients were randomized in each arm and the median follow-up was less than 4 years. There was no statistical difference between the two groups even though 6-year disease-free survival was higher for patients treated with HDC (80%, compared with 60% for patients treated with standard regimen). A statistical improvement in terms of disease-free survival ($P = 0.008$) and a favourable trend in

---

Table 10.3 Results of the LNH87-2 protocol.[29,30] The LNH-87-2 trial compared high dose therapy with autologous bone marrow transplantation with sequential consolidation chemotherapy in 541 patients in complete remission after ACVB induction chemotherapy. A total of 236 patients were considered to have a high–intermediate or high risk according to the International Prognostic Index

	Sequential consolidation chemotherapy (%)	High dose therapy with autologous bone marrow transplantation (%)	*p* value
All randomized patients			
8-year disease-free survival	52	56	NS
8-year overall survival	64	65	NS
Poor-risk patients			
5-year disease-free survival	39	59	0.01
5-year overall survival	52	65	0.06
Poor-risk patients			
8-year disease-free survival	39	55	0.02
8-year overall survival	49	64	0.04

terms of progression-free survival ($P = 0.08$) for intermediate–high- plus high-risk patients assigned to HDC were observed. However, the number of the patients included in this trial was low, the median follow-up (at time of publication) was short and 29% of the patients assigned to HDC did not receive it. The same conclusions and remarks may be applied to the European Organization for Research and Treatment of Cancer (EORTC) trial recently presented as an abstract.[32] In this trial, the median follow-up was 3 years, only 59% received the planned treatment, and more than two-thirds of the patients did not have a poor prognosis according to the IPI criteria.

Following abbreviated standard induction therapy

Several randomized studies have explored the use of HDC as part of the induction regimen and compared it with a conventional chemotherapy regimen. In the recently completed LNH-93 trial, 370 patients with poor risk according to the age-adjusted IPI were randomized at diagnosis to receive standard therapy with ACVB followed by sequential chemotherapy,[33] or three cycles of abbreviated induction therapy followed by HDC with the BEAM regimen.[34] In the standard chemotherapy arm, only patients who reached a CR continue with sequential chemotherapy, other patients being treated with a salvage regimen and, if they respond, they may receive HDC. In the HDC arm, all patients received the HDC, even in case of poor response to the abbreviated standard chemotherapy. In the initial analysis of this trial, patients who underwent full-course conventional ACVB induction chemotherapy had a better outcome than patients who received early HDC. With a median follow-up of 3 years, the event-free survival and overall survival were 54% and 63% for patients treated with conventional chemotherapy and 41% and 47% for patients receiving early HDC, respectively (both differences statistically significant with P values of 0.01 and 0.003, respectively).[34]

In another trial with a similar design, the German High-Grade Lymphoma Study Group randomized young patients with high LDH levels to receive either five cycles of standard induction therapy or three cycles followed by HDC.[35] In the first report of this study, the 2-year overall survival was similar in the two arms.

Both of these studies failed to confirm an advantage for high dose therapy delivered as part of the induction regimen. However, the induction therapy delivered before HDC was less intensive than that administered with the conventional intensive chemotherapy in the control arm. In both studies patients went in to HDC very early in the course of the treatment, just after three cycles of chemotherapy; even if they responded to this short therapy, they probably did not reach a good complete response and the quality of the response before HDC may be a very important parameter as demonstrated in relapsing patients. The conclusion of these trials favoured the attainment of a good CR before going to HDC.

Upfront high dose induction therapy

Another approach for the treatment of these high-risk patients was to intensify their initial induction therapy.[36,37] In a recent study from Milan, 98 patients with B cell lymphoma without bone marrow involvement but with a bulky tumour or an advanced stage were randomized to receive standard chemotherapy or high dose sequential therapy followed by autologous transplant.[37] Patients treated with HDT had a statistically longer event-free survival: 7-year event-free survival of 76%, compared with 49% for patients treated with standard induction. However, overall survival was not significantly different. One bias in this trial was the fact that partial response to standard therapy was defined as an event and that patients not responding to the allocated treatment were allowed to cross over. Moreover, the results of this high dose sequential therapy regimen were never reproduced.

In recent years, the development of peripheral stem cell reinfusion has allowed the delivery of repeated cycles of intensive chemotherapy in order to increase the dose intensity of induction regimens.[38,39] Whether this approach has a benefit for high-risk lymphoma patients is a question that merits its comparison with standard treatment and other dose-intensive induction regimens that can be administered without peripheral stem cell reinfusion.[33,36]

Conclusion

In conclusion, the use of HDC in the first-line treatment of patients who have aggressive lymphoma with adverse prognosis still needs to be clarified. In our opinion, the results of the LNH87-2 study indicate that HDC as a consolidation is recommended in poor-prognosis patients achieving a CR or a very good partial response after a full induction therapy. Other indications have to be tested in controlled randomized studies, as outlined in the above-cited consensus conference.[11] It may also be interesting to stratify cases not only using the IPI but also according to the different histological entities (B cell versus T cell, mediastinal large cell with sclerosis, anaplastic large cell lymphoma, etc.) since it appears likely that the outcome of patients with these different entities is somewhat different.[40,41] New biological prognostic factors may also help in identifying patients who may benefit from this intensification.[42]

HIGH DOSE CHEMOTHERAPY IN PATIENTS WITH PARTIAL RESPONSE AT THE END OF THE FIRST TREATMENT

Some studies have examined the role of HDC in patients whose response to initial standard therapy was judged insufficient. However, this setting is not very well defined and the results are difficult to interpret. These patients correspond to at least four situations: those with a true partial response at the end of the planned treatment, i.e. patients in whom lymphoma cells persist in bone marrow or some residual sites; those whose tumour regrows soon after the end of the treatment, i.e. refractory disease; those responding slowly to the initial treatment but who may reach a CR at the end; those in CRu with persisting masses of unknown significance. Patents in CRu have a disease-free survival not different from those in true CR[33,43,44] and no study concludes in favour of intensifying treatment for these patients. If PET scanning is able to show residual tumour, it may be interesting to consider these patients as true partial responders and then to intensify their therapy, but such a study has not been realized yet.[45]

Slow-responding patients may be defined as patients with a slow reduction of the tumour volume during chemotherapy or those with persisting tumour on gallium scan or PET scan fixation after two or three courses of chemotherapy. The first group of patients, those with a slow decrease in radiological abnormalities, may not have such a poor outcome if they reach a CR or a CRu at the end of the treatment. To intensify therapy in the middle of its planned course because of these persisting radiological abnormalities is no more justified than treatment intensification for patients with CRu. One randomized study realized in this setting shows similar results for patients who continued with the planned treatment and those whose treatment was intensified.[46] Another study randomized clinically partially responding patients into continuing chemotherapy with the DHAP regimen or HDC with the BEAC regimen and showed a non-statistically significant longer progression-free survival for patients receiving HDC.[47] However, the number of patients in these studies was limited (69 and 49, respectively), impairing a general conclusion. Furthermore, the criteria used to define partial response were not uniformly defined and accepted. It seems that patients with persisting tumour on fixation on gallium scan or PET scan after a few chemotherapy courses have a much higher risk of failure.[45] High dose chemotherapy will be a logical choice for them, but no randomized trial has been conducted in this setting yet.

The only indication for HDC therapy in partial response may be for patients with a true partial response at the end of the initial treatment. However, no randomized study has been done in this setting and only phase II reports or compilations of registries of selected patients have been presented. These reports have showed a benefit for patients whose treatment was intensified in PR.[48]

HIGH DOSE CHEMOTHERAPY IN PATIENTS WITH NON-DLCL AGGRESSIVE LYMPHOMAS

The data presented earlier were obtained in trials that included patients with so-called aggressive lymphomas, which are diffuse large B-cell lymphomas in 80% of cases. These results may be applied to other lymphomas with aggressive behaviour, such as mantle cell lymphoma, Burkitt's lymphoma or peripheral T cell lymphomas with little modification of results.

Mantle cell lymphoma

Mantle cell lymphoma patients have an especially poor outcome, even with their initial clinical indolent presentation, because sustained long-term remission is rarely achieved with conventional treatment and refractoriness to chemotherapy leads to short survival.[49] Reports of HDC with autologous bone marrow transplant in mantle cell lymphoma have been rather disappointing.[50,51] Other recent studies using peripheral blood stem cells showed that a high rate of complete remission can be obtained, and some studies have indicated that good long-term disease-free and overall survival may be achieved with this treatment.[52–54] The experience reported in these short series suggests, however, that the best benefit can be obtained when HDC is performed early in the disease course in patients who have achieved a good response to first-line chemotherapy. A randomized European study testing HDC after

induction therapy is now being performed in mantle cell lymphoma.

Lymphoblastic lymphoma

Although lymphoblastic lymphoma is a rare disease in adult patients, several studies have been performed using HDC during the first-line therapy or at relapse.[55,56] A report from the EBMT evaluated this therapeutic approach in 214 patients and indicated that some relapsing patients can achieve long-term survival with this treatment.[57] Randomized studies are ongoing but, because of the low incidence of this lymphoma, they may never conclude. Results obtained for adult patients with acute lymphoblastic leukemia with a T cell phenotype have also failed to demonstrate the therapeutic value of HDC.[58] Whether the use of peripheral blood stem cells may modify these findings remains therefore to be determined, especially if these patients with lymphoblastic lymphoma were treated with intensive leukemia-like chemotherapy. Allogeneic stem cell transplantation may also be considered in this setting but its efficacy has not been determined in a randomized trial.

Burkitt's lymphoma

Several reports have included variable numbers of this particular aggressive subtype. However, the optimal therapeutic approach for adults with Burkitt's lymphoma has still to be defined and there is no evidence for a role of high dose therapy in untreated patients.[59,60] In partially responding or relapsing patients, HDC has clearly been of benefit in a small subset of patients, but its use is frequently hampered by bone marrow and central nervous system disease dissemination.[60]

Peripheral T-cell lymphoma

Several reports have included patients with peripheral T cell lymphoma, which has been shown to be a more aggressive disease than B cell diffuse large cell lymphoma.[40] It has been proposed that some patients with this lymphoma may particularly benefit from HDC,[61] although these findings have not been demonstrated in a randomized trial.

OPEN QUESTIONS REGARDING THE OPTIMAL HDC MODALITIES IN LYMPHOMA PATIENTS

Is peripheral blood progenitor preferable to bone marrow?

Although most studies were performed with stem cells harvested from bone marrow until the end of the 1980s, the use of mobilized peripheral blood stem cells has been increasing since the beginning of the last decade. The ease of peripheral blood progenitor collection in lymphoma patients, the faster haemopoietic recovery after peripheral blood stem cell infusion compared with bone marrow and the ability to harvest peripheral stem cells in patients who have received previous pelvic radiotherapy all constituted strong advantages favouring the use of peripheral blood stem cells.[62] However, only a few studies were performed to compare bone marrow with peripheral blood as the origin of the stem cells. One randomized trial included 58 patients with lymphoma (non-Hodgkin's and Hodgkin's) and demonstrated a substantial benefit for haematological recovery in patients receiving peripheral blood stem cells, for both neutrophils (11 days versus 14 days, $P = 0.005$) and platelets (16 days versus 23 days, $P = 0.02$).[63] Recently, 227 non-Hodgkin's lymphoma patients who received HDC with peripheral blood stem cell transplantation and who were registered in the EBMT database were pair-matched with the same number of patients who received bone marrow cells.[23] Interestingly, the number of toxic deaths was found to be similar in both groups (13.6% with peripheral blood stem cells versus 13.7% with bone marrow). The long-term outcome was similar in the two groups for both

progression-free and overall survival, indicating that there is a significant difference in the therapeutic use of each stem cell source.

Therefore, the adherence to the practice of using peripheral blood stem cells is largely based on this product's ability to hasten haemopoietic recovery rather than on established and demonstrated clinical superiority, either for a decreased incidence of lethal toxicity or for the improvement of long-term survival.

Are peripheral blood stem cells less contaminated with tumour cell than bone marrow stem cells?

Tumour cell contamination of the graft has been a logical worry for physicians administering autologous cells to lymphoma patients. Follicular lymphoma can be considered as a paradigm for this issue, given the frequency of bone marrow involvement in this disease and the presence of a molecular marker in tumour cells which can be detected using the very sensitive polymerase chain reaction (PCR). A study evaluated the growth of tumour cells in the haemopoietic harvest in lymphoma patients and found that patients with detectable tumour cells had a worse outcome than those without tumour cell growth.[64] These data supported the notion that tumour cells reinfused into the patient might contribute to the relapse. On the other hand, one may argue that patients who became PCR negative after purging could have a more favourable outcome because of a lower percentage of marrow involvement and a higher sensitivity of tumour cells to chemotherapy. The positive influence of bone marrow graft purging was not supported by a comparison of registry data[65] and therefore still remains a matter of debate.

Is there a role for stem cell selection?

When using autologous peripheral blood stem cells, both positive and negative selection can be performed on the harvest before reinfusion. Patients transplanted with selected peripheral CD34+ cells seem to engraft well, with an eventual minor delay in platelet recovery in comparison with patients reinfused with unselected cells.[66] In addition, many studies have demonstrated that these selection processes can deplete the graft of tumour cells by a factor of 2–4 log.[67] However, there are no established data supporting a clinical benefit for the use of these expensive and somewhat cumbersome techniques. At the time of writing, stem cell selection remains an investigative procedure that should be reserved for clinical trials.

In vivo, monoclonal antibody therapy was able to purge the harvest in patients with follicular lymphoma.[68] However, so far no study has shown that this may be applied to patients who have a more aggressive lymphoma.

Is there a best conditioning regimen in lymphoma patients?

Autologous transplant has been performed with several different chemotherapy regimens (Table 10.4) and with the use of total body irradiation combined with cyclophosphamide and etoposide.[71] This later modality has been mostly used for indolent and low-grade lymphoma, while chemotherapy alone is more popular for aggressive lymphoma subtypes. At present, no randomized comparison has been performed between these different preparative regimens. The CBV regimen and the BEAM regimen may have the same therapeutic value, and regimens that include total body irradiation have not been proved to be superior to chemotherapy-alone regimens, particularly in aggressive lymphomas.[71]

Is there a place for allogeneic stem cell in HDC for lymphoma patients?

High dose chemotherapy with allogeneic stem cell transplantation has two theoretical advantages over HDC with autologous stem cell

Table 10.4 Intensive chemotherapy regimens most frequently used for high dose therapy in lymphoma patients

Regimen	Drug	Dose (mg/m²)
CBV*	Cyclophosphamide	6000
	Carmustine	300
	Etoposide	1000
BEAM†	Carmustine	300
	Etoposide	800
	Cytarabine	800
	Melphalan	140
BEAC	Carmustine	300
	Etoposide	800
	Cytarabine	800
	Cyclophosphamide	5600
ICE	Ifosfamide	9000
	Carboplatinum	1500
	Etoposide	1500

*A reinforced CBV regimen is sometimes used with increased dose of the initial drugs[69] or with the addition of mitoxantrone (30–60 mg/m²).[70]
†Doses of etoposide and cytarabine can also be increased up to two-fold.

transplant: lymphoma cells do not contaminate stem cells and a graft-versus-lymphoma effect may increase the therapeutic effect. Numerous studies have been devoted to resistant indolent lymphomas[72] and a few included aggressive lymphomas. None of these randomized trial permits any conclusions but the higher toxic death rate did not counterbalance the lower relapse rate in most of the studies, resulting in a lower survival in patients treated with HDC and allogeneic transplant.[73] The small successes achieved in patients who relapsed after autologous cell transplant were, however, encouraging,[74] as was the lesser toxicity observed with non-myeloablative conditioning regimens.[75] Definitive answers on the place of this technique need further studies.[11]

FUTURE DIRECTIONS FOR AUTOLOGOUS TRANSPLANTATION IN LYMPHOMA PATIENTS

Although lymphoma constitutes one of the haematological malignancies in which HDC has contributed to therapeutic advances in the last two decades, many patients still relapse after this treatment. Several ways have been recently explored to decrease the number of relapses. Some studies are evaluating the possibility of using repeated HDC cycles supported with stem cells, either as tandem transplant[76] or with sequential high-dose non-myeloablative regimens.[38,39] The tandem transplant approach should be strictly monitored because it may expose patients to additional immunosuppression and toxicities.[77] The eventual benefits of these modalities remain to be established in prospective randomized studies and they may not be recommended outside clinical trials.

The use of radiolabelled antibodies targeted against tumour cells has been also explored, with very encouraging results in association with HDC.[78] Rituximab, a non-labelled monoclonal antibody, has a proven efficacy in indolent and aggressive lymphoma.[79,80] It has been associated with disappearance of lymphoma cells from blood and bone marrow, even in the absence of complete response.[81] Thus, it may be used to purge the blood before the stem cell collection. Trials are running to test this hypothesis and the first results showed that rituximab effectively depleted the blood of lymphoma cells; however, the clinical efficacy on the reduction of post-transplant relapses has not yet been demonstrated.[68]

Finally, specific or non-specific immunotherapy in the minimal residual state achieved after HDC should also be considered. The possibility of inducing an autologous immune reaction mimicking the graft-versus-host reaction observed in the allogeneic setting has been investigated with some preliminary interesting results.[82] Administration of cytokines, such as interferon or interleukin-2,[83] as well as monoclonal antibodies targeting tumour cells, after transplant is worth testing. Additional reinfusion of activated or educated autologous stem cells can also be tested, as well as the combination of allogeneic T cell and autologous stem cell reinfusion.[84]

REFERENCES

1. Jaffe ES, Harris NL, Diebold J et al. World Health Organization Classification of lymphomas: a work in progress. Ann Oncol 1998;9:25–30.
2. Jaffe ES, Harris NL, Stein H, Vardiman JW. World Health Organization classification of tumours: pathology and genetics of tumours of the hematopoietic and lymphoid tissues. Lyon, IARC, 2001.
3. The Non-Hodgkin's Lymphoma Classification Project. A clinical trial of the International Lymphoma Study Group classification of non-Hodgkin's lymphoma. Blood 1997;89:3909–18.
4. Armitage JO, Weisenburger DD. New approach to classifying non-Hodgkin's lymphomas: clinical features of the major histologic subtypes. J Clin Oncol 1998;16:2780–95.
5. Coiffier B. Non-Hodgkin's lymphomas. In: Cavalli F, Hansen HH, Kaye SB, editors. Textbook of medical oncology. London: Martin Dunitz Ltd, 1999.
6. The International Non-Hodgkin's Lymphoma Prognostic Factors Project. A predictive model for aggressive non-Hodgkin's lymphoma. N Engl J Med 1993;329:987–94.
7. Shipp MA. Prognostic factors in aggressive non-Hodgkin's lymphoma: who has high-risk disease? Blood 1994;83:1165–73.
8. Appelbaum FR, Herzig GP, Ziegler JL et al. Successful engraftment of cryopreserved autologous bone marrow in patients with malignant lymphoma. Blood 1978;52:85–95.
9. Philip T, Armitage JO, Spitzer G et al. High-dose therapy and autologous bone marrow transplantation after failure of conventional chemotherapy in adults with intermediate-grade or high-grade non-Hodgkin's lymphoma. N Engl J Med 1987; 316:1493–8.
10. Philip T, Guglielmi C, Hagenbeek A et al. Autologous bone marrow transplantation as

compared with salvage chemotherapy in relapses of chemotherapy-sensitive non Hodgkin's lymphoma. N Engl J Med 1995;333:1540–5.

11. Shipp MA, Abeloff MD, Antman KH et al. International Consensus Conference on High-Dose Therapy with Hematopoietic Stem Cell Transplantation in Aggressive Non-Hodgkin's Lymphomas: report of the jury. J Clin Oncol 1999;17:423–9.

12. Ketterer N, Espinouse D, Chomarat M et al. Infections following peripheral blood progenitor cell transplantation for lymphoproliferative malignancies: etiology and potential risk factors. Am J Med 1999;106:191–7.

13. Ketterer N, Sonet A, Dumontet C et al. Toxicities after peripheral blood progenitor cell transplantation for lymphoid malignancies: analysis of 300 cases in a single institution. Bone Marrow Transplant 1999;23:1309–15.

14. Gratwohl A, Passweg J, Baldomero H et al. Blood and marrow transplantation activity in Europe 1997. Bone Marrow Transplant 1999;24:231–45.

15. Takvorian T, Canellos GP, Ritz J et al. Prolonged disease-free survival after autologous bone marrow transplantation in patients with non-Hodgkin's lymphoma with a poor prognosis. N Engl J Med 1987;316:1499–505.

16. Vose JM, Armitage JO, Bierman PJ et al. Salvage therapy for relapsed or refractory non-Hodgkin's lymphoma utilizing autologous bone marrow transplantation. Am J Med 1989;87:285–8.

17. Petersen FB, Appelbaum FR, Hill R et al. Autologous marrow transplantation for malignant lymphoma. A report of 101 cases from Seattle. J Clin Oncol 1990;8:638–47.

18. Bosly A, Coffier B, Gisselbrecht C et al. Bone marrow transplantation prolongs survival after relapse in aggressive lymphoma patients treated with the LNH-84 regimen. J Clin Oncol 1992;10:1615–23.

19. Blay JY, Gomez F, Sebban C et al. The International Prognostic Index correlates to survival in patients with aggressive lymphoma in relapse: analysis of the Parma trial. Blood 1998;92:3562–8.

20. Vose JM, Anderson JR, Kessinger A et al. High-dose chemotherapy and autologous hematopoietic stem-cell transplantation for aggressive non-Hodgkin's lymphoma. J Clin Oncol 1993;11:1846–51.

21. Conde E, Sierra J, Iriondo A et al. Prognostic factors in patients who received autologous bone marrow transplantation for non-Hodgkin's lymphoma. Report of 104 patients from the Spanish cooperative group GEL/TAMO. Bone Marrow Transplant 1994;14:279–86.

22. Mills W, Chopra R, Mcmillan A et al. BEAM chemotherapy and autologous bone marrow transplantation for patients with relapsed or refractory non-Hodgkin's lymphoma. J Clin Oncol 1995;13:588–95.

23. Majolino I, Pearce R, Taghipour G et al. Peripheral blood stem cell transplantation versus autologous bone marrow transplantation in Hodgkin's and non-Hodgkin's lymphomas: a new matched-pair analysis of the European Group for Blood and Marrow Transplantation Registry data. J Clin Oncol 1997;15:509–17.

24. Guglielmi C, Gomez F, Philip T et al. Time to relapse has prognostic value in patients with aggressive lymphoma enrolled onto the Parma trial. J Clin Oncol 1998;16:3264–9.

25. Bosly A, Sonnet A, Salles G et al. Superiority of late over early intensification in relapsing/refractory aggressive non-Hodgkin's lymphoma: a randomized study from the GELA: LNH-RP93. Blood 1997;90(suppl 1):594 (abstract).

26. Coiffier B, Philip T, Burnett AK et al. Consensus Conference on Intensive Chemotherapy plus Hematopoietic Stem Cell Transplantation in Malignancies, Lyon, France, June 4–6, 1993. J Clin Oncol 1994;12:226–31.

27. Vose JM, Rowlings PA, Lazarus HM et al. Multivariate analysis of autotransplantations for patients with aggressive non-Hodgkin's lymphoma failing primary induction therapy. Blood 1997;90(suppl 1):594 (abstract).

28. Haïoun C, Lepage E, Gisselbrecht C et al. Comparison of autologous bone marrow transplantation with sequential chemotherapy for intermediate-grade and high-grade non-Hodgkin's lymphoma in first complete remission. A study of 464 patients. J Clin Oncol 1994;12:2543–51.

29. Haïoun C, Lepage E, Gisselbrecht C et al. Benefit of autologous bone marrow transplantation over sequential chemotherapy in poor-risk aggressive non-Hodgkin's lymphoma. Updated results of the prospective study LNH87-2. J Clin Oncol 1997;15:1131–7.

30. Haïoun C, Lepage E, Gisselbrecht C et al. Survival benefit of high-dose therapy over

sequential chemotherapy in poor-risk aggressive non-Hodgkin's lymphoma. Final analysis of the prospective LNH87-2 protocol, a Groupe d'Etude des Lymphomes de L'Adulte study. J Clin Oncol 2000;18:3025–30.

31. Santini G, Salvagno L, Leoni P et al. VACOP-B versus VACOP-B plus autologous bone marrow transplantation for advanced diffuse non-Hodgkin's lymphoma: results of a prospective randomized trial by the Non-Hodgkin's Lymphoma Cooperative Study Group. J Clin Oncol 1998;16:2796–802.

32. Kluin-Nelemans J-C, Zagonel V, Anastaso-poulou A et al. Standard chemotherapy with or without high-dose chemotherapy for aggressive non-Hodgkin's lymphoma: randomized phase II EORTC study. J Natl Cancer Inst 2001;93:22–30.

33. Coiffier B. Fourteen years of high-dose CHOP (ACVB regimen): preliminary conclusions about the treatment of aggressive-lymphoma patients. Ann Oncol 1995;6:211–17.

34. Reyes F, Lepage E, Morel P et al. Failure of first-line inductive high-dose chemotherapy in poor-risk patients with aggressive lymphoma: updated results of the randomized LNH93-3 study. Blood 1997;90(suppl 1):594 (abstract).

35. Kaiser U, Uebelacker I, Havemann K. High dose chemotherapy with autologous stem cell trans-plantation in high grade NHL: first analysis of a randomized multicenter study. Bone Marrow Transplant 1998;21(suppl 1):177.

36. Shipp MA, Neuberg D, Janicek M et al. High-dose CHOP as initial therapy for patients with poor-prognosis aggressive non-Hodgkin's lym-phoma: a dose-finding pilot study. J Clin Oncol 1995;13:2916–23.

37. Gianni AM, Bregni M, Siena S et al. High-dose chemotherapy and autologous bone marrow transplantation compared with MACOP-B in aggressive B-cell lymphoma. N Engl J Med 1997; 336:1290–7.

38. Shea TC, Mason JR, Storniolo AM et al. High-dose carboplatin chemotherapy with GM-CSF and peripheral blood progenitor cell support: a model for delivering repeated cycles of dose-intensive therapy. Cancer Treat Rev 1993;19: 11–20.

39. Stoppa AM, Bouabdallah R, Chabannon C et al. Intensive sequential chemotherapy with repeated blood stem-cell support for untreated poor-prognosis non-Hodgkin's lymphoma. J Clin Oncol 1997;15:1722–9.

40. Gisselbrecht C, Gaulard P, Lepage E et al. Prognostic significance of T-cell phenotype in aggressive non-Hodgkin's lymphomas. Blood 1998;92:76–82.

41. Tilly H, Gaulard P, Lepage E et al. Primary anaplastic large-cell lymphoma in adults: clinical presentation, immunophenotype, and outcome. Blood 1997;90:3727–34.

42. Salles G. Towards new prognostic factors in dif-fuse large cell non-Hodgkin's lymphoma. Ann Oncol 1996;7:993–6.

43. Surbone A, Longo DL, DeVita VT et al. Residual abdominal masses in aggressive non-Hodgkin's lymphoma after combination chemotherapy: sig-nificance and management. J Clin Oncol 1988; 6:1832–7.

44. Cheson BD, Horning SJ, Coiffier B et al. Report of an International Workshop to standardize response criteria for non-Hodgkin's lymphomas. J Clin Oncol 1999;17:1244–53.

45. Coiffier B. How to interpret the radiological abnormalities that persist after treatment in non-Hodgkin's lymphoma patients? Ann Oncol 1999;10:1141–3.

46. Verdonck LF, Van Putten W, Hagenbeek A et al. Comparison of CHOP chemotherapy with autol-ogous bone marrow transplantation for slowly responding patients with aggressive non-Hodgkin's lymphoma. N Engl J Med 1995;332: 1045–51.

47. Martelli M, Vignetti M, Zinzani PL et al. High-dose chemotherapy followed by autologous bone marrow transplantation versus dexametha-sone, cisplatin, and cytarabine in aggressive non-Hodgkin's lymphoma with partial response to front-line chemotherapy. A prospective random-ized Italian multicenter study. J Clin Oncol 1996; 14:534–43.

48. Haïoun C, Lepage E, Gisselbrecht C et al. High-dose therapy followed by stem cell transplanta-tion in partial response after first-line induction therapy for aggressive non-Hodgkin's lym-phoma. Ann Oncol 1998;9:5–8.

49. Coiffier B. Which treatment for mantle-cell lym-phoma patients in 1998? J Clin Oncol 1998; 16:3–5.

50. Stewart DA, Vose JM, Weisenburger DD et al. The role of high-dose therapy and autologous hematopoietic stem cell transplantation for man-tle cell lymphoma. Ann Oncol 1995;6:263–6.

51. Freedman AS, Neuberg D, Gribben JG et al. High-dose chemoradiotherapy and anti-B-cell

monoclonal antibody purged autologous bone marrow transplantation in mantle-cell lymphoma: no evidence for long-term remission. J Clin Oncol 1998;16:13–18.

52. Haas R, Brittinger G, Meusers P et al. Myeloablative therapy with blood stem cell transplantation is effective in mantle cell lymphoma. Leukemia 1996;10:1975–9.

53. Ketterer N, Salles G, Espinouse D et al. Intensive therapy with peripheral stem cell transplantation in 16 patients with mantle cell lymphoma. Ann Oncol 1997;8:701–4.

54. Kroger N, Hoffknecht M, Dreger P et al. Long-term disease-free survival of patients with advanced mantle-cell lymphoma following high-dose chemotherapy. Bone Marrow Transplant 1998;21:55–7.

55. Milpied N, Gaillard F, Moreau P et al. High-dose therapy with stem cell transplantation for mantle cell lymphoma: results and prognostic factors. A single center experience. Bone Marrow Transplant 1998;22:645–50.

56. Bouabdallah R, Xerri L, Bardou VJ et al. Role of induction chemotherapy and bone marrow transplantation in adult lymphoblastic lymphoma: a report on 62 patients from a single center. Ann Oncol 1998;9:619–25.

57. Sweetenham JW, Pearce R, Philip T et al. High-dose therapy and autologous bone marrow transplantation for intermediate and high grade non-Hodgkin's lymphoma in patients aged 55 years and over: results from the European Group for Bone Marrow Transplantation. Bone Marrow Transplant 1994;14:981–7.

58. Boucheix C, David B, Sebban C et al. Immunophenotype of adult acute lymphoblastic leukemia, clinical parameters, and outcome: an analysis of a prospective trial including 562 tested patients (LALA87). French Group on Therapy for Adult Acute Lymphoblastic Leukemia. Blood 1994;84:1603–12.

59. Patte C, Michon J, Frappaz D et al. Therapy of Burkitt and other B-cell acute lymphoblastic leukaemia and lymphoma: experience with the LMB protocols of the SFOP (French Paediatric Oncology Society) in children and adults. Clin Haematol 1994;7:339–48.

60. Sweetenham JW, Pearce R, Taghipour G et al. Adult Burkitt's and Burkitt-like non-Hodgkin's lymphoma: outcome for patients treated with high-dose therapy and autologous stem-cell transplantation in first remission or at relapse.

Results from the European Group for Blood and Marrow Transplantation. J Clin Oncol 1996;14:2465–72.

61. Vose JM, Peterson C, Bierman PJ et al. Comparison of high-dose therapy and autologous bone marrow transplantation for T-cell and B-cell non-Hodgkin's lymphomas. Blood 1990;76:424–31.

62. Kessinger A. Consensus Conference on High-Dose Therapy with Hematopoietic Stem Cell Transplantation in Diffuse Large-Cell Lymphoma: type of cells, optimal mobilization of stem cells. Positive and negative selection. Ann Oncol 1998;9:23–30.

63. Schmitz N, Linch DC, Dreger P et al. Randomised trial of filgrastim-mobilised peripheral blood progenitor cell transplantation versus autologous bone-marrow transplantation in lymphoma patients. Lancet 1996;347:353–7.

64. Sharp JG, Kessinger A, Mann S et al. Outcome of high-dose therapy and autologous transplantation in non-Hodgkin's lymphoma based the presence of tumor in the marrow or infused hematopoietic harvest. J Clin Oncol 1996;14:214–19.

65. Williams CD, Goldstone AH, Pearce RM et al. Purging of bone marrow in autologous bone marrow transplantation for non-Hodgkin's lymphoma. A case-matched comparison with unpurged cases by the European Blood and Marrow Transplant Lymphoma Registry. J Clin Oncol 1996;14:2454–64.

66. Brugger W, Scheding S, Bock T et al. Purging of peripheral blood progenitor cell autografts and treatment of minimal residual disease. Stem Cells 1997;15:159–65.

67. Gorin NC, Lopez M, Laporte JP et al. Preparation and successful engraftment of purified CD34+ bone marrow progenitor cells in patients with non-Hodgkin's lymphoma. Blood 1995;85:1647–54.

68. Salles G, Moillet I, Charlot C et al. In vivo purging with rituximab before autologous peripheral blood progenitor cell transplantation in lymphoma patients. Blood 1999;94.

69. Wheeler C, Antin JH, Churchill WH et al. Cyclophosphamide, carmustine, and etoposide with autologous bone marrow transplantation in refractory Hodgkin's disease and non-Hodgkin's lymphoma: a dose-finding study. J Clin Oncol 1990;8:648–56.

70. Attal M, Canal P, Schlaifer D et al. Escalating

dose of mitoxantrone with high-dose cyclophosphamide, carmustine, and etoposide in patients with refractory lymphoma undergoing autologous bone marrow transplantation. J Clin Oncol 1994;12:141–8.

71. Mounier N, Gisselbrecht C. Conditioning regimens before transplantation in patients with aggressive non-Hodgkin's lymphoma. Ann Oncol 1998;9:15–21.

72. Van Besien K, Sobocinski K, Rowlings PA et al. Allogeneic bone marrow transplantation for low-grade lymphoma. Blood 1998;92:1832–6.

73. Chopra R, Goldstone AH, Pearce R et al. Autologous versus allogeneic bone marrow transplantation for non-Hodgkin's lymphoma: a case–controlled analysis of the European Bone Marrow Transplant group registry data. J Clin Oncol 1992;10:1690–5.

74. Tsai T, Goodman S, Saez R et al. Allogeneic bone marrow transplantation in patients who relapse after autologous transplantation. Bone Marrow Transplant 1997;20:859–63.

75. Khouri IF, Keating M, Korbling M et al. Transplant-lite: induction of graft-versus-malignancy using fludarabine-based nonablative chemotherapy and allogeneic blood progenitor cell transplantation as treatment for lymphoid malignancies. J Clin Oncol 1998;16:2817–24.

76. Vandenberghe E, Pearce R, Taghipour G et al. Role of a second transplant in the management of poor-prognosis lymphomas: a report from the European Blood and Bone Marrow Registry. J Clin Oncol 1997;15:1595–600.

77. Haïoun C, Gisselbrecht C, Quesnel B et al. Double autotransplant as first line consolidative treatment in poor-risk aggressive lymphoma: a

pilot study of 31 patients. Bone Marrow Transplant 1998;21(suppl 1):174.

78. Press OW, Eary JF, Appelbaum FR et al. Phase II trial of I-131-B1 (anti-CD20) antibody therapy with autologous stem cell transplantation for relapsed B cell lymphomas. Lancet 1995;346:336–40.

79. McLaughlin P, Grillo-Lopez AJ, Link BK et al. Rituximab chimeric anti-CD20 monoclonal antibody therapy for relapsed indolent lymphoma: half of patients respond to a four-dose treatment program. J Clin Oncol 1998;16:2825–33.

80. Coiffier B, Haïoun C, Ketterer N et al. Rituximab (anti-CD20 monoclonal antibody) for the treatment of patients with relapsing or refractory aggressive lymphoma. A multicenter phase II study. Blood 1998;92:1927–32.

81. Lopez-Guillermo A, Cabanillas F, McLaughlin P et al. The clinical significance of molecular response in indolent follicular lymphomas. Blood 1998;91:2955–60.

82. Gryn J, Johnson E, Goldman N et al. The treatment of relapsed or refractory intermediate grade non-Hodgkin's lymphoma with autologous bone marrow transplantation followed by cyclosporine and interferon. Bone Marrow Transplant 1997;19:221–6.

83. Slavin S, Nagler A. Immunotherapy in conjunction with autologous and allogeneic blood or marrow transplantation in lymphoma. Ann Oncol 1998;9:31–9.

84. Guillaume T, Rubinstein DB, Symann M. Immune reconstitution and immunotherapy after autologous hematopoietic stem cell transplantation. Blood 1998;92:1471–90.

11

High dose chemotherapy in ovarian cancer

Jonathan A Ledermann and Ruth Herd

CONTENTS   Background • What is the evidence for a dose effect in the treatment of ovarian cancer? • High dose chemotherapy in advanced ovarian cancer • High dose chemotherapy as initial treatment for ovarian cancer • Multicycle high dose chemotherapy • Randomized trials – the future • Conclusions

BACKGROUND

Ovarian cancer is the fourth most common female cancer and accounts for 6% of all cancer deaths in women. Its incidence rises rapidly over the age of 30 years; 20% of cases occur in women under 50 years and approximately 50% of cases are in women under 65 years of age. Early stages of the disease are often asymptomatic and, at the time of diagnosis, the majority of women have advanced disease. Surgery has an important diagnostic and therapeutic role in ovarian cancer. Removal of the ovaries, fallopian tubes, uterus, omentum and other large masses is followed by chemotherapy; the survival rate is better in patients with only a small amount of residual disease after tumour debulking surgery.[1] Chemotherapy plays an important role in the management of advanced disease: tumour responses are seen in the majority of patients with residual disease, or those in whom debulking surgery is not possible. However, there is uncertainty about the value of chemotherapy in early FIGO (Federation International of Gynaecological Oncologists) stage I tumours.

Over the last 25 years many new drugs have been introduced to treat advanced ovarian cancer. Platinum-based drugs (cisplatin or carboplatin) are the most active single agents, with tumour responses occurring in 70–80% of patients; in 40–50% of cases these responses are complete. Cisplatin is more active than single alkylating agents such as melphalan, chlorambucil or cyclophosphamide. Combination therapy with cisplatin and cyclophosphamide, or this combination plus doxorubicin (Adriamycin) (CAP), was the standard treatment for advanced ovarian cancer for many years.[2,3] There seems to be equivalence between cisplatin and carboplatin,[4,5] and the latter has lower toxicity. However, combination therapies with carboplatin have to be carefully designed because it is myelosuppressive. Mature data from randomized trials have shown that approximately 25–30% of patients with advanced ovarian cancer can be expected to survive 5 years.[6] Recently taxanes have been incorporated into the treatment of ovarian cancer. The activity of paclitaxel (Taxol) in platinum-resistant relapsed disease[7] has led to its introduction into 'first-line' therapy. Response and survival with cisplatin and paclitaxel (Taxol) appear to be superior to standard cisplatin and cyclophosphamide.[8,9] Many would regard six cycles of cisplatin or carboplatin and paclitaxel as the standard therapy for ovarian cancer.

Many patients will enter a complete remission following surgery and chemotherapy but will relapse after a median interval of approximately 18 months from diagnosis. In these patients, residual microscopic disease remains resistant to standard doses of drugs. Prolongation of chemotherapy has not been shown to improve survival.[10,11] Drug resistance remains the major obstacle to successful therapy, and escalation of the dose of therapy is one way of overcoming this.

WHAT IS THE EVIDENCE FOR A DOSE EFFECT IN THE TREATMENT OF OVARIAN CANCER?

Experimental data from in vitro and animal models have demonstrated that tumour response is related to the dose of drug and that resistance to treatment is reduced by dose escalation. The application of this approach to ovarian cancer depends on demonstrating a dose–response effect for chemotherapy and depends on being able to escalate the dose of active drugs without excessive normal tissue damage. Levin and Hyrnuik[12] have carried out retrospective analyses of the effect of (platinum) dose intensity in ovarian cancer. Their data, taken from the results from more than 30 randomized trials, demonstrated a significant correlation between the dose intensity, measured as drug delivery ($mg/m^2/week$), and response and survival.[13,14] However, as the range of the 'standard' cisplatin doses used was 30–110%, one may conclude only that lower doses are less good, rather than 'more is better'.

Several randomized trials have been conducted over the last decade in the expectation that increases in dose above the amount used in standard therapy might improve outcome. These studies (Table 11.1) did not use doses of drugs that lead to the profound myelosuppression that necessitates intensive support with haemopoietic growth factors or autologous bone marrow or peripheral blood stem cell transplantation. Most of the studies that used higher doses of platinum reported an increase in the response rate, but this rarely had an effect on survival. In one example, a study from Kaye et al.[16] was initially reported as showing a survival benefit in patients receiving cisplatin $100 \, mg/m^2$ compared with $50 \, mg/m^2$. Both groups received the same dose of cyclophosphamide. However, an updated analysis at 4 years showed a less marked difference.[22] Neurotoxicity in the high dose arm was significant, and it was concluded that an intermediate dose of $75 \, mg/m^2$ should be recommended. In the other studies the intended dose of cisplatin or carboplatin was approximately doubled without showing any survival benefit. In practice, delivered dose is often less than the intended dose. Gore et al.[19] compared four cycles of carboplatin AUC 12 with six cycles of carboplatin AUC 6. The intended dose increase was 33% but the received dose increase was 22%. Two studies[17,18] examined dose density, the same dose given over a different time. There was no significant difference in response, or progression-free or overall survival.

In summary, none of these prospective studies have shown a benefit of dose escalation in the treatment of ovarian cancer. However, selection of patients may have biased the results: in many of the studies patients had residual bulky disease, a known adverse factor for response and survival. Having said this, a two-fold increment in dose is unlikely to be significant. In vitro data suggest that a five-fold increase in dose is required to produce a significant effect.[23] The maximum dose of cisplatin that has been given is $200 \, mg/m^2$: the response rate was high but non-haematological (neuro-) toxicity was marked.[24]

Alkylating agents and carboplatin are active drugs in ovarian cancer that can be significantly escalated. Over a wide dose range myelotoxicity is dose limiting; provided that the patient's bone marrow can be supported, significantly higher doses can be given. High dose chemotherapy (HDC) with autologous bone marrow transplantation (ABMT) or peripheral blood stem cell transplantation (PBSCT) is an approach that should be considered in ovarian cancer because it is a disease with a high response rate to chemotherapy and one in which a proportion of cases are cured with conventional doses of drugs.

Trial	No. of patients	Regimen	Response (%)	Median survival (months)
Ngan et al. (1989)[15]	50	Cis 60 mg/m^2; 3–4 weeks	30	NA
		Cis 120 mg/m^2; 3–4 weeks	55	NA
Kaye et al. (1992)[16]	159	Cis 50 mg/m^2; 3 weeks × 6	34	17
		Cis 100 mg/m^2; 3 weeks × 6	61	29
Colombo et al. (1993)[17]	296	Cis 50 mg/m^2; weekly × 9	66	36
		Cis 75 mg/m^2; 3 weeks × 6	61	33
McGuire et al. (1995)[18]†	458	Cis 50 mg/m^2; 3 weeks × 8	65	21
		Cis 100 mg/m^2; 3 weeks × 4	59	24
Gore et al. (1996)[19]	241	Carbo AUC 6; 4 weeks × 6	57	NSD
		Carbo AUC 12; 4 weeks × 4	63	NSD
Conte et al. (1996)[20]	145	Cis 50 mg/m^2; 4 weeks × 6	61	24
		Cis 100 mg/m^2; 4 weeks × 6	57	29
Jakobsen et al. (1997)[21]	222	Carbo AUC 4; 4 weeks × 6	15*	19
		Carbo AUC 8; 4 weeks × 6	16*	19

Table 11.1 Randomized trials of platinum dose

AUC, Area under curve; Carbo, carboplatin; Cis, cisplatin; NA, not available; NSD, no significant difference.
†Dose density study.
‡Pathological complete response (only 50% had 'second-look' operation).

HIGH DOSE CHEMOTHERAPY IN ADVANCED OVARIAN CANCER

Most experimental therapies begin in patients who have refractory disease. This group comprises patients who fail to respond or progress during first-line therapy with platinum (primary resistance), or those who have relapsed on one or more occasions and are unresponsive to conventional doses of further agents. Numerous reports have appeared in the literature since the early 1980s describing a variety of regimens in a small series of heterogeneous cases. Shpall et al. have comprehensively reviewed many of these early studies.[25] High dose melphalan, cyclophosphamide, thiotepa and carboplatin are the most commonly used drugs. High dose intraperitoneal cisplatin was used by the group from Duke University[26] but this led to severe renal toxicity unless given by infusion over several days. Mitoxantrone and etoposide (VP-16) are two other drugs that have been employed in some regimens.

Our knowledge of high dose chemotherapy in refractory ovarian cancer is summarized in Table 11.2. There are theoretical reasons to suppose that synergy exists between high dose cisplatin and thiotepa with cyclophosphamide. The results from a Duke University study of this combination, supported by ABMT, produced response rates in 75% of patients with refractory ovarian cancer. The median response was 6 months (range 3–9 months) and toxicity was significant.[26] Cisplatin is now rarely used

Table 11.2 High dose chemotherapy in refractory ovarian cancer

Trial	No. of patients	Regimen	Response	Median duration (months)
Mulder et al. (1989)[27]	11 (8 micro/ minimal, 3 bulky)	Cyclophosphamide 7 g/m^2 Etoposide 0.9 or 1.0 g/m^2	6/8 (micro) (75%) 0/3 (bulky) (0%)	15 –
Shpall et al. (1990)[26]	12 (8 evaluated)	Cyclophosphamide 5.6 g/m^2 Thiotepa 300 mg/m^2 Cisplatin (ip) 165 mg/m^2	6/8 (75%)	NA
Broun et al. (1994)[28]	9 (8 evaluated)	Carboplatin 1500 mg/m^2 Ifosfamide 7.5–10 g/m^2	7/8 (88%)	6

ip, Intraperitoneal; NA, not available.

because the dose of carboplatin can be escalated more without incurring as much non-haematological toxicity. Stiff et al.[29,30] used carboplatin with high dose mitoxantrone and cyclophosphamide in patients with ovarian cancer. In a phase II study the response rate was 84% in patients with platinum-refractory disease. The median progression-free survival (PFS) was 5.1 months. Their experience has since been expanded[31] to include the results of treatment of 100 patients who received one or three regimens. Sixty-six per cent had 'platinum-resistant' disease and 61% had disease with a tumour bulk of $\geqslant 1$ cm. They had been previously treated with a median of two regimens (range one to six). The median PFS and overall survival (OS) were 7 and 13 months, respectively. A stepwise Cox proportional hazards model identified tumour bulk and cisplatin sensitivity as the best predictors of PFS. Age was an additional factor predicting OS. For 20 patients with platinum-sensitive disease $\leqslant 1$ cm in bulk, the median PFS was 19 months and the OS 30 months.

Thus, caution is needed in determining the usefulness of HDC. Prognostic variables that have been so important in predicting long-term survival of newly diagnosed ovarian cancer[32] are equally relevant in the group of patients with relapsed disease undergoing HDC. In a much older study, Mulder et al.[27] selected a group of patients with persistent ovarian cancer after induction chemotherapy and treated them with high dose cyclophosphamide and etoposide with ABMT. Complete responses were seen in six patients, five confirmed pathologically, out of eight patients who had disease that was $\leqslant 2$ cm in bulk. The median response duration was 15 months.

Several lessons have been learned from the studies of relapsed ovarian cancer. Firstly, a number of agents can be administered safely in high doses, supported by ABMT or PBSCT. Response rates are high but the duration of remission is often short. Pretreatment prognostic factors such as tumour bulk and platinum sensitivity have a marked effect on outcome. Analysis of two large transplant registries [American Bone Marrow Transplant Registry (ABMTR) and European Blood and

Marrow Transplant Group (EBMT)] support these findings. Patients with chemosensitive disease and small tumour bulk were the only ones who appeared to receive benefit from the treatment.[33,34]

HIGH DOSE CHEMOTHERAPY AS INITIAL TREATMENT FOR OVARIAN CANCER

Given the high relapse rate following conventional treatment it would seem reasonable to study the effect of consolidating the response to first-line therapy with HDC. This has now been explored by several groups in a phase II non-randomized setting (Table 11.3). In a retrospective series Viens et al.[35] published the results of treating 35 patients, 19 of whom had disease of ≤2 cm at the end of first-line platinum-based chemotherapy. In this group, high dose melphalan (140–200 mg/m²) was supported by ABMT. The duration of response was short but better in those who had ≤2 cm residual disease. However, three out 35 patients died as a result of the procedure. A further publication from the Marseille group, using drug combination regimens that included carboplatin, VP-16 and thiotepa, reported a projected 3-year PFS of 52.5%.[36]

Benedetti-Panici et al.[36] entered previously untreated patients with FIGO stage III–IV ovarian carcinoma into a study of HDC. Twenty patients aged less than 55 years with tumours less than 0.5–2.0 cm after primary surgery were enrolled. Two induction courses of intensive dose cisplatin (160 mg/m²) and cyclophosphamide were followed by one cycle of very high dose chemotherapy consisting of cisplatin 100 mg/m², etoposide 650 mg/m² and carboplatin 1800 mg/m², supported by ABMT and PBSCT, cells for the latter being obtained during the induction therapy. The toxicity from the very high dose chemotherapy proved to be acceptable and manageable. The pathological response rate was 84% (37% CR). The median follow-up from enrolment was 48 months, and the PFS and OS at 4 years were 57% and 62% respectively.

The largest experience has come from the group in Clermont-Ferrand who reported the results of high dose consolidation therapy after primary chemotherapy in 53 patients.[38] Women underwent surgery, followed by platinum-based chemotherapy and a 'second-look' laparotomy at the end of treatment. One patient treated in relapse was included. This was a cohort study in which the number of cisplatin-containing cycles varied from three to 24 (median six) and the median interval between 'second-look' surgery and HDC was 5 months (range 1–10). Patients were divided into two groups: 31 in clinical remission, of whom 19 were in complete pathological remission, and 22 who had further debulking surgery at the end of chemotherapy. In 18 of these tumour debulking was complete or bulk was reduced to <2 cm. In the first 23 patients, high dose melphalan (140 mg/m²) was given. The remainder were given carboplatin 1600 mg/m² and cyclophosphamide 6.4 g/m² over 4 days. Haematological support was by ABMT in the early part of this study and PBSCT more recently. There was one toxic death.

The results were published in 1997 with a mean follow-up of more than 7 years. The 5-year OS from diagnosis was 59.9% (median 65.8 months) and the DFS was 23.6% (median 30.4 months). The division of patients into two groups at high dose therapy was based on known prognostic factors. Twenty out of 31 patients in the consolidation group had <2 cm residual disease, or complete removal of bulk disease at the first laparotomy. In this group, the 5-year OS and DFS were 71.2% and 26.9%, respectively. There was no difference in outcome between patients treated with melphalan and those treated with the combination of carboplatin and cyclophosphamide.

Long-term survival depends on several prognostic factors such as stage, grade, tumour bulk after primary surgery and type of response documented at 'second-look' surgery.[32,41] Legros et al.[38] have divided their patients into two broad groups to reflect the importance of these parameters. The results in both groups are impressive when compared with conventional therapy

Table 11.3 High dose chemotherapy as initial treatment			
Group	**No. of patients**	**Regimen (no. of patients)**	**Outcome**
Viens et al. (1990)[35]	35	Platinum-based → Mel + ABMT	OS 47% at 54 months
Benedetti-Panici et al. (1995)[36]	20	Cis/Cyclo × 2 → Cis/Etop/Carbo + PBSCT/ABMT	RR 84% pCR 37% pPR (microscopic) 26% pPR (macroscopic) 21% PFS 57% at 4 years; OS 62% at 4 years
Viens et al. (1995)[37]	28	Cis → Mel (3) or Cyclo/Mel (9) or Carbo/Etop/Mel (12) or Thio/Cyclo/Carbo (4)	PFS 52.5% OS 72.5% at 3 years
Legros et al. (1997)[38]	53	Cis/Dox/Cyclo → Mel + ABMT (23) or Carbo/Cyclo + PBSCT (30)	OS 59.9% at 5 years DFS 23.6% at 5 years (OS 74.2%; DFS 32.8% in 19 patients with pCR at second surgery)
Sequential high dose			
Fennelly et al. (1995)[39]	16	Cyclo/Paclitax × 2 Carbo/Cyclo × 4 + PBSCT	RR 100% (38.5% pCR; 46% microscopic residuum)
Wandt et al. (1999)[40]	21	Cyclo × 1 Carbo × 2 + PBSCT Carbo/Etop/Mel × 1 + PBSCT	RR 100% (57% CR 43% PR) MS 36.5 months

ABMT, autologous bone marrow transplantation; Carbo, carboplatin; Cis, cisplatin; CR, complete response; Cyclo, cyclophosphamide; DFS, disease-free survival; Dox, doxorubicin; Etop, etoposide; Mel, melphalan; MS, median survival; OS, overall survival; p, pathological; Paclitax, paclitaxel; PBSCT, peripheral blood stem cell transplantation; PFS, progression-free survival; PR, partial response; RR, response rate; Thio, thiotepa.

and knowledge about prognostic factors. However, the DFS figures show that a large proportion of patients relapse after HDC. It was encouraging that many of these patients had a further response to chemotherapy; only three patients had a second high dose procedure.

The EBMT has recently analysed the outcome of 254 patients entered onto the ovarian cancer solid tumour registry from 39 centres between 1982 and 1996.[34] These patients were given HDC

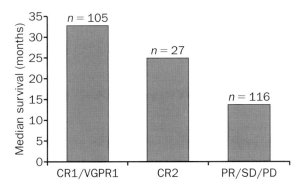

Figure 11.1
Survival (months) of patients following high dose chemotherapy from EBMT registry. CR1, First clinical remission (CR); CR2, second CR; PD, progressive disease; PR, partial response; SD, stable disease; VGPR1, very good partial response (microscopic disease at second-look surgery); $n = 254$ (six patients unknown).

either as consolidation therapy, or as part of a relapse protocol. Most received melphalan or carboplatin, or a combination (86%) supported by ABMT or PBSCT. One hundred and five patients underwent HDC in complete remission, or very good partial response with microscopic disease. Only 25% of patients were known to have no or microscopic disease after initial surgery; but in 20% the tumour status was unknown. Twenty-seven patients underwent high dose therapy in second remission and more than 50% were given the treatment in the presence of bulky disease after conventional chemotherapy. Patient outcome is summarized in Fig. 11.1. The median survival of patients treated in remission was 33 months, which was significantly better than a remission of 14 months seen in other groups ($P = 0.0001$). Many of these patients had drug-resistant relapse. The durability of remission was longer after transplantation in patients treated in first remission than in second remission: the median DFS was 18 months compared with 9 months ($P = 0.005$).[34]

Comparison of the outcome with conventional therapy is difficult, as the registry data are collected retrospectively; patients are a selected group and not all data on prognostic factors are available. Nevertheless, the survival results in patients with stage III or IV disease provide encouragement for the further study of HDC. With a median follow-up of 76 months from diagnosis, the median DFS and OS in stage III disease transplanted in remission are 42 and 59 months, respectively, and for stage IV disease 26 and 40 months. These data lend further support to the view that HDC should only be given as part of first-line therapy to patients with small volume drug-sensitive disease.

MULTICYCLE HIGH DOSE CHEMOTHERAPY

In most series patients have been given high dose consolidation therapy. This is the simplest approach and is based on eradicating small amounts of residual disease that are resistant to conventional doses but sensitive to higher ones. We know relatively little about the extent to which resistance is induced by chemotherapy, or the magnitude of resistance in the clinical setting. However, the single administration of a high dose after lower dose therapy may not make best use of the active agents that are available. Thus it has been suggested that it would be better to use the most active agents in as high a dose as possible early in the treatment of cancers.[42,43] Furthermore, the evidence from tumour kinetic modelling (Norton–Simon hypothesis) suggests that therapy is likely to be more successful if repeated cycles of active drugs are given.[44,45] Whilst in vitro chemotherapy data are able to demonstrate a dose–response relationship in ovarian cancer, it is difficult to escalate the dose of an individual drug more than four- or five-fold in the clinic. Taking all these considerations together, it could be better to use multiple cycles of HDC rather than single doses, even if some compromise on dose is made so that cycles can be repeated at short intervals.

Two studies have addressed this concept in the treatment of ovarian cancer. In the first, Fennelly et al.[39] used escalating doses of paclitaxel in patients treated with multiple cycles of cyclophosphamide and high dose carboplatin and cyclophosphamide. Two cycles of cyclophosphamide $(3.0 \, g/m^2)$ were given with paclitaxel $(150–300 \, mg/m^2)$. Following peripheral blood stem cell harvests, patients were given four cycles of high dose carboplatin $(1000 \, mg/m^2)$ and cyclophosphamide $(1500 \, mg/m^2)$ (platinum–cyclophosphamide combinations are frequently used, as there is in vitro evidence of synergy[40]). Each cycle was supported by PBSCT and G-CSF. Sixteen patients with previously untreated advanced poor-prognosis ovarian cancer were entered and 12 completed all six cycles. The overall response rate was 100%, with 38.5% of patients achieving a complete pathological remission. Six patients were left with only microscopic residual disease.

A similar approach has been adopted by Wandt et al.[46] In this study the majority of patients received cyclophosphamide $(6 \, g/m^2)$ followed by three further PBSC-supported cycles. Two cycles of carboplatin $(1600–1800 \, mg/m^2)$ were followed by a cycle of carboplatin $(1600 \, mg/m^2)$, etoposide $(1600 \, mg/m^2)$ and melphalan $(140 \, mg/m^2)$. Twenty-one patients with previously untreated ovarian cancer were entered on to the study; eight patients received paclitaxel $(175 \, mg/m^2)$ with each cycle. Patients all had poor-prognosis disease; five had inoperable tumour at the outset. The overall response rate was 100%, with 57% experiencing complete remissions. The median PFS at the time of reporting, with a median follow-up of just under 2 years, was 25 months, which is encouraging in this group of patients. The toxicity of this approach was acceptable. Ototoxicity was not seen in patients who received a median carboplatin dose of 'AUC' 20 (median 17–22). Severe grade 3 or 4 infections occurred in 7% of cycles but there were no treatment-related deaths. A considerable part of the treatment programme could be managed in the daycare setting with brief inpatient stays.

RANDOMIZED TRIALS – THE FUTURE

Over the last 15 years it has become clear that ovarian cancer is a chemosensitive disease and that response rates can be augmented by dose intensification. Phase I and II trials, cohort series and registry data have shown that many drugs are active in this setting. However, the duration of response is in many series short. It is clear that patients treated in relapse, or with persistent disease after conventional treatment, have a shorter duration of response than those treated in first remission.[34,38] However, even amongst a group of patients treated with first-line chemotherapy, one might expect differences in outcome because several powerful prognostic factors have been clearly defined in patients receiving conventional dose chemotherapy.[32,41] Whether these apply to the same extent in patients receiving HDC is unclear.

A true benefit of HDC can be demonstrated only in a prospective randomized trial. Several trials have started; only one has completed recruitment. In 1995 the French–Italian Group d'Investigateurs Nationaux pour l'Etude des Cancers Ovariens (GINECO) group opened a study in which a single high dose consolidation therapy with carboplatin and cyclophosphamide was compared with conventional doses of the drug in patients with minimal residual disease or pathological complete remission after conventional platinum-based chemotherapy (Table 11.4). This trial has recruited 102 patients and preliminary results were reported in 2001. The DFS was 11 months following conventional therapy and 22 months after HDC $(P = 0.03)$.[47] Survival data are not yet available. A similar approach was adopted by the Gynecologic Oncology Group (GOG) group who opened their study (trial no. 164) in 1996. In this trial patients who have responded to four to six cycles of cisplatin/paclitaxel ($\leqslant 1$ cm residual disease) were randomized to either six more cycles of carboplatin/paclitaxel or a single HDC cycle of carboplatin, cyclophosphamide and mitoxantrone (see Stiff et al.[29]).

This trial has been prematurely closed due to poor accrual. There are several reasons why this

Table 11.4 Randomized trials of high dose chemotherapy in ovarian cancer

Group	Type	Standard	Intensive
Consolidation studies			
GOG no. 164	Post-induction Carbo/Paclitax 4–6 <1 cm disease at SLO	Carbo/Paclitax × 6	HD Carbo/Cyclo/Mitox × 1
Netherlands NWAST	Clinical CR post platinum- based chemotherapy	Carbo/Cyclo × 3	HD Carbo/Cyclo/Thio × 1
GINECO	Platinum-based induction CR or small volume disease at SLO	Carbo/Cyclo × 3	HD Carbo/Cyclo × 1
First-line high dose			
Rome: Catholic University	Macroscopic disease	Carbo/Paclitax × 2 → IDS Carb/Paclitax × 4	Esc. Carbo/Epi/Paclitax × 2 → IDS HD Carbo/Ifos/Paclitax × 1 HD Carbo/Etop/Mel × 1
FINOVA	Surgery ≤2 cm residual disease	Cis/Paclitax × 6	Cis/Paclitax × 3 (if no PD) → HD Carbo/Cyclo/Mitox × 1
EBMT (OVCAT)	Surgery ≤2 cm residual disease	Cis or Carbo/Paclitax × 6	Cyclo/Paclitax × 2 → HD Carbo/Paclitax × 2 HD Carbo/Mel/Paclitax × 1
AGO (OVAR-2)	Surgery, any residual disease	Cis or Carbo/Paclitax × 6	Cyclo/Paclitax × 2 → HD Carbo/Paclitax × 2 HD Carbo/Mel × 1

Carbo, carboplatin; Cis, cisplatin; Cyclo, cyclophosphamide; Etop, etoposide; Esc., escalated dose; HD, high dose; IDS, interval debulking surgery; Ifos, ifosfamide; Mel, melphalan; Mitox, mitoxantrone; Paclitax, paclitaxel; SLO, second-look operation.

might have occurred. Firstly, patients often find the concept of randomization into a trial harder if it does not take place at the outset. Secondly, those women committed to a study such as this might feel disappointed if they were offered the conventional arm at randomization. This is partly because at the time of randomization, having undergone conventional chemotherapy, they may have strong views about any further treatment. Furthermore, previous studies have shown no difference in outcome between five and 10 cycles of treatment.[10] It is likely that

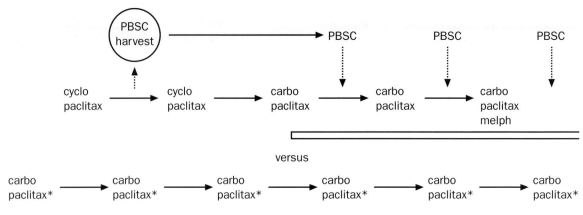

Figure 11.2
EBMT trial of sequential high dose chemotherapy for ovarian cancer (OVACT). *High dose:* cyclo, cyclophosphamide 4 g/m^2; carbo, carboplatin AUC 20; paclitax, paclitaxel 200 mg/m^2; melph, melphalan 140 mg/m^2. *Standard dose:* cisplatin 75 mg/m^2 or carboplatin AUC 5; paclitaxel 175 mg/m^2; *doxorubicin or epirubicin may be added if standard in some centres.

some potential registrants may have opted for high dose therapy out of the study if it was available.

The Finnish (FINOVA) group performed a similar trial to the GOG, although randomization took place at the outset. Patients with stage III and ≤2 cm residual disease were randomized to six cycles of paclitaxel and cisplatin, or three cycles followed by high dose cyclophosphamide (120 mg/kg over 4 days), carboplatin (1500 mg/m^2 over 4 days) and mitoxantrone (75 mg/m^2). This was preceded by high dose cyclophosphamide (3.0 g/m^2) and paclitaxel (175 mg/m^2) to mobilize peripheral blood stem cells. Reassessment in both arms of the trial occurred after three cycles. Patients progressing in either arm were removed from the study. Recruitment to this trial was slow and the trial closed prematurely.

The EBMT have adopted a different approach using multicycle high dose treatment after initial surgery. The high dose regimen (Fig. 11.2) that has been adopted is a minor modification of the protocol of Wandt et al.[46] Etoposide has been omitted and the dose of paclitaxel has been increased to 200 mg/m^2. The control arm of this study is standard platinum/paclitaxel, with either carboplatin or cisplatin selected by the centre. Those centres wishing to add an anthracycline, which some believe has an additional effect, may do so if it is their declared policy. Patients with advanced stage III or IV disease may enter but the disease must be ≤2 cm maximum diameter at the end of surgery. In total, the study will need 300 patients to demonstrate an absolute benefit of 20% in the 2-year PFS. The largest difference in survival is likely to be seen in patients in a better-prognosis group, and for this reason patients with ≤2 cm residual disease only are included. A very similar trial is being run by a German group that also allows patients with larger volume disease to be included. The paclitaxel dose is slightly higher, at 250 mg/m^2. Both trials opened in 1998 and were accruing slowly. The trials merged in December 2001, and the new study HIDOC-EIS (High Dose Ovarian Cancer-European Intergroup Study) currently has 115 patients in the study.

CONCLUSIONS

Ovarian cancer is a very chemosensitive solid tumour. There is no doubt that the response rate can be increased by escalating the dose of drugs that are active in this disease. It is clear without evidence from randomized studies that HDC is of no value in patients who have demonstrable chemoresistance or in those who have bulky residual disease. Cohort and registry data suggest that HDC may have a role in first-line treatment. Consolidation therapy and multiple sequential high dose therapy are both being investigated in randomized trials. There can be no role for high dose therapy outside a clinical trial at the moment. It is essential that these trials are completed soon and that they contain a sufficient number of patients to detect any real effect for this toxic and costly therapy.

REFERENCES

1. Griffiths CT. Surgical resection of tumour bulk in the primary treatment of ovarian carcinoma. Natl Cancer Inst Monographs 1975;42:101–4.
2. Gruppo Interregionale Cooperativo Oncologico Ginecologia. Long term results of a randomised trial comparing cisplatin with cisplatin and cyclophosphamide with cisplatin, cyclophosphamide and adriamycin in advanced ovarian cancer. Gynecol Oncol 1992;45:115–17.
3. Omura GA, Bundy BN, Berek JS, Currey S, Delgado G, Mortel R. Randomised trial of cyclophosphamide plus cisplatin with or without doxorubicin in ovarian carcinoma: a Gynecologic Oncology Group study. J Clin Oncol 1989;7:457–65.
4. Mangioni C, Bolis G, Pecorelli S et al. Randomized trial in advanced ovarian cancer comparing cisplatin and carboplatin. J Natl Cancer Inst 1989;81(19): 1464–71.
5. Taylor AE, Wiltshaw E, Gore ME, Fryatt I, Fisher C. Long-term follow-up of the first randomized study of cisplatin versus carboplatin for advanced epithelial ovarian cancer. J Clin Oncol 1994;12(10):2066–70.
6. Ovarian Cancer Meta-Analysis Project. Cyclophosphamide plus cisplatin versus cyclophosphamide, doxorubicin, and cisplatin chemotherapy of ovarian carcinoma: a meta-analysis. J Clin Oncol 1991;9(9):1668–74.
7. Trimble EL, Adams JD, Vena D et al. Paclitaxel for platinum-refractory ovarian cancer: results from the first 1,000 patients registered to National Cancer Institute Treatment Referral Center 9103. J Clin Oncol 1993;11(12):2405–10.
8. McGuire WP, Hoskins WJ, Brady MF et al. Cyclophosphamide and cisplatin compared with paclitaxel and cisplatin in patients with stage III and stage IV ovarian cancer. N Engl J Med 1996;334:1–6.
9. Piccart MJ, Bertelsen K, James K et al. Randomized intergroup trial of cisplatin-paclitaxel versus cisplatin-cyclophosphamide in women with advanced epithelial ovarian cancer: three-year results. J Natl Cancer Inst 2000;92: 699–708.
10. Hakes TB, Chalas E, Hoskins WJ et al. Randomised prospective trial of 5 versus 10 cycles of cyclophosphamide, doxorubicin and cisplatin in advanced ovarian carcinoma. Gynecol Oncol 1992;45:284–9.
11. Lambert HE, Rustin GJ, Gregory WM, Nelstrop AE. A randomized trial of five versus eight courses of cisplatin or carboplatin in advanced epithelial ovarian carcinoma. A North Thames Ovary Group Study. Ann Oncol 1997;8(4): 327–33.
12. Levin L, Hryniuk WM. Dose intensity analysis of chemotherapy regimens in ovarian carcinoma. J Clin Oncol 1987;5:756–67.
13. Levin L, Simon R, Hryniuk W. Importance of multiagent chemotherapy regimens in ovarian carcinoma: dose intensity analysis. J Natl Cancer Inst 1993;85:1732–42.
14. Levin L. Chemotherapy Options in Ovarian Carcinoma – a Dose Intensity Perspective. London: Chapman & Hall; 1995.
15. Ngan HY, Choo YC, Cheung M et al. A randomized study of high-dose versus low-dose cis-platinum combined with cyclophosphamide in the treatment of advanced ovarian cancer. Hong Kong Ovarian Carcinoma Study Group. Chemotherapy 1989;35(3):221–7.
16. Kaye SB, Lewis CR, Paul J et al. Randomised study of two doses of cisplatin with cyclophosphamide in epithelial ovarian cancer. Lancet 1992;340:329–33.
17. Colombo N, Pittelli M, Parma G et al. Cisplatin dose-intensity in advanced ovarian cancer: a randomized trial of dose-intense versus standard dose cisplatin monochemotherapy. Proc ASCO 1993;12:(abstract 255).
18. McGuire WP, Hoskins WJ, Brady MF et al. Assessment of dose-intensive therapy in suboptimally debulked ovarian cancer: a Gynecologic

Oncology Group study. J Clin Oncol 1995;13(7): 1589–99.

19. Gore M, Mainwaring P, MacFarlane V et al. A randomised trial of high-versus standard-dose carboplatin in patients with advanced epithelial ovarian cancer. Proc ASCO 1996;15:284:(abstract 769).

20. Conte PF, Bruzzone M, Carnino F et al. High-dose versus low-dose cisplatin in combination with cyclophosphamide and epidoxorubicin in suboptimal ovarian cancer: a randomized study of the Gruppo Oncologico Nord-Ovest. J Clin Oncol 1996;14(2):351–6.

21. Jakobsen A, Bertelsen K, Andersen JE et al. Dose-effect study of carboplatin in ovarian cancer: a Danish Ovarian Cancer Group study. J Clin Oncol 1997;15(1):193–8.

22. Kaye SB, Paul J, Cassidy J et al. Mature results of a randomised trial of two doses of cisplatin for the treatment of ovarian cancer. J Clin Oncol 1996;14:2113–19.

23. Behrens BC, Hamilton TC, Masuda H et al. Characterization of a cis-diamminedichloro-platinum(II)-resistant human ovarian cancer cell line and its use in evaluation of platinum analogues. Cancer Res 1987;47(2):414–18.

24. Ozols RF, Ostchega Y, Myers CE, Young RC. High-dose cisplatin in hypertonic saline in refractory ovarian cancer. J Clin Oncol 1985;3(9):1246–50.

25. Shpall E, Stemmer S, Bearman S et al. High dose chemotherapy with autologous bone marrow support for the treatment of epithelial ovarian cancer. In: Markman M, Hoskins WJ, eds. Cancer of the Ovary. New York: Raven Press; 1993: 327–38.

26. Shpall EJ, Clarke-Pearson D, Soper JT et al. High-dose alkylating agent chemotherapy with autologous bone marrow support in patients with stage III/IV epithelial ovarian cancer. Gynecol Oncol 1990;38(3):386–91.

27. Mulder PO, Willemse PH, Aalders JG et al. High-dose chemotherapy with autologous bone marrow transplantation in patients with refractory ovarian cancer. Eur J Cancer Clin Oncol 1989;25(4):645–9.

28. Broun ER, Belinson JL, Berek JS et al. Salvage therapy for recurrent and refractory ovarian cancer with high-dose chemotherapy and autologous bone marrow support: a Gynecologic Oncology Group pilot study. Gynecol Oncol 1994;54(2):142–6.

29. Stiff PJ, McKenzie RS, Alberts DS et al. Phase I clinical and pharmacokinetic study of high-dose mitoxantrone combined with carboplatin, cyclophosphamide, and autologous bone marrow rescue: high response rate for refractory ovarian carcinoma. J Clin Oncol 1994;12(1): 176–83.

30. Stiff P, Bayer R, Camarda M et al. A phase II trial of high-dose mitoxantrone, carboplatin, and cyclophosphamide with autologous bone marrow rescue for recurrent epithelial ovarian carcinoma: analysis of risk factors for clinical outcome. Gynecol Oncol 1995;57(3):278–85.

31. Stiff PJ, Bayer R, Kerger C et al. High-dose chemotherapy with autologous transplantation for persistent/relapsed ovarian cancer: a multivariate analysis of survival for 100 consecutively treated patients. J Clin Oncol 1997;15(4):1309–17.

32. Neijt JP, ten Bokkel Huinink WW, van der Burg MEL et al. Long term survival in ovarian cancer: mature data from The Netherlands Joint Study Group for Ovarian Cancer. Eur J Cancer 1991;27:1367–72.

33. Stiff PJ, Veum-Stone J, Lazarus HM et al. High-dose chemotherapy and autologous stem-cell transplantation for ovarian cancer: an autologous blood and marrow transplant registry report. Ann Intern Med 2000;133(7):504–15.

34. Ledermann JA, Herd R, Maraninchi D et al. High-dose chemotherapy for ovarian carcinoma: long-term results from the Solid Tumour Registry of the European Group for Blood and Marrow Transplantation (EBMT). Ann Oncol 2001;12:693–9.

35. Viens P, Maraninchi D, Legros M et al. High dose melphalan and autologous marrow rescue in advanced epithelial ovarian carcinomas: a retrospective analysis of 35 patients treated in France. Bone Marrow Transplant 1990;5(4): 227–33.

36. Benedetti-Panici P, Greggi S, Scambia G et al. High-dose chemotherapy with autologous peripheral stem cell support in advanced ovarian cancer. Ann Med 1995;27(1):133–8.

37. Viens P, Gravis G, Blaise D et al. High dose chemotherapy (HDC) with bone marrow rescue for patients with FIGO stage III or IV common epithelial ovarian carcinoma responding to first-line treatment. Proc ASCO 1995;14:285 (abstract 811).

38. Legros M, Dauplat J, Fleury J et al. High-dose chemotherapy with hematopoietic rescue in

patients with stage III to IV ovarian cancer: long-term results. J Clin Oncol 1997;15(4):1302–8.

39. Fennelly D, Schneider J, Spriggs D et al. Dose escalation of paclitaxel with high-dose cyclophosphamide, with analysis of progenitor-cell mobilization and hematologic support of advanced ovarian cancer patients receiving rapidly sequenced high-dose carboplatin/cyclophosphamide courses. J Clin Oncol 1995; 13(5):1160–6.

40. Lidor YJ, Shpall EJ, Peters WP, Bast RC, Jr. Synergistic cytoxicity of different alkylating agents for epithelial ovarian cancer. Int J Cancer 1991;49(5):704–10.

41. Marsoni S, Torri V, Valsecchi MG et al. Prognostic factors in advanced epithelial ovarian cancer. (Gruppo Interregionale Cooperativo di Oncologia Ginecologia (GICOG)). Br J Cancer 1990;62(3):444–50.

42. Coldman AJ, Goldie JH. Impact of dose-intense chemotherapy on the development of permanent drug resistance. Semin Oncol 1987;14(4 suppl 4):29–33.

43. Gianni AM, Bonadonna G. High dose chemo-radiotherapy for sensitive tumors: is sequential better than concurrent drug delivery? Eur J Cancer Clin Oncol 1989;25(7):1027–30.

44. Norton L, Simon R. Tumour size, sensitivity to therapy and the design of treatment protocols. Cancer Treat Rep 1977;61:1307–17.

45. Norton L, Simon R. The Norton–Simon hypothesis revisited. Cancer Treat Rep 1986;70(1):163–9.

46. Wandt H, Birkmann J, Denzel T et al. Sequential cycles of high-dose chemotherapy with dose escalation of carboplatin with or without pacli-taxel supported by G-CSF mobilized peripheral blood progenitor cells: a phase I/II study in advanced ovarian cancer. Bone Marrow Transplant 1999;23(8):763–70.

47. Cure H, Battista J, Guastalla M et al. Phase III randomised trial of high dose chemotherapy (HDC) and peripheral blood stem cell (PBSC) support as consolidation in patients with responsive low-burden advanced ovarian cancer: preliminary results of a GINECO/FNCLCC/ SFGM-TC study. Proc Am Soc Clin Oncol 2001;20:204a (abstract 815).

12

High dose chemotherapy in breast cancer

John Crown

CONTENTS Background: chemotherapy of breast cancer – theory and practice • Chemotherapy dose–response effect • Haematopoietic support of high dose chemotherapy • High dose chemotherapy strategies • Single-arm trials of high dose chemotherapy with autograft support in breast cancer • Randomized trials of high dose chemotherapy with autograft support in breast cancer • Critical analysis of the literature of randomized trials of high dose chemotherapy in breast cancer • Research priorities and future directions

BACKGROUND: CHEMOTHERAPY OF BREAST CANCER – THEORY AND PRACTICE

Breast cancer is the classic example of a partially chemotherapy-sensitive neoplasm. Modern combination regimens will produce objective responses in the majority of patients with locally advanced or metastatic disease. This can result in substantial amelioration of the distressing symptoms of cancer and also produces a degree of survival prolongation, which is probably of the order of magnitude of 1–2 years. Some patients who are close to death, with impending failure of crucial organ systems, will be restored to reasonably good health and will go on to live for months, or in some cases for years. Most responses are partial, however, and are temporary in all but exceptional cases. Durable complete remission is rare to the point of being anecdotal.[1,2]

Adjuvant chemotherapy given to patients with earlier-stage disease has a greater survival impact and may contribute to cure.[3] This is consistent with the results of the classic experiments of Skipper and Schabel, which suggested that

- tumours grew exponentially with a constant growth rate,
- chemotherapy killed a constant proportion of cells and
- there was an invariably inverse relationship between the size of a tumour and its curability by chemotherapy.

Their model had profound implications for the concept of adjuvant systemic therapy and appeared to be particularly relevant to breast cancer therapeutics.[4] While several generations of studies have confirmed that adjuvant chemotherapy has a beneficial impact in patients with both node-positive and node-negative breast cancer, the impact is less than might have been expected on the basis of the Skipper–Schabel model.[5]

Norton and Simon proposed an alternative paradigm for tumour growth kinetics, and one which went some considerable distance to explaining why the impact of chemotherapy had been less than might have been anticipated on the basis of the exponential model. These researchers hypothesized that tumours grew and regressed according to Gompertzian kinetics.

The essential feature of Gompertzian growth is that the growth rate is not constant as had been predicted by Skipper and Schabel; rather, growth rate varies inversely with the size of the tumour. Thus, large tumours have lower growth fractions than smaller ones, and hence are less sensitive to cytotoxic drugs. Norton and Simon also proposed that the cell-kill induced by a chemotherapy drug was directly related to the size of the dose and to the growth rate of the unperturbed tumour at that point in its growth curve.[6]

This model had important therapeutic implications. Norton and Simon proposed that patients with overt cancer should first be treated with 'induction' chemotherapy to reduce their tumour burden, which would place them in the more sensitive phase of their growth curve. At this point tumour eradication might be attempted. Paradoxically, the same rapid regrowth that enhances cytotoxicity of smaller populations could, in the case of very small amounts of residual cancer cells, also make tumour eradication more difficult, in that the small numbers of cells which might survive a given cycle of treatment would undergo rapid, but wholly clinically inapparent, regrowth prior to the next cycle. Because of this, it was suggested that the late phase of the treatment should be 'intensified'. Several randomized trials have tested this hypothesis. The Cancer and Leukaemia Group B study (CALGB) randomized patients with node-positive breast cancer to receive either doxorubicin-containing chemotherapy as late intensification, or further CMF (cyclophosphamide, methotrexate, and 5-fluorouracil)[7] following a phase of CMF induction. The Italian GOIRC group performed a similar study in patients with metastases.[8] Both studies showed advantages for cross-over late-intensification therapy.

Further support for the Norton–Simon model came from the work of Buzzoni, Bonadonna and colleagues, who tested alternating putatively non-cross-resistant chemotherapy (an approach based on the Goldie–Coldman hypothesis)[9] versus the sequential administration of the same regimens, in node-positive breast cancer. Sequential chemotherapy was found to be significantly superior.[10]

CHEMOTHERAPY DOSE–RESPONSE EFFECT

The frustrating phenomenon of partial chemotherapy sensitivity prompted the exploration of dose escalation or intensification in the therapy of both early- and late-stage breast cancer. A substantial body of experimental evidence suggests that a relationship exists between the concentration of a drug to which a cancer cell is exposed and the likelihood that the cell will be killed.[11] In these experiments, substantial dose escalation (typically of a log order of magnitude) was required to fully eradicate cancers. This degree of dose escalation would be difficult to achieve in routine clinical practice due to toxicity. Therefore it is scarcely surprising that in the clinic, minor degrees of dose escalation within the 'conventional' range have had a modest and inconsistent effect on survival.

The concept of dose intensity relates to dose per unit time. Some retrospective studies have suggested that there is a relationship between dose intensity and survival in breast cancer.[12] The currently available colony stimulating factors (CSF) facilitate a degree of dose escalation, but thrombocytopenia and cumulative myelosuppression limit their impact.[13]

Proving the benefit of escalating therapy beyond standard parameters requires exacting studies. Retrospective studies which have suggested the existence of a relationship between dose and anti-cancer effect do not prove causality. It is possible that those patients who were able to tolerate high dose therapy were those who were fitter and with a good performance status as a result of having better prognosis/less aggressive disease. Similarly, the results of single-arm studies of moderately intensified therapy in both early- and late-stage breast cancer may possibly be explained on the basis of case selection.[14]

A number of prospective random assignment clinical trials have now addressed the issue of moderate dose escalation or intensification in the treatment of either metastatic or early-stage breast cancer. These studies have produced inconsistent results. In general, higher response rates are reported for the higher dose arms in metastatic disease, but any impact on survival is limited. In the adjuvant therapy of early-stage disease, the effects on survival are also seen to be inconsistent.[15–22] However, one conclusion that can be reached on the basis of these studies is that arbitrary reductions below standard dose should be avoided.

HAEMATOPOIETIC SUPPORT OF HIGH DOSE CHEMOTHERAPY

The technique of bone marrow harvesting, cryopreservation and reinfusion as a form of support for intensive chemotherapy or radiotherapy has been investigated extensively over the last 30 years.[15] This technology allowed for a degree of dose escalation which approximated the dose levels which were necessary for cure in experimental systems. In early studies, very high dose chemotherapy with bone marrow autograft support was reported to produce exceptionally high rates of complete remission in patients with relapsed metastatic breast cancer,[16] at the cost of significant levels of treatment-related morbidity and mortality.

The introduction of the haemopoietic CSFs had a powerful impact on the field of autograft-supported high dose chemotherapy (HDC). The administration of CSF following marrow reinfusion resulted in a dramatic abbreviation of the period of neutropenia, and a consequent fall in mortality.[17] More importantly, it was also discovered that the administration of CSF to patients, either at steady state or following myelosuppressive chemotherapy, resulted in the mobilization of large numbers of haematopoietic progenitors into the peripheral blood.[18] These peripheral blood progenitor cells (PBPC) could in turn be harvested by leukapheresis, and used as a substitute for autologous bone marrow (ABM). They were demonstrated to be superior to growth factors

alone, or to marrow in prospective random assignment trials.[19,20] The dramatic improvement in the toxicity profile of HDC now allowed a more systematic investigation of this modality in a number of clinical settings, including high-risk early-stage and overtly metastatic breast cancer. Eddy surveyed the global single-arm literature of chemotherapy in breast cancer and reported that HDC with autograft support produced complete remission more than four times more frequently than did conventionally dosed therapy. It is widely accepted that high dose therapy is indeed more active than low dose therapy, i.e. it produces more frequent and more complete responses. Investigators have attempted to harness this activity using one or other of a number of different high dose strategies. Before studying the history of HDC in breast cancer, I will first discuss these strategies.

HIGH DOSE CHEMOTHERAPY STRATEGIES

Primary high dose chemotherapy

In this strategy, HDC is administered as one (or uncommonly, two or more) definitive cycles of 'stand-alone' treatment to patients with cancer. This approach predominated in early studies and toxicity in these early programs was substantial. These regimens produced high rates of usually short-lived response in patients with metastatic breast cancer. In these first-generation trials, it was noted that patients who underwent this treatment for chemotherapy-resistant cancer had very poor outcomes.[21] Primary HDC has had rather little investigation, due primarily to the early and widespread acceptance of the late-intensification model.[22]

Late intensification

This model is based on an application of the Norton–Simon hypotheses. As outlined above, these researchers suggested that curative chemotherapy should consist of a phase of induction treatment, which would induce response. The resulting tumour would be smaller and with a higher growth fraction, rendering it more sensitive to chemotherapy. It would, however, have a propensity for rapid regrowth according to the principles of Gompertzian mechanics. In order to ensure eradication of the 'left-shifted' tumour, it should now be treated with a 'clinically tolerable dose intensification'. As has been mentioned, the types of intensification which were available in the 1970s, when the Norton–Simon model was first formulated, were not in fact very intensive. The use of marrow or peripheral blood progenitor autografting allowed a much more substantial degree of dose escalation and, during the 1980s, late intensification became the most widespread application of HDC.

Several other rationales were advanced in support of the 'conventional dose induction, high dose consolidation model'. It was proposed that the cytoreduction which was achieved by conventional chemotherapy might increase the ability of the subsequent high dose cycle to eradicate the cancer, by presenting it with a smaller tumour burden.

In addition, as early studies of HDC in a variety of disease types had indicated that it seldom produced cures in patients with disease that was resistant to conventional chemotherapy, the early conventionally dosed induction phase of the programme would allow the identification of those patients whose cancer was resistant. Thus, conventional chemotherapy would act as an in vivo chemosensitivity assay, which would predict which patients would benefit from HDC. Conventional chemotherapy might also improve the performance status of patients with advanced cancer prior to their being subjected to high dose treatment. In the USA, it also was argued that it allowed for a period of time in which insurance cover for the high dose could be negotiated.

The only precise validation for this model would come from a random assignment trial in which primary HDC was compared to the use of the same regimen as intensification following conventional therapy. None have as yet been carried out, but a historical comparison of identical HDC regimens with or without induction did not suggest a major benefit for the induction therapy approach.[31,32]

High dose sequential therapy

In an attempt to deal with the clonal heterogeneity predicted by Goldie and Coldman, Gianni and colleagues treated patients with a number of different single agents given in sequence at, or close to, maximum dose. This innovative strategy enabled very high doses of drugs to be delivered in a fashion which minimized overlapping toxicity. High dose sequential therapy has produced highly promising results in the treatment of aggressive lymphoma[23] and high-risk stage II breast cancer,[24] and in metastatic breast cancer. A principal theoretical argument against the high dose sequential approach is that single cycles of therapy have not been shown to be an efficient means of eradicating cells which are sensitive to those agents.

Multi-cycle high dose chemotherapy

The multi-cycle high dose chemotherapy model (MCHDC) has its origins both in a critical analysis of the general development of clinical chemotherapy theory and practice, and in an alternative interpretation of the Norton–Simon model, which was proposed by Crown and Norton.[25]

When viewed in the context of the curative therapy programmes which have evolved for lymphoma, Hodgkin's disease, early-stage breast cancer and testicular germ cell cancer, the induction/consolidation and high dose sequential programmes look very odd. Curative chemotherapy has generally involved the identification of highly active regimens, and then the application of a sufficient number of cycles of those regimens to achieve tumour eradication. Thus, in the early MOPP programme of chemotherapy for Hodgkin's disease from the

United States National Cancer Institute, patients achieved remission after an average of three cycles of therapy. It is thus reasonable to assume that the cure rate in this series would have been low if only a single cycle of MOPP had been administered. Similarly, is it not possible that single applications of HDC would not represent the optimal use for this technology in patients with breast cancer? Should we not instead try to administer multiple high dose cycles?

Another observation that emerged in early chemotherapy studies in Hodgkin's disease was the finding that pretreatment with relatively ineffective therapy compromised the ability of subsequent active combination regimens to effect cure. This flawed strategy is exactly what the late-intensification model of HDC does.

It can thus be argued that primary single-cycle HDC, late-intensification HDC and high dose sequential therapy all represent substantial departures from classic chemotherapy theory and practice. Multi-cycle HDC, on the other hand, appears to be more consistent with successful precedents.

The original Norton–Simon interpretations of the kinetics of tumour growth and chemotherapy-induced regression were that tumour regression was directly related both to the dose of drug administered, and to the growth rate of the unperturbed tumour at the time of treatment. It was nowhere stated that the dose–response relationship only existed for the late, intensified part of therapy. Rather, the greatest curative impact of intensified therapy might be at a time of minimal residual disease. As has been discussed, at the time of the formulation of these recommendations, it would not have been feasible to administer multiple cycles of highly intensive therapy.

A further consideration is that the Norton–Simon model emphasizes the potential for accelerated regrowth of surviving cells in between cycles of effective therapy. This acceleration would, according to the model, have its greatest impact in patients who harboured very small, subclinical populations of cells. Thus, according to this interpretation of tumour kinetics, the inter-cycle interval between such

high dose treatments might be of crucial importance. The essential difference between MCHDC and high dose sequential chemotherapy is that the latter attempts to overcome drug resistance by introducing a number of different drugs and regimens, whereas MCHDC is designed to ensure that the therapeutic effects of 'effective' therapy are maximized by administering an optimum number of cycles.

Investigators in New York demonstrated the feasibility of accelerated progenitor-supported MCHDC in breast and ovarian cancer.[26] Conventional dose induction therapy might in theory allow the proliferation of those cells which are resistant to conventional doses and sensitive only to high doses. Thus, the later application of HDC might result in the high dose therapy 'confronting' a higher burden of cancer than it would have done had it been applied at the outset.

SINGLE-ARM TRIALS OF HIGH-DOSE CHEMOTHERAPY WITH AUTOGRAFT SUPPORT IN BREAST CANCER

Metastatic disease

Only a small number of trials explored primary high dose therapy as initial treatment for metastatic disease. The group at Duke University treated newly diagnosed patients with metastatic disease with a single cycle of high dose cyclophosphamide, BCNU and cisplatin. Fifty-four per cent of patients achieved a complete remission and one quarter of these remissions were durable at 5 years.

Patients in studies of late-intensification HDC, on the other hand, were typically treated with four and six cycles of anthracycline-containing induction therapy. Those patients who had achieved either a partial or complete response were then 'consolidated' with single (or in a few cases) tandem cycles of high dose therapy. In most of these studies, 50–70% of patients responded to the induction component, and proceeded to 'transplant'. Overall, approximately 50–70% of patients achieved a complete response (CR) following both phases of therapy. The great majority of these remissions ended in relapse, but a proportion, approximately a quarter (i.e. 10–15% of patients subjected to the induction–consolidation approach), remained in CR for 5 years.

The 'high dose sequential' model has also had little study in metastatic breast cancer. Patrone and colleagues treated patients with stage IV disease with a regimen which was similar to that employed by Gianni. Again, a small proportion of patients achieved durable remissions.[27]

The approach of accelerated MCHDC was studied by investigators at Memorial Sloan-Kettering Cancer Center in New York. Patients in a state of ongoing response following conventional chemotherapy were treated with a sequence of high dose single alkylating agents. In the first trial, 42 patients received tandem cycles of cyclophosphamide followed by tandem cycles of autograft-supported thiotepa. There were no treatment-related deaths, and overall, 20% of patients achieved prolonged remission.[28] In a second trial, the therapy was further intensified, by substituting autograft-supported high dose melphalan for one of the cyclophosphamide cycles. The regimen was active but toxic, and three of 17 patients died from an unanticipated syndrome of fulminant interstitial pneumonitis. A fourth patient developed late leukaemia. Five patients, however, remained alive and in continued remission at up to 5 years from treatment.[29]

While historical comparisons seem to suggest a substantial survival advantage compared to conventional chemotherapy,[30] the possibility that case selection bias might be an important contributory factor to the apparent success of HDC in this setting mandated prospective random assignment trials.[31]

Adjuvant treatment of high-risk early-stage disease

Peters and colleagues treated patients with breast cancer involving at least 10 axillary lymph nodes with an aggressive doxorubicin-based regimen followed by a single cycle of high dose late-intensification chemotherapy supported by an autograft of bone marrow or peripheral blood. These authors reported that 70% of patients remained free of relapse at 5 years. Interestingly, many of the relapses were loco-regional recurrences and occurred before the routine introduction of radiotherapy consolidation.[32] Gianni and colleagues studied 'high dose sequential chemotherapy' (see below) in patients with stage II breast cancer involving 10 or more axillary lymph nodes. In their study, 65% of patients remained free of relapse.[33]

RANDOMIZED TRIALS OF HIGH DOSE CHEMOTHERAPY WITH AUTOGRAFT SUPPORT IN BREAST CANCER

Metastatic disease

Four random assignment trials comparing HDC to conventionally dosed therapy have been carried out in patients with overtly metastatic breast cancer. Three utilized the late-intensification approach and were either negative or ambiguous.

Peters and colleagues treated patients with metastatic disease with four cycles of an aggressive doxorubicin-based regimen.[34] Patients who achieved CR were randomized to receive HDC as intensification, or to observation. Patients who were randomized to observation were then treated with the same high dose regimen at the time of relapse. Those patients who achieved partial response or stable disease following induction proceeded automatically to high dose therapy. Interestingly, 15% of this latter group were converted to long-term remission. Of the randomized patients, those who received the consolidative 'transplant' had significantly prolonged disease-free survival compared to those who were observed. Paradoxically, those who received the 'salvage' high dose therapy had superior survival.

The French PEGASE cooperative group randomized patients who were in an ongoing state of response to induction therapy to receive either further conventional therapy or a single high dose cycle.[35] Patients who received the high dose had a statistically significantly prolonged duration of response but not of survival. At 5 years of follow-up, the difference in relapse-free survival had disappeared.

Stadtmauer and colleagues randomized patients who were in an ongoing state of response to conventional therapy to receive either further conventional therapy or a single high dose cycle. No advantage for high dose was demonstrated in either disease-free or overall survival.[36]

The sole randomized trial which addressed the relative merits of primary MCHDC over conventional chemotherapy was conducted by Bezwoda and colleagues.[37] However, following investigations, the high-dose studies of this investigator[37-38] were found to be invalid.[39,40]

Adjuvant treatment of early-stage breast high-risk disease

At the time of writing, the results of five randomized trials in which the role of HDC in the treatment of high-risk early-stage breast cancer was studied have been reported. In four of these studies, the strategy of late intensification was studied.

In the Scandinavian study by Berg et al.,[41] patients with high risk disease were randomly assigned to receive either FEC chemotherapy followed by a single high dose cycle or, in the 'low dose' arm, individually tailored doses of FEC chemotherapy. Patients in the low dose arm in fact received substantially higher doses of anthracycline, cyclophosphamide and 5-fluourouracil than did patients in the high dose arm. This study was negative, but it was in fact a comparison between two high dose strategies, and as such contributes little to the debate concerning the merits of high dose therapy.[41]

The Cancer and Leukaemia Group B (CALGB) attempted to validate the earlier-cited[22] adjuvant single-arm study in a large random assignment trial. Patients received aggressive doxorubicin-based induction, followed by either high dose cisplatin, BCNU, cyclophosphamide with an autograft, or lower but still aggressive doses of the same triplet with filgrastim support. At a very early follow-up (less than 3 years), no advantage was seen for the high dose treatment, Patients on the high dose arm of this study had an unusually high (8%) rate of treatment-related mortality. It is tempting to speculate that this study might in fact have been positive if a more typical rate of toxic death (generally 1–2% in other trials) had occurred.[42] Two other very small studies in which late-intensification HDC was compared to conventionally dosed therapy were also negative.[43,44]

As has been mentioned, the fifth trial, conducted by Bezwoda and colleagues,[38] which used the alternative model of primary multi-cycle (two cycles in this case) HDC, has been invalidated on the basis of research irregularities.[39,40]

CRITICAL ANALYSIS OF THE LITERATURE OF RANDOMIZED TRIALS OF HIGH DOSE CHEMOTHERAPY IN BREAST CANCER

Single-cycle late intensification cannot be regarded as an evidence-based approach for patients with either metastatic or multi-node positive breast cancer. The only trial of primary MCHDC in metastatic disease, as previously stated, has been called into doubt. Thus the randomized literature to date may point to the direction in which future investigations should proceed, but does not justify routine use.

RESEARCH PRIORITIES AND FUTURE DIRECTIONS

The lack of positive results from credible first-generation random assignment trials of high-versus conventionally-dosed chemotherapy for any breast cancer indication, together with the revelations of research fraud in the South African studies pose real difficulties for the future of this field. The results of current, ongoing random assignment trials will be key determinants of the direction of future investigative efforts in the field of dose-intensive chemotherapy. In the event that these studies demonstrate meaningful clinical benefits for the high dose approach, two broad strategies will need to be addressed in successor trials:

- Attempts will have to be made to improve on this treatment. The impacts of new high dose regimens versus existing programmes, engineered versus unmanipulated autograft products,[45,46] adjuvant immunotherapy,[47] gene therapy,[48] multiple versus single high dose cycles, and late-intensification versus high dose sequential and primary high dose chemotherapy strategies could all be studied. Anti-angiogenesis factors might usefully be employed to maintain HDC-induced remissions.[49] Allogeneic transplantation is also under investigation.[50]
- There have also been substantial advances in conventionally dosed therapy in recent years. Thus, some current control groups may be considered suboptimal by the time that current random assignment trials might produce positive results.[51]

Even if the current studies are negative, the possibility would still have to be entertained that the high dose arms of current studies could be improved on. In the case of breast cancer, will these trials confirm an emerging suspicion that late intensification, the dominant strategy in the current studies, is not the optimal use of this technology after all?

REFERENCES

1. Cold S, Jensen NV, Brincker H, Rose C. The influence of chemotherapy on survival after recurrence in breast cancer – a population-based study of patients treated in the 1950s, 1960s and the 1970s. Eur J Cancer 1993;29A:1146–52.
2. Greenberg PAC, Hortobagyi GN, Smith TL et al. Long-term follow-up of patients with complete remission following combination chemotherapy for metastatic breast cancer. J Clin Oncol 1996;14: 2197–205.
3. Early Breast Cancer Trialist's Collaborative Group. Systemic treatment of early breast cancer by hormonal, cytotoxic or immune therapy: 133 randomized trials involving 31,000 recurrences and 24,000 deaths among 75,000 women. Lancet 1992;339:1–15.
4. Skipper HE, Schabel FM. Quantitative and cytokinetic studies in experimental tumor systems. In: Holland J, Frei FE, editors. Cancer Medicine. Philadelphia: Lea and Febiger, 1988: 663–84.
5. Norton L, Simon R. The Norton–Simon hypothesis revisited. Cancer Treat Rep 1986;70:163–9.
6. Norton L, Simon R, Brereton HD et al. Predicting the course of Gompertzian growth. Nature 1976;264:542–5.
7. Perloff M, Norton L, Korzun AH et al. Post surgical adjuvant chemotherapy of stage II breast carcinoma with or without crossover to a non-cross-resistant regimen: a Cancer and Leukemia Group B Study. J Clin Oncol 1996;14:1589–98.
8. Cocconi G, Bisagni G, Bacchi M et al. A comparison of continuation versus late intensification followed by discontinuation of chemotherapy in advanced breast cancer. A prospective randomized trial of the Italian Oncology Group for Clinical Research (G.O.I.R.C.). Ann Oncol 1990;1(1):36–44.
9. Goldie J, Coldman AJ. A mathematical model for relating the drug sensitivity of tumors to their spontaneous mutation rate. Cancer Treat Rep 1979;63:1727–73.
10. Buzzoni R, Bonnadonna G, Vallagussa P et al. Adjuvant chemotherapy with doxorubicin plus cyclophosphamide, methotrexate, and flurouracil in the treatment of resectable breast cancer with more than 3 positive axillary nodes. J Clin Oncol 1994;9:2134–40.
11. Teicher BA, Holden SA, Cucchi CA et al. Combination thiotepa and cyclophosphamide in vivo and in vitro. Cancer Res 1988;48:94–100.
12. Hryniuk W, Bush H. The importance of dose intensity in chemotherapy of metastatic breast cancer. J Clin Oncol 1984;2:81–8.
13. O'Dwyer PJ, LaCreta FP, Schilder R et al. Phase I trial of thiotepa in combination with recombinant human granulocyte–macrophage colony-stimulating factor. J Clin Oncol 1992;10:1352–8.
14. Bronchud MH, Howell A, Crowther D et al. The use of granulocyte colony-stimulating factor to increase the intensity of treatment with doxorubicin in patients with advanced breast and ovarian cancer. Br J Cancer 1989;60:121–5.
15. Lazarus H, Reed MD, Spitzer TR et al. High-dose

iv thiotepa and cryopreserved autologous bone marrow transplantation for therapy of refractory cancer. Cancer Treat Rep 1987;71:689–95.

16. Eder JP, Antman K, Peters WP et al. High-dose combination alkylating agent chemotherapy with autologous marrow support for metastatic breast cancer. J Clin Oncol 1986;4:1592–7.

17. Peters WP, Rosner G, Ross M et al. Comparative effects of granulocyte–macrophage colony-stimulating factor (GM-CSF) and granulocyte colony-stimulating factor (G-CSF) on priming peripheral blood progenitor cells for use with autologous bone marrow after high-dose chemotherapy. Blood 1993;81:1709–19.

18. Socinski MA, Elias A, Schnipper L, Cannistra SA, Antman KH, Griffin JD. Granulocyte–macrophage colony-stimulating factor expands the circulating haemopoietic progenitor cell compartment in man. Lancet 1988;i:1194–8.

19. Beyer J, Schwella N, Zingsem J et al. Bone marrow versus peripheral blood stem cells as rescue after high-dose chemotherapy. Blood 1993; 82(suppl 1):454 (abstract).

20. Kritz A, Crown J, Motzer R. Beneficial impact of peripheral blood progenitor cells in patients with metastatic breast cancer treated with high-dose chemotherapy plus GM-CSF: a randomized trial. Cancer 1993;71:2515–21.

21. Eder JP, Antman K, Peters WP et al. High-dose combination alkylating agent chemotherapy with autologous marrow support for metastatic breast cancer. J Clin Oncol 1986;4:1592–7.

22. Peters WP, Shpall EJ, Jones RB et al. High-dose combination alkylating agents with bone marrow support as initial treatment for metastatic breast cancer. J Clin Oncol 1988;6:1368–76.

23. Gianni AM, Bregni M, Siena S et al. High-dose chemotherapy and autologous bone marrow transplantation compared with MACOP-B in aggressive B-cell lymphoma. N Engl J Med 1997;336(18):1290–7.

24. Gianni AM, Siena S, Bregni M et al. Growth factor supported high-dose sequential adjuvant chemotherapy in breast cancer with >10 positive nodes. Proc ASCO 1992;11:60.

25. Crown J, Norton L. Potential strategies for improving the results of high-dose chemotherapy in patients with metastatic breast cancer. Ann Oncol 1995;6(suppl 4): 21–6.

26. Crown J, Wasserheit C, Hakes T et al. Rapid delivery of multiple high-dose chemotherapy courses with G-CSF and peripheral blood-derived haemopoietic progenitor cells. J Natl Cancer Inst 1992;84:1935–6.

27. Patrone F, Ballestrero A, Ferrando F et al. Four-step high-dose sequential chemotherapy with double hematopoietic progenitor-cell rescue for metastatic breast cancer. J Clin Oncol 1995;13: 840–6.

28. Vahdat L, Raptis G, Fennelly D et al. Rapidly cycled courses of high-dose alkylating agents supported by filgrastim and peripheral blood progenitor cells in patients with metastatic breast cancer. Clin Cancer Res 1995;1:1267–73.

29. Crown J, Raptis G, Vahdat L et al. Rapid administration of sequential high-dose cyclophosphamide, melphalan, thiotepa supported by filgrastim and peripheral blood progenitors in patients with metastatic breast cancer: a novel and very active treatment strategy. Proc ASCO 1994;13:110 (abstract).

30. Antman K, Ayash L, Elias A et al. A phase II study of high-dose cyclophosphamide, thiotepa, and carboplatin with autologous marrow support in women with measurable advanced breast cancer responding to standard-dose therapy. J Clin Oncol 1992;10:102–10.

31. Rahman ZU, Frye DK, Buzdar AU. Impact of selection process on response rate and long-term survival of potential high-dose chemotherapy candidates treated with standard-dose doxorubicin-containing chemotherapy in patients with metastatic breast cancer. J Clin Oncol 1997;15: 3171–7.

32. Peters WP, Ross M, Vredenburgh JJ et al. High-dose chemotherapy and autologous bone marrow support as consolidation after standard-dose adjuvant therapy for high risk primary breast cancer. J Clin Oncol 1993;11: 1132–44.

33. Gianni AM, Siena S, Bregni M et al. Growth factor supported high-dose sequential adjuvant chemotherapy in breast cancer with >10 positive nodes. Proc ASCO 1992;11:60.

34. Peters WP, Jones RB, Vredenburgh J et al. A large, prospective, randomized trial of high-dose combination alkylating agents (CBP) with autologous cellular support as consolidation for patients with metastatic breast cancer achieving complete remission after intensive doxorubicin-based induction therapy (AFM). Proc ASCO 1996;15:121.

35. Lotz J-P, Cure H, Janvier M et al. and the PEGASE Group. High-dose chemotherapy (HD-CT) with hematopoietic stem cell transplantation

(HSCT) for metastatic breast cancer: results of the French Protocol Pegase 04. Proc ASCO 1999;18:43 (abstract).

36. Stadtmauer EA, O'Neill A, Goldstein LJ et al. Phase III randomized trial of high-dose chemotherapy (HDC) and stem cell support (SCT) shows no difference in overall survival or severe toxicity compared to maintenance chemotherapy with cyclophosphamide, methotrexate and 5-fluorouracil (CMF) for women with metastatic breast cancer who are responding to conventional induction chemotherapy: The Philadelphia Intergroup Study (PBT-01). Proc ASCO 1999;18:1 (abstract).

37. Bezwoda WR, Seymour L, Dansey RD. High-dose chemotherapy with hematopoietic rescue as primary treatment for metastatic breast cancer: a randomised trial. J Clin Oncol 1995;13: 2483–9.

38. Bezwoda WR. Randomised, controlled trial of high dose chemotherapy (HD-CNVp) vs. standard dose (CAF) chemotherapy for high risk, surgically treated, primary breast cancer. Proc Am Soc Clin Oncol 1999;18:2 (abstract).

39. Weiss RB, Rifkin RM, Stewart FM et al. High-dose chemotherapy for high-risk primary breast cancer: an on-site review of the Bezwoda study. Lancet 2000; 355:999–1003.

40. Weiss RB, Gill GG, Hudis CA. An on-site audit of the South African trial of high-dose chemotherapy for metastatic breast cancer and associated publications. J Clin Oncol 2001;19: 2771–7.

41 The Scandinavian Breast Cancer Study Group 9401. Results from a randomized adjuvant breast cancer study with high-dose chemotherapy with CTC$_b$ supported by autologous bone marrow stem cells versus dose escalated and tailored FEC therapy. Proc ASCO 1999;2 (abstract).

42. Peters W, Rosner G, Vredenburgh J et al. for CALGB, SWOG and NCIC. A prospective, randomized comparison of two doses of combination alkylating agents as consolidation after CAF in high-risk primary breast cancer involving ten or more axillary lymph nodes: preliminary results of CALGB 9082/SWOG 9114/NCIC MA-13. Proc ASCO 1999;18:1 (abstract).

43. Hortobagyi GN, Buzdar AU, Theriault RL et al. Randomized trial of high-dose chemotherapy and blood cell autografts for high-risk primary breast carcinoma. J Natl Cancer Inst 2000;92(3):225–33.

44. Rodenhuis S, Richel DJ, van der Wall E et al. Randomised trial of high-dose chemotherapy and haemopoietic progenitor–cell support in operable breast cancer with extensive axillary lymph-node involvement. Lancet 1998;352: 515–21.

45. Brugger W, Heimfeld S, Berenson RJ, Mertelsmann R, Kanz L. Reconstitution of hematopoiesis after high-dose chemotherapy by autologous progenitor cells generated ex vivo. N Engl J Med 1995;333:283–7.

46. Shpall EJ, Jones RB, Bearman SI et al. Transplantation of enriched CD34-positive autologous marrow into breast cancer patients following high-dose chemotherapy: influence of CD34-positive peripheral-blood progenitors and growth factors on engraftment. J Clin Oncol 1994;12:28–36.

47. Kennedy MJ, Vogelzang G, Beveridge R et al. Phase I trial of intravenous cyclosporine to induce graft versus host disease in women undergoing autologous bone marrow transplantation for breast cancer. J Clin Oncol 1993;11: 478–84.

48. Hesdorffer C, Ayello J, Ward M et al. Phase I trial of retroviral-mediated transfer of the human MDR1 gene as marrow chemoprotection in patients undergoing high-dose chemotherapy and autologous stem-cell transplantation. J Clin Oncol 1998;16:165–72.

49. O'Reilly MS, Holmgren L, Chen C, Folkman J. Angiostatin induces and sustains dormancy of human primary tumors in mice. Nature Med 1996;2(6):689–92.

50. Ueno N, Rondón G, Mirza NQ. Allogeneic peripheral-blood progenitor-cell transplantation for poor-risk patients with metastatic breast cancer. J Clin Oncol 1998;16:986–93.

51. Chan S, Friedrichs K, Noel D et al. Prospective randomized trial of docetaxel versus doxorubicin in patients with metastatic breast cancer. J Clin Oncol 1999;17:2341–54.

13

High dose chemotherapy in sarcomas: science, fiction or science fiction?

Caroline Seynaeve and Jaap Verweij

CONTENTS Introduction • Soft tissue sarcomas • The Ewing's family of tumours • Conclusion

INTRODUCTION

Adult sarcomas constitute an interesting group of mesenchymal neoplasms accounting for only ±1% of adult malignancies. This group of rare diseases is characterized by a striking heterogeneity in morphology (both in subtype and grade; intra- and inter-lesional), tissue origin, site and location (superficial or deep) of the primary tumour, and clinical behaviour and outcome, resulting in a complexity that is unique to solid tumours. Over the last decade widespread use of immunohistochemistry, developments in cytogenetics and the introduction of modern molecular techniques have provided the basis for more accurate and therefore more reproducible classification. This has allowed for the identification of new entities and questioned the existence of old entities (e.g. haemangiopericytoma), resulting in a better understanding of the biology of the disease, which certainly will advance in the new millennium. At present, the recognized groups of entities are: soft tissue sarcomas (STS) comprising the majority of histological subtypes; bone sarcomas (osteo/chondrosarcomas); the round-cell sarcoma group including the Ewing's family of tumours (EFT), which consists of bone/extraosseous Ewing's sarcoma (ES), peripheral primitive neuroectodermal tumour

(pPNET), Askin tumour and atypical Ewing's sarcoma; and desmoplastic round-cell tumours (DSRCT).

The best opportunity for cure and long-term survival in localized STS still remains oncologically radical surgery with or without radiotherapy. Prognostic factors that have been identified in localized STS are tumour grade, specific subtypes, size or volume, location (superficial/deep) and radical surgery.[1–5] Over the last decade, important shifts in local therapy have emerged, consisting of both limb salvage strategies (sophisticated surgical procedures, perfusion techniques), as well as newer techniques of radiotherapy. These all aim to improve local control; nevertheless, many of these tumours tend to metastasize early and haematogenously. As a result, more than 50% of patients will die from metastatic disease. Therefore, the value of adjuvant chemotherapy has to be examined further. Patients with high-grade STS should be informed of the rationale behind adjuvant therapy and, where possible, be included in appropriate study protocols. When STS present with metastatic disease, systemic chemotherapy offers the best hope of disease control, symptom palliation and prolonged survival. As there are only modest gains in survival with the use of the current chemotherapeutic armamentarium, and new and better drugs are not immediately on the horizon, current chemotherapeutic strategies have focused on the use of available standard agents either optimizing the schedule and/or intensifying the dose.

In contrast to STS, the EFT is considered a systemic disease regardless of apparent stage, whereby standard treatment consists of upfront multiagent chemotherapy, adequate local (surgical and/or radiological) therapy and consolidation chemotherapy. The addition of multiagent chemotherapy to local therapy has considerably improved the outcome in small volume, localized disease. However, patients who are diagnosed with bulky disease (>100 ml or 8 cm^2) still have a poor long-term outcome with a 5-year disease-free survival (DFS) and overall survival (OS) of only 15% and 38%, respectively. Patients with metastatic disease at presentation have an even worse prognosis, with less than 10% surviving longer than 3 years.[6,7] For the two latter groups, therefore, better treatment strategies are needed.

The most easily understood rationale for the use of high dose chemotherapy (HDC) can be summarized as 'more is better'. The scientific basis for this hypothesis includes the expectation that increasing the dose will successfully overcome relative drug resistance. Preclinical data clearly support this view, at least for selected drugs such as alkylating agents, and in some cell systems.[8,9] Demonstrably increased cell kill due to increased drug exposure is termed 'dose–response' and HDC is the translation of this laboratory observation into the clinic. The introduction of better supportive measures and the clinical use of growth factors have allowed intensification of treatment. Furthermore, with the development of the modern bone marrow and/or stem cell transplantation techniques, it has become possible to study the value of HDC regimens. The most commonly used approach is to administer induction standard dose chemotherapy aiming at achieving a partial or complete response (PR, CR), which is then followed by one or two cycles of HDC. The theoretical basis therefore can be found in the log-kill model of Skipper et al.[10] that assumes that several cycles of chemotherapy will reduce the total tumour load, and that the subsequent administration of HDC will 'mop up' remaining sensitive cells. Further support can be found in the Gompertzian model of tumour growth, hypothesizing that a smaller tumour will have a relatively high growth fraction and therefore greater sensitivity to cell cycle specific agents.[11] Because of the low long-term cure rate achieved with conventional therapy, as mentioned above, there has been interest in exploring the use of HDC in poor-outcome subgroups of STS and EFT.

In view of the above, the optimal approach to sarcoma consists of the initial delineation of an overall therapeutic strategy, preferably patient tailored on the basis of specific biology and sensitivity of the disease, by means of a multimodal and interdisciplinary team of clinicians experienced in this field. On the one hand, this results in better long-term outcome for the individual patient,[12-14] while on the other it is the only potential route to further therapeutic advances. Because such an approach is only achievable in a specialized centre, referral of patients is encouraged.

In this chapter we will summarize current knowledge of conventional and intensified chemotherapy regimens and review the rationale and results of HDC for STS and EFT respectively. Some conclusions on its current use and directions for the studies that should be done for further evaluation are discussed, emphasizing the importance of treating patients as much as possible within the content of controlled clinical trials.

SOFT TISSUE SARCOMAS

Conventional chemotherapy: activity and dose–response relationship

Over recent decades, a variety of different chemotherapeutic agents have been studied in STS. Unfortunately, most have demonstrated only marginal activity, with response rates as

Table 13.1 Single-agent activity of chemotherapeutic drugs in soft tissue sarcoma

Agent	Dose	First line (%)	Second line (%)
Doxorubicin	>60 mg/m^2	19–23	17
Epirubicin	>150 g/m^2	18–29	–
Ifosfamide	>6 g/m^2	19–28	8–35
Dacarbazine	>1000 mg/m^2	–	17–18

low as 10% or less. Only three drugs have been identified as showing a reproducible response rate of approximately 20%: doxorubicin, ifosfamide, and dacarbazine (Table 13.1). However, it has to be noted that due to the growing awareness of the important heterogeneity in tumour characteristics and prognostic factors, it becomes increasingly difficult to make clear statements on the value of a specific drug for treatment of (a subtype of) STS on the basis of the published results. Usually, early clinical studies include a very heterogeneous group of patients (chemotherapy naive/pretreated, bone/soft tissue sarcomas), which largely biases outcome. In the experience of the European Organization for Research and Treatment of Cancer (EORTC), results of well-designed phase II studies were not reproducible in subsequent randomized phase III studies.[15] More recent data on the poor response rate to anthracycline-containing chemotherapy of leiomyosarcomas, particularly gastrointestinal stromal tumours (GIST), indicate that the various prognostic factors and the fraction of histological subtypes enrolled in a study, especially in non-randomized studies, should be taken into account when interpreting the data.[16] Moreover, over recent years, response assessments have increasingly been performed by means of more sophisticated and accurate imaging techniques (e.g. computerized tomography, magnetic resonance imaging, positron emission tomography: CT, MRI, PET), while quality control measures such as independent

response review have been implemented. These factors are thought to have contributed to the generally observed reduction in response rates over the decades. Therefore, we would recommend using only results of relatively recent, large and/or randomized studies, with stratification for known prognostic factors and histological subtypes, in decision-making processes.

Some of the favourable prognostic factors for response to anthracycline-based chemotherapy in advanced STS are good performance status, young age, absence of liver metastases, high histopathological grade and liposarcoma. In addition, good performance status, absence of liver metastases, low histopathological grade, long disease-free interval and young age have been identified as favourable prognostic factors for survival.[16]

Single-agent therapy
In general, the activity of doxorubicin is estimated to be approximately 20%.[17,18] At increasing doses, doxorubicin produces higher response rates; it seems to be necessary to try to achieve a dose intensity of at least 70 mg/m^2 every 3 weeks in order to obtain an optimal chance of response (25–30%).[19,20] Exploring the dose–response curve at doses higher than 90 g/m^2 has been limited by the cardiotoxicity of doxorubicin. In an attempt to reduce these side effects without compromising activity, epirubicin has been investigated. However, at the higher doses this drug caused similar cardiotoxicity and evidence for a dose–response

relationship has been lacking.[21,22] Other anthracycline analogues have not shown an advantage over doxorubicin.

The activity of ifosfamide has been confirmed in several studies from the late 1970s onwards. A dose–response relationship for the drug has been suggested, with response rates below 15% at a dose of 5–6 g/m^2, increasing to 20–25% at doses of approximately 10 g/m^2. That response rates may vary considerably, not only between studies performed in different institutions, but also between studies performed by the same cooperative group, is demonstrated by two consecutive randomized studies performed by the EORTC. In a first study investigating ifosfamide versus cyclophosphamide, ifosfamide 5 g/m^2 was administered over 24 h, yielding an overall response rate of 18%, being 23% in chemo-naive patients. In a consecutive study enrolling 101 patients, the same ifosfamide regimen resulted in a response rate of only 11% as first line, and 6% as second line. The high percentage of patients with leiomyosarcoma in the second study has been suggested to partly explain the difference in response rates. In the same study, the high-dose ifosfamide regimen (3 g/m^2/day, days 1–3) yielded a response rate of 28% in first line, and only 8% in second line. The latter is not different from the response rate of standard dose ifosfamide in second line.[23] The subsequent study investigating a regimen of 12 g/m^2 administered as a continuous infusion over 3 days showed only a 15% overall response rate at the cost of an unacceptable rate of major toxicity.[24] At higher doses of ifosfamide, nephrotoxicity and myelosuppression became the dose-limiting side effects.

Combination regimens

Major randomized studies investigating combination regimens in first-line therapy are shown in Table 13.2. The Eastern Cooperative Oncology Group (ECOG) randomly compared the activity of three different schedules: doxorubicin 80 mg/m^2, doxorubicin 60 mg/m^2 with ifosfamide 7500 mg/m^2 and the combination of doxorubicin (40 mg/m^2) with cisplatin and mitomycin. The response rates were higher for the combination arms, being 20% (CR 2%), 34% (CR 3%), and 32% (CR 7%), respectively. However, no significant survival differences were observed.[26] The EORTC studied the activity of either doxorubicin 75 mg/m^2, or doxorubicin/ifosfamide or CYVADIC (cyclophosphamide, doxorubicin, dacarbazine) in 663 patients. At interim analysis, CYVADIC showed no advantage over the other treatment modalities and accrual to this arm was closed prematurely. No differences in response rates, remission duration or OS were observed.[27] In an intergroup study [Cancer and Leukaemia Group B (CALGB)/SWOG], patients were randomized to either doxorubicin/dacarbazine or MAID doxorubicin/ifosfamide/dacarbazine (DOX/IFOS/DTIC), given over 4 days. Because of unacceptable toxicity and a decreased dose density, the doses in the MAID regimen were adjusted. The response rate in the IFOS-containing arm was significantly higher (32% versus 17%), but this did not translate into an improved survival.[28] The conclusions from these studies are that combination chemotherapy regimens produced higher response rates and more toxicity, but did not improve the complete response rate, the time to failure or survival. Therefore, doxorubicin 75–80 mg/m^2 still may be considered the standard regimen against which new therapeutic regimens will need to be tested.

Intensified regimens

In consecutive phase II and III studies, the EORTC investigated a doxorubicin/ifosfamide regimen intensifying the doxorubicin dose (75 mg/m^2) supported by granulocyte–macrophage colony stimulating factor (GM-CSF). While the phase II study showed a high response rate of 45% (10% CR) and suggested a longer median OS compared with previous experiences, in a subsequent randomized phase III study the intensified regimen was not superior to the conventional doxorubicin/ifosfamide (50 mg/5 g) regimen with respect to response rate, progression-free survival and OS. It has been suggested that the different types of GM-CSF (*Escherichia coli*, yeast) that have been used in the two studies may partly

Table 13.2 Soft tissue sarcomas: randomized studies of combination regimens*

Group/regimen	No. of evaluated patients	Schedule* (days)	Dose (mg/m²)	Response rate (%)	CR (%)	Overall response (months)	Reference
ECOG							
Dox	112	1	70	19			Borden et al. (1987)[25]
Dox/DTIC	110	1–5	60/1250	30			
ECOG				(P = 0.03)		(NS)	
Dox	90	1	80	20	2	9	Edmonson et al. (1993)[26]
Dox/Ifos	88	1–2	60/7500	34	3	12	
Dox/CDDP/MMC	84	1	40/60/8	32	7		
SWOG/CALGB				(P = 0.005)		(NS)	
Dox/DTIC	186	1–4	60/1000	17	2	13.3	Antman et al. (1993)[28]
Dox/Ifos/DTIC	77	1–4	60/7500/1000	32	2	11.9	
	111	1–4	60/6000/1000				
EORTC							
Dox	263	1	75	23	2	12	Santoro et al. (1995)[27]
Dox/Ifos	258	1	50/5000	28	3	12.8	
CYVADIC	142	1	500/1.4/50/750	28	4	11.8	
EORTC						(NS)	
Dox/Ifos	262	1	50/5000	20	4		Tursz et al. (1997)[29]
Dox/Ifos		1	75/5000	21	2		
Belgrado						(P = 0.001)	
Epi	45	1–3/4 weeks	180	29	2	(0% at 3 years)	Jelic et al. (1997)[30]
Epi/CDDP	54	1–5/4 weeks	180/120	54	13	(11% at 3 years)	

*In none of the studies was a haematological growth factor used; schedule repeated every 3 weeks unless otherwise mentioned. CALGB, Cancer and Leukemia Group B; CDDP, cisplatin; CR, complete response; CYVADIC, cyclophosphamide/vincristine/doxorubicin/dacarbazine; Dox, doxorubicin; DTIC, dacarbazine; ECOG, Eastern Cooperative Oncology Group; EORTC, European Organization for Research and Treatment of Cancer. Epi, epirubicin; Ifos, ifosfamide; MMC, mitomycin C; OS, overall survival; SWOG, Southwestern Oncology Group.

explain the apparent differences in results.[29,31] In another, non-randomized phase II study the combination of doxorubicin (75 and 90 mg/m^2) and ifosfamide (10 g/m^2) with the support of G-CSF was investigated at the MD Anderson Cancer Center.[32] At the time of the last analysis (79 evaluable patients) the reported overall objective response rate was 65% (CR 9%), varying from 76% for patients with primary tumours only, to 52% for those with metastatic disease. Breakdown of activity by histology demonstrated a response rate of 60% in malignant fibrous histiocytoma ($n = 20$), 100% in synovial sarcoma ($n = 14$), and 46% in non-gastrointestinal leiomyosarcoma, supporting the suggestion by others that synovial sarcomas may be quite chemosensitive, while leiomyosarcomas are relatively chemo-insensitive.[33] Although this regimen has not been studied in a randomized setting, it seems to be an active regimen that may be used in appropriate clinical situations.

Other intensified regimens that have been investigated are: epirubicin in combination with ifosfamide, varying the dose of both drugs either up to 120 mg/m^2 or 12 500 mg/m^2, respectively, etoposide/ifosfamide in different schedules and doses, and the combination of cisplatin with either doxorubicin/ifosfamide or epirubicin.[21] Some of these studies have shown unexpectedly high response rates, but in general without significantly prolonged OS. However, some conclusions may be drawn from these studies. First, achieving CR seems important for improved survival, and increasing dose intensity may increase the CR rate. Second, it has to be kept in mind that encouraging results from non-randomized phase II studies should not be taken for granted, and should be confirmed in sufficiently powered phase III trials, avoiding bias in patient selection.

High dose chemotherapy

In view of the suggested dose–response relationships of the active drugs for STS, and given the availability of haemopoietic support by means of growth factors, HDC regimens with peripheral blood stem cell transplantation (PBSCT) and/or autologous bone marrow transplantation (ABMT) rescue have been explored by some investigators in poor-prognosis STS. So far, however, the literature is inconclusive and no appropriately designed controlled randomized studies have been performed (Table 13.3). Although apparently high response rates are obtained with HDC, even in heterogeneous groups of STS patients, there are as yet no consistent data suggesting an improved survival. Moreover, in view of the data emerging on varying chemosensitivity for different subtypes of STS, HDC should not be offered to any STS patient for whom further standard therapy is not available. In order to be able to make a real assessment of the value of HDC in STS, randomized studies involving those patients most likely to benefit from this strategy should be carried out. It is the task of the international research community to cooperate and properly design studies in which eligible patients may be included.

THE EWING'S FAMILY OF TUMOURS

The Ewing's family of tumours is characterized by small, round, blue, glycogen-containing malignant cells that exhibit degrees of neural differentiation. The differential diagnosis includes metastatic carcinoma (particularly neuro-endocrine carcinomas), neurogenic sarcoma, and lymphoma. Immunohistochemical markers allow for the differentiation of ES and PNETs, and Askin tumours, while cytogenetic studies reveal that a characteristic t(11,22) (q24;q12) translocation fusing the EWS and FLI-1 genes is shared by these tumours. Molecular analysis also allows for the distinction from other small blue round-cell tumours (SRCT) such as rhabdomyosarcoma and intra-abdominal desmoplastic SRCT. Whilst the latter entity shares the same t(11,22) translocation, but fuses the EWS with the WT1 gene, there are some indications that they are equally sensitive to Ewing's-type therapy.[41,42]

While EFTs respond well to radiotherapy,

Table 13.3 Sarcomas: high dose chemotherapy regimens

Regimen*	No. of patients	Schedule (days)	Dose (mg/m²)	Support	RR (%)	Complete response, CR (%)	Overall survival (months)	Reference
HDC: CTX/Thio + either CDDP/carbo/melphalan	23 (6 ET)		Variable	ABMT			5.1	Samuels et al. (1989)[34]
Melphalan based or VIC ± TBI	9 ev/22 (11 RMS)		Variable	ABMT	66		19 26 (CR) (32% at 5 years)	Dumontet et al. (1992)[35]
DTIC/CTX + TBI + either: Dox (n = 7)/CTX-CDDP-ETO (n = 4) Melphalan (n = 1)/ CIE (n = 1)	13 (3 RMS)			PBSC	54	23	7.5	Lessinger et al. (1994)[36]
ETO/Ifos/CDDP (VIC) as consolidation post response	35 (24 STS)	1–5	1000/9000/200	ABMT	32	23	26 (34% at 3 years)	Bouhour et al. (1996)[37]
Epi/Ifos	11	1–2	120/17.500	PBSCT	64		NA	Reichardt et al. (1998)[38]
Dox/Ifos	18	1–4	75/8000–16 000	PBSCT	50	22	13	Bokemeyer et al. (1987)[39]
Various HDC regimens, EBMT Registry	280 STS (208 RMS)		Variable	PBSC or ABMT			(19% at 5 years) (31% at 5 years) (for CRs)	Rosti et al. (1996)[40]

ABMT, autologous bone marrow transplantation; Carbo, Carboplatin; CDDP, cisplatin; CIE, carboplatin/ifosfamide/etoposide; CTX, cyclophosphamide; Dox, doxorubicin; DTIC, dacarbazine; EBMT, European Blood and Bone Marrow Transplantation Registry; Epi, epirubicin; ETO, etoposide; HDC, high dose chemotherapy; Ifos, ifosfamide; NA, not available; OS, overall survival; PBSCT, peripheral blood stem cell transplantation; RR, response rate; TBI, total body irradiation; Thio, thiothepa; VIC, etoposide/ifosfamide/cisplatin.

resulting in local control rates of 50–80%, over 90% of patients receiving only local therapy relapsed and died of metastatic disease within 2–5 years of therapy. Since the 1970s, intensive multiagent cytotoxic therapy has increased survival rates to 55–65% in localized, and to 30% in metastatic, disease, and thereby has become the backbone of treatment.

Prognostic factors

The most powerful consistently poor prognostic factors for EFTs are metastases at diagnosis (particularly bone/bone marrow metastases), poor histological response to chemotherapy and large volume of local disease (>100 ml, >8 cm²). A young age at presentation has been identified as a good prognostic factor in some series, whereas other analyses failed to confirm this. It has also been suggested that rather than age at diagnosis, the way the disease is treated, with less dose-intensive therapies for the older patient group, may be important for outcome. Whether pelvic localization is a truly unfavourable prognostic factor, or reflects the difficulty and thus the importance of radical local therapy, remains to be further elucidated. Other poor prognostic features that have been identified include increased LDH, neural features and short disease-free interval.[21]

Conventional therapy and dose intensity

Over the last 30 years, a number of studies have been performed by different cooperative groups. Long-term results from the first Intergroup Ewing's Sarcoma Study (IESS1) in 342 localized ES patients indicated that VACA chemotherapy (vincristine, actinomycin, cyclophosphamide, doxorubicin) following radiotherapy was superior to both VAC (vincristine, actinomycin, cyclophosphamide) or VAC with lung irradiation, showing 5-year DFS of 60%, 24% and 44%, respectively, demonstrating the activity of doxorubicin in this disease.[43] In a subsequent study, two different VACA sched-

ules were investigated: on the one hand a high dose intermittent regimen consisting of intensified chemotherapy (at that time) and giving the doxorubicin from the beginning; on the other a moderate dose given continuously. The former regimen was by far superior, improving the DFS from 48% to 68%, and OS from 53% to 77% ($P = 0.02$, and $P = 0.05$, respectively).[44]

A British cooperative group examined a different approach, studying the role of surgery in multimodality therapy. They did not identify a benefit for the group of patients undergoing surgery, in addition to VACA chemotherapy and radiotherapy. In this study, OS at 10 years was significantly better in patients without metastases, being 37% for localized tumours versus 9% for metastatic disease.[45] In the subsequent study (ET2), cyclophosphamide was replaced by ifosfamide in the so-called IVAD (VAIA) and IVA regimens, resulting in a 5-year DFS of 56% and OS of 62%. For patients without metastases the 5-year DFS was 62% compared with 23% for patients with metastatic disease at presentation. The 5-year DFS of 62% is clearly better than the 37% in the former ET1 trial, suggesting superiority of ifosfamide over cyclophosphamide.[46]

The VACA combination was intensively studied by a German collaborative group (CESS81), first as induction chemotherapy, and then with intercalation of local therapy. The 10-year DFS and OS were 53% and 56% respectively.[47] In the follow-up study, VAIA was administered and local therapy was intensified by means of more often (and earlier) surgery and hyper-fractionated radiotherapy. At 8-year follow-up, the DFS and OS were 67 and 69%, respectively. Analysing the data of both studies together, there is evidence that ifosfamide regimens are superior over cyclophosphamide chemotherapy, showing for example an improved OS of large bulky tumours of 66%, as compared with 31% in CESS81.[48] This is in concordance with the data of the ET2 study.

The Children's Cancer Group and Pediatric Oncology Group performed a randomized study of VACA versus the combination of VACA + ifosfamide/etoposide (IE), given in an alternating schedule. Local therapy was intercalated. The 3-year event-free survival was significantly better for VACA + IE, being 69% versus 50%, and the OS of 80% was similarly better for VACA + IE. A group of the US National Cancer Institute also studied a regimen of VAC + IE, and reported an EFS and OS at 5 years of 42% and 45%, respectively.[49]

In summary, with multiagent chemotherapy, 5-year survival rates in localized disease are now 55–65% and in metastatic disease up to 35%.

High dose chemotherapy

The recognition that some patients have very little chance of long-term survival with conventional approaches has prompted the scientific community to study the value of HDC. Hence, EFT meets generally accepted criteria for considering this type of therapy. First, it is sensitive both to radiation and to those classes of chemotherapy that have myelosuppression as their dose-limiting toxicity. Second, a dose–response effect has been shown for several drugs (and radiation) in EFT. Small studies have suggested some benefit in poor-prognosis EFT, while others failed to demonstrate a gain for patients undergoing HDC. However, well-designed randomized studies have not yet been performed.

Table 13.4 reviews the studies that have been performed to date involving at least 15 patients.[6,50–57] The European BMT Solid Tumour Registry (EBMT) has reported on 63 EFT patients in first or second complete remission who have received megatherapy with either PBSCT or ABMT rescue. Patients consolidated in first or second complete remission respectively achieved a 5-year DFS of 21% and 32%. Favourable outcome was limited to patients relapsing after localized disease.[6] Atra et al.[51] reported on a combination of busulfan/melphalan, given as consolidation therapy either in first or second complete remission. With a follow-up of 2 years, 13 (72%) patients remained in complete remission, which compared favourably to

historical controls.[51] A report from an international study performed in Germany, the UK and Austria, on 47 EFT patients receiving HDC, did not show superiority of HDC compared with patients not receiving megatherapy.[54]

Overall, there are some indications from the literature that consolidation therapy by HDC and PSCT/ABMT rescue may contribute to an improved outcome in poor-risk EFT patients, while other studies failed to confirm this benefit. Therefore, in the absence of randomized studies, we cannot draw conclusions on the real value of HDC in EFT.

Recently a randomized study by a European International Ewing working group (Euro-Ewing) was activated. This study will compare high dose therapy with standard maintenance therapy in intermediate-risk patients. Patients with poor-risk disease will be enrolled on an aggressive high dose experimental therapy which may be consolidated with lung irradiation.

CONCLUSION

For patients with STS, higher chemotherapy doses appear to increase response rates. Ifosfamide and doxorubicin, in particular, have clinically relevant dose–response relationships. However, dose-intensified regimens do not lead to an improvement in OS for the patient group as a whole. For patients with widespread metastatic disease requiring palliative therapy, transplant regimens do not seem to offer sufficient activity in meaningfully influencing survival, but they do add toxicity. However, those patients who can be rendered tumour-free by first-line therapy consisting of a multimodal approach, or those who have limited metastatic disease (such as resectable pulmonary metastases), may well be a subset that benefits from a dose-intensified regimen. This approach needs to be investigated in randomized studies. Prognostic factors may be of help in the design of such studies. Until then, HDC cannot be considered standard treatment for STS.

For the EFT, the value of high dose regimens

Table 13.4 High dose regimens in Ewing's tumours

Regimen	No. of patients	Dose	Setting	Support	Event-free survival	Overall survival	Reference
EBMT '82–'92 Variable, 93% melphalan	63 ET	Variable	First CR 32, Second CR 31	ABMT/ PSCT or both (6)	(5-year) CR1 21% CR2 32%		Ladenstein et al. (1995)[6]
Busulfan/ melphalan	16 ET	600 mg/m², 140 mg/m²	First CR 16, Second CR 10	PSCT 49%	(3-year) 71%	(3-year) (1996)[50]	Volteau-Couanet et al. (1996)[50]
Busulfan/ melphalan	18 ET	16 mg/kg, 140–160 mg/m²	First CR 12, Second CR 4	PSCT/ ABMT	(2-year) 72%		Atra et al. (1997)[51]
Busulfan/VP16/ thiothepa	33 ET	16 mg/kg, 1200 mg/m², 300 mg/m²	CR/major PR	PSCT			Tienghi et al. (1997)[52]
CDDP/VP16/CTX (evtl. × 2)	16 ET	150/900/4500 mg/m²	Consolidation	PSCT	proj. DFS 50%, 4-year		Casado et al. (1998)[53]
Melphalan-based + TBI 51% double ME (30%)	32 ET (24/32) 14	1–3/4 weeks, 1–5/4 weeks	45% in CR 30% in PR 4% PD	PSCT/ ABMT	(4-year) 15%		Paulussen et al. (1998)[54]
Melphalan/ETO + TBI double ME + lung irradiation	39 ET M1, early relapse	120/1800 mg/m²		PSCT		(3.5-year) 31%	Pape et al. (1999)[55]
Melphalan/ETO + TBI + IL-2	25 ET M1, early relapse	120/1800 mg/m²		PSCT	(5-year) 34%		Laws et al. (1999)[56]
Melphalan-based conventional consolidation	52 RMS 44 RMS		Consolidation	PSCT/ ABMT	29.7% (3-year) 19.2%	40% (3-year) 27.7%	Carli et al. (1999)[57]

CR, complete response; ET, Ewing's tumour; ME, melphalan/etoposide; PD, progressive disease; PR, partial response; RMS, rhabdomyosarcoma; TBI, total body irradiation; VP16, etoposide. See Tables 13.2 and 13.3 for other abbreviations.

remains unclear. While patients in first partial or first/second complete remission might benefit from HDC, the real value of this approach can only be determined by randomized studies.

Finally, because of the rarity and heterogeneity of these diseases, randomized studies can only be performed by close collaboration of the several cooperative groups. In this way, it may be possible to answer some of these questions within a realistic time frame. Moreover, it must be appreciated by physicians that their patients' interests are best served by participation in clinical trials.

REFERENCES

1. Pisters PWT, Leung DHY, Woodruff J et al. Analysis of prognostic factors in 1,041 patients with localized soft tissue sarcomas of the extremities. J Clin Oncol 1996;14:1679–89.
2. Coindre J-M, Terrier P, Binh Bui N et al. Prognostic factors in adult patients with locally controlled soft tissue sarcoma: a study of 546 patients from the French Federation of Cancer Centers Sarcoma Group. J Clin Oncol 1996;14: 869–77.
3. Le Doussal V, Coindre J-M, Leroux A et al. Prognostic factors for patients with localized primary malignant fibrous histiocytoma. Cancer 1996;77:1823–30.
4. Jenkins MP, Alvaranga JC, Thomas JM. The management of retroperitoneal soft tissue sarcomas. Eur J Cancer 1996;32:622–6.
5. Kilpatrick SE, Doyon J, Choong PFM et al. The clinicopathologic spectrum of myxoid and round cell liposarcoma. Cancer 1996;77:1450–8.
6. Ladenstein R, Lasset C, Pinkerton R et al. Impact of megatherapy in children with high-risk Ewing's tumours in complete remission: a report from the EBMT Solid Tumour Registry. Bone Marrow Transplant 1995;15:697–705.
7. Verrill MW, Judson IR, Harmer CL et al. Ewing's sarcoma and primitive neuro-ectodermal tumor in adults: are they different from Ewing's sarcoma and primitive neuroectodermal tumor in children? J Clin Oncol 1997;15:2611–21.
8. Frei E III, Canellos G. Dose: a critical factor in cancer chemotherapy. Am J Med 1980;69:585–94.
9. Frei E III. Pharmacologic strategies for high-dose chemotherapy. In: Armitage JO, Antman KH, editors. High-dose cancer therapy. Baltimore: Williams & Wilkins, 1995:3–16.
10. Skipper H, Schnabel FJ, Wilcox W. Experimental evaluation of potential anticancer agents. On the criteria and kinetics associated with 'curability' of experimental leukemia. Cancer Chemother Rep 1964;35:1–111.
11. Norton L, Simon R, Brereton J et al. Predicting the course of Gompertzian growth. Nature 1976;264:542–5.
12. Pollock RE, Karnell LH, Menck HR et al. The national cancer data base report on soft tissue sarcoma. Cancer 1996;78:2247–57.
13. Verweij J, Mouridsen HT, Nielsen OS et al. The present state of the art in chemotherapy for STS in adults: the EORTC point of view. Hematology 1995;20:193–201.
14. Patel SR, Benjamin RS. Preference in Sarcomas II. Hemato/Oncology Clinics of Natl America 1995;9(4):xi–xii.
15. Van Glabbeke M, van Oosterom AT, Azzarelli A et al. We do need to confirm the results of small chemotherapy trials in advanced soft tissue sarcoma with randomised studies: the experience of the EORTC/STBSG. Proc Ann Meeting Conn Tissue Oncol Soc, Vancouver, 1998;(4):1.
16. Van Glabbeke M, van Oosterom AT, Oosterhuis JW et al. Prognostic factors for the outcome of chemotherapy in advanced soft tissue sarcoma: an analysis of 2185 patients treated with anthracyclin-containing first line regimens. A EORTC/STBSG study. J Clin Oncol 1999;17:150–7.
17. Verweij J, van Oosterom AT, Somers R et al. Chemotherapy in the multi-disciplinary approach to soft tissue sarcomas. Ann Oncol 1992;3(suppl):75–80.
18. Dombernowsky P, Mouridsen H, Nielsen OS et al. A phase III study comparing adriamycin versus two schedules of high dose epirubicin in advanced soft tissue sarcoma. Proc ASCO 1995; 15:515 (abstract).
19. Steward WP. Chemotherapy for metastatic soft tissue sarcomas. In: Verweij J, Pinedo HM, Suit HD, editors. Soft tissue sarcomas: present achievements and future prospects. Norwell, MA: Kluwer Academic Publishers, 1997: 157–72.
20. Reichardt P, Verweij J, Crowther D. Current controversies in cancer: should high-dose chemotherapy be used in the treatment of soft tissue sarcoma? Eur J Cancer 1997;33:1351–60.
21. Seynaeve C, Verweij J. High-dose chemotherapy

in adult sarcomas: no standard yet. Semin Oncol 1999;26:119–33.

22. Nielsen OS, Dombernowsky P, Mouridsen H et al. High dose epirubicin is not an alternative to standard dose doxorubicin in the treatment of advanced soft tissue sarcoma. Br J Cancer 1999;78:1634–9.

23. Van Oosterom AT, Krzemienlecki K, Nielsen OS et al. Randomised phase II study of the EORTC Soft Tissue and Bone Sarcoma group comparing two different ifosfamide regimens in chemotherapy untreated advanced STS patients. Proc ASCO 1997;18:1787 (abstract).

24. Nielsen OS, Judson I, van Hoesel Q et al. Effect of high dose ifosfamide in advanced soft tissue sarcomas. A multicenter phase II study of the EORTC soft tissue and bone sarcoma group. Eur J Cancer, 2000;36:61–7.

25. Borden EC, Amato DA, Rosenbaum CH et al. Randomised comparison of three adriamycin regimens for metastatic soft tissue sarcomas. J Clin Oncol 1987;5:840–50.

26. Edmonson JH, Ryan LM, Blum RH et al. Randomised comparison of doxorubicin alone versus ifosfamide plus doxorubicin or mitomycin, doxorubicin, and cisplatin against advanced soft tissue sarcomas. J Clin Oncol 1993;11:1269–75.

27. Santoro A, Tursz T, Mouridsen H et al. Doxorubicin versus CyVADIC versus doxorubicin plus ifosfamide in first-line treatment of advanced soft tissue sarcomas: a randomised study of the EORTC/STBSG. J Clin Oncol 1995; 13:1537–45.

28. Antman K, Crowly J, Paulursuli SP et al. An intergroup phase III randomised study of doxorubicin and dacarbazine with or without ifosfamide and Mesna in advanced soft tissue and bone sarcomas. J Clin Oncol 1993;117:1270–85.

29. Tursz T, Verweij J, Judson I et al. Is high-dose chemotherapy of interest in advanced soft tissue sarcomas? An EORTC randomised phase III trial. Proc ASCO 1996;15:337 (abstract).

30. Jelic S, Kovcin V, Milanovic N et al. Randomised study of high-dose epirubicin versus high-dose epirubicin-cisplatin chemotherapy for advanced STS. Eur J Cancer 1997;33:220–5.

31. Steward WP, Verweij J, Somers R et al. GM-CSF allows safe escalation of dose-intensity of chemotherapy in metastatic adult STS: a study of the EORTC/STBSG. J Clin Oncol 1993;11: 15–21.

32. Patel SR, Vadhan-Raj S, Burgess MA et al. Results of 2 consecutive trials of dose-intensive chemotherapy with doxorubicin and ifosfamide in patients with sarcomas. Am J Clin Oncol 1998;21:317–21.

33. Patel SR, Benjamin RS. New chemotherapeutic strategies for soft tissue sarcomas. Semin Surg Oncol 1999;17:47–51.

34. Samuels B, Elias A, Vogelzang N et al. High dose chemotherapy with ABMT for refractory sarcoma. Proc ASCO 1989;30:1086 (abstract).

35. Dumontet C, Biron P, Bouffet E et al. High dose chemotherapy with ABMT in STS. A report of 22 cases. Bone Marrow Transplant 1992;10:405–8.

36. Kessinger A, Petersen K, Bishop M et al. High dose therapy with autologous hematopoietic stem cell rescue for patients with metastatic STS. Proc ASCO 1994;13:1674 (abstract).

37. Bouhour D, Biron P, Blay JY. High dose chemotherapy (HDCT) with autologous hematopoietic stem cell support for STS of adults. Proceedings of the Annual Meeting of the Connective Tissue Oncology Society 1996, Toronto, Canada (abstract).

38. Reichardt P, Tilgner J, Hohenberger P et al. Dose-intensive chemotherapy with ifosfamide, epirubicin, and filgrastim for adult patients with metastatic or locally advanced soft tissue sarcoma: a phase II study. J Clin Oncol 1998;16: 1438–43.

39. Bokemeyer C, Franzke A, Hartman JT et al. A phase I/II study of sequential, dose-escalated, high dose ifosfamide plus doxorubicin with PBSC support for the treatment of patients with advanced STS. Cancer 1997;80:1221–7.

40. Rosti G, Philip T, Chauvin F et al. European group for blood and marrow transplantation (EBMT) registry in solid tumours: 12 years of experience. Bone Marrow Transplant 1996;17:469 (abstract).

41. De Saint Aubain Somerhausen N, Fletcher CDM. Soft tissue sarcomas: an update. Eur J Surg Oncol 1999;25:215–20.

42. Lawlor ER, Mathers JA, Bainbridge T et al. Peripheral primitive neuroectodermal tumours in adults: documentation by molecular analysis. J Clin Oncol 1998;16:1150–7.

43. Nesbit ME, Gehan EA, Burgert EO et al. Multimodal therapy for the management of primary nonmetastatic Ewing's sarcoma of bone: a long-term follow-up of the first intergroup study. J Clin Oncol 1990;8:1664–74.

44. Burgert EO, Nesbit ME, Garnsey LA et al. Multimodal therapy for the management of non-pelvic, localized Ewing's sarcoma of bone: intergroup study IESS-II. J Clin Oncol 1990;8:1514–24.

45. Craft AW, Cotterill SJ, Bullimore JA et al. Long-term results from the first IKCCSG Ewing's tumour study (ET-1). Eur J Cancer 1997;33:1061–9.

46. Craft A, Cotterill S, Malcolm A et al. Ifosfamide containing chemotherapy in Ewing's sarcoma: the second United Kingdom Children's Cancer Study Group and the Medical Research Council Ewing's Tumor Study. J Clin Oncol 1998;16:3628–33.

47. Sauer HR, Jurgens H, Burgers JM et al. Prognostic factors in the treatment of Ewing's sarcoma. The Ewing's sarcoma study group of the German Society of Pediatric Oncology (CESS 81). Radiother Oncol 1987;10:101–10.

48. Paulussen M, Ahrens S, Burdach S et al. Primary metastatic Ewing tumours. Survival analysis of 171 patients from the EICESS studies. Ann Oncol 1998;9:275–81.

49. Wexler LH, DeLaney TF, Tsokos M et al. Ifosfamide and etoposide plus vincristine, doxorubicin, and cyclophosphamide for newly diagnosed Ewing's sarcoma family of tumours. Cancer 1996;78:901–11.

50. Volteau-Couanet D, Oberlin O, Benhamou E et al. High efficiency of busulfan-melphalan as consolidation in metastatic Ewing's sarcoma. Bone Marrow Transplant 1996;17(suppl 1):463 (abstract).

51. Atra A, Whelan JS, Calvagna V et al. High-dose busulphan/melphalan with autologous stem cell rescue in Ewing's sarcoma. Bone Marrow Transplant 1997;2:843–6.

52. Tienghi A, Vertogen B, Rosti G. Intensive mobilizing induction chemotherapy followed by high-dose chemotherapy with PBSC rescue in young adults with high risk Ewing's sarcoma. Proc ASCO 1997;16:498 (abstract).

53. Casado A, Martin M, Garcia-Carbonero Y et al. High-dose DICEP chemotherapy with or without PBSC support as consolidation treatment in young adults with high risk Ewing's sarcoma and PNET. Preliminary results. Proc ASCO 1998;17:520 (abstract).

54. Paulussen M, Ahrens S, Braun-Munzinger G et al. High dose therapy with stem cell rescue in EICESS patients with metastatic Ewing tumours. Bone Marrow Transplant 1998;21(suppl 1):68–70.

55. Pape H, Laws HJ, Burdach S et al. Radiotherapy and high-dose chemotherapy in advanced Ewing's tumours. Strahlenther Onkol 1999;175:484–7.

56. Laws HJ, Burdach S, van Kaick B et al. Multimodality diagnostics and megatherapy in poor prognosis Ewing's tumour patients. A single center report. Strahlenther Onkol 1999;175:488–94.

57. Carli M, Colombatti R, Oberlin O et al. High-dose melphalan with autologous stem-cell rescue in metastatic rhabdomyosarcoma. J Clin Oncol 1999;17:2796–803.

14

Dose intensification and small cell lung cancer

Rhada Bhaskaran, Mark Middleton, Paul Burt, Ron Stout and Nicholas Thatcher

CONTENTS Introduction • Retrospective analyses of dose intensity • Intensive induction, early intensification • Late intensification • Accelerated chemotherapy • New approaches • Summary

INTRODUCTION

The clinical value of dose intensification in small cell lung cancer (SCLC) has recently been the subject of a number of randomized controlled trials. Preclinical models, particularly the work of Skipper and Schabel, established the relationship between dose factors and tumour response. The work indicated that the dose–response curve for the majority of anti-tumour agents was usually steep in the linear phase. Importantly, from these data, it was determined that a dose reduction of the order of 20% could lead to a reduction of cure of 50% or more. In contrast, a two-fold increase in the dose could lead to a 10-fold increase in tumour cell kill.[1–5] Skipper also reported a retrospective analysis of the original data,[6] which indicated that dose intensity affects the degree of response achieved (complete versus partial, i.e. proportion of cures), whereas cumulative dose correlates more with survival time in animals in whom the tumour is not eradicated.

The older clinical reports, which in general showed no relationship between total dose, dose intensity and survival, were analysed on planned protocol doses rather than the actual dose received by the patient. As many of the 'high dose intensity' regimens had doses reduced due to patient toxicity, the received dose intensity in these trials was almost always less than in the standard arm. Therefore in many of these studies the relationship between dose intensity and survival was not adequately assessed.

Nevertheless SCLC is a very chemosensitive tumour and somatic models predict the probability of developing drug resistance with time.[5,7] These models suggest that the probability of developing drug resistance due to random mutations in later dosing is greatly reduced by higher initial doses of chemotherapy. In addition, dose-intensive regimens should reduce tumour growth between treatments, possibly fewer mutants will arise during chemotherapy and long-term remissions or cures should be more frequent. It would make sense, then, to treat with maximal chemotherapy doses in the first instance, with the shortest possible intervals between treatments.

RETROSPECTIVE ANALYSES OF DOSE INTENSITY

There have been a number of retrospective analyses of the relationship between dose intensity (defined as mg/m^2 per week) and outcome. The meta-analysis by Klasa et al.[8] in 1991 examined 60 published studies. Increased dose intensity in the CAVE (cyclophosphamide, doxorubicin, vincristine, etoposide) and CAE (cyclophosphamide, doxorubicin, etoposide) regimens correlated positively with median survival in extensive-stage disease but this was not so with the CAV (cyclophosphamide, doxorubicin, vincristine) regimen. Another study of extensive-stage patients who received CAV-type regimens at conventional doses or at a higher dose intensity reported significantly better 1-year survival rates (32% versus 12%) and overall survival with the higher dose intensity.[9] A recent analysis of two consecutive phase II studies in 131 limited-stage patients has been reported. The two studies used the same four drugs (etoposide, cyclophosphamide, doxorubicin, cisplatin) in an alternating radiotherapy chemotherapy schedule. The 5-year survival rate was 25% for the higher initial doses of cisplatin and cyclophosphamide but only 9% ($P < 0.01$) for the other patients treated with lower doses.[10]

If toxicity requires dose modification it may be better to maintain the dose but increase the interval between chemotherapy courses rather than reduce the dose, which is common practice.[11] The Manchester group has examined the combination of ifosfamide, carboplatin and etoposide with mid-course vincristine (VICE) in three consecutive phase II studies totalling 166 patients. Inclusion criteria required a reasonable performance status, but both limited and extensive stage were accepted.[12–14] An important policy was that no dose reduction over a total of six chemotherapy courses was adopted. Survival rates of 30% or more were seen with a minimum follow-up of 2 years. Further analysis has demonstrated a 5-year survival rate of 19% with a minimum follow-up of 4.5 years.[15,16] The dose intensity was maintained with this policy of dose delay rather than dose reduction. Despite the myelotoxicity, most of the patients received all six courses of chemotherapy at full dose. However, when cisplatin was alternated with carboplatin, fewer courses were given, a lower percentage of patients received all six courses and there was increased toxicity, mainly due to renal impairment.[13] Table 14.1 shows that the protocol dose intensity can be maintained with this policy both over the first three and also subsequent cycles. If both dose delay and dose reduction are practised, the relative dose intensity is reduced, as in the London study.[17] Again, when only four courses of chemotherapy were given together with dose reduction, a poorer 2-year survival rate was obtained even though a similar population of patients was treated.[18] Despite the bone marrow toxicity of the VICE regimen, the patients' performance status and disease-related symptoms improved rapidly.[12–16] These parameters of therapeutic efficacy are rarely reported for intensive regimens and should be considered alongside the conventional grading of haematological and other toxicities, which are usually transient.

INTENSIVE INDUCTION, EARLY INTENSIFICATION

It would appear logical to treat an extremely sensitive tumour like SCLC with early high dose therapy before drug resistance could develop. The earlier studies arose from the trial of Cohen et al., which reported significantly improved response rate and survival when the dose of cyclophosphamide was increased from 0.5 to 1 g/m^2, lomustine from 50 to 100 mg/m^2, and methotrexate from 10 to 15 mg/m^2.[19] However, the standard arm of this trial would now be considered suboptimal in terms of dose. These earlier studies mainly used cyclophosphamide and etoposide and are summarized in Tables 14.2 and 14.3. On occasions, very high doses were used together with bone marrow transplantation. While higher complete response rates were seen in certain circumstances, none of these other studies showed an improvement in survival. As a result of these studies, Souhami and Ruiz De Elvira[30] concluded that no firm conclusions could be drawn about potential survival benefit with an increasing intensity of treatment.

Table 14.1 Dose intensity VICE-type chemotherapy

Regimen	RDI		Patients receiving all 6 courses	Survival		Reference
	1–3 courses	4–6 courses		Median (months)	2 years (%)	
VICE	1	1	74	14	33	Thatcher et al. (1989)[12]
VIC/PE†	1	0.77	68	14	30	Prendiville et al. (1990)[13]
VICE†	1	0.86	72	16	31	Prendiville et al. (1994)[14]
RMH‡	0.92	0.66	72	13	22	Smith et al. (1990)[17]
WSLCG†	–	–	only 4 courses	10	11	Hatton et al. (1995)[18]

C, carboplatin; E, etoposide; I, ifosfamide; P, cisplatin; RDI, relative dose intensity; RMH, Royal Marsden Hospital, London; V, vincristine; VICE, ifosfamide + carboplatin + etoposide + mid-course vincristine; WSLCG, West of Scotland Cancer Group.
†Intercalated radiotherapy used.
‡Dose reduction practised.

A more recent randomized study examined higher doses of cisplatin and etoposide in extensive disease, with a higher dose intensity being planned for just the first two cycles. Despite treatment delays which resulted in lower than planned dose rate intensity in the high dose arm, dose intensity remained 46% higher than the standard treatment arm.[35] Both complete response and median survival were similar in both arms, with higher treatment-related toxicity in the high dose arm.

A prospective French trial of a four-drug regimen (cisplatin, cyclophosphamide, etoposide, doxorubicin), which was based on an earlier retrospective study,[10] randomized patients to receive higher or lower initial doses of cisplatin and cyclophosphamide. This was followed by five cycles of standard therapy with three intercalated courses of radiotherapy. In this study the initial doses of cyclophosphamide and cisplatin were 20–25% higher than the standard regimen. The 2-year survival rate was 43% for the higher dose group, compared with 26% for the lower dose chemotherapy group ($P = 0.02$).[34]

LATE INTENSIFICATION

As the growth fraction of a tumour may increase as the tumour responds to treatment, the intensity of therapy which results in regression may be insufficient to sustain a tumour response. Norton and Simon therefore suggest that chemotherapy should be intensified as soon as possible for as long as possible after standard induction treatment.[36] The success of late intensification in haematological malignancies with bone marrow transplantation, etc., encouraged the use of a similar approach in chemoresponsive tumours such as SCLC. A

Table 14.2 Intensive induction for small cell lung cancer: phase II studies

Regimen (mg/m²) unless otherwise stated	No. of patients		Response		Survival		Reference
	LS	ES	CR (%)	PR (%)	Median (months)	2 years (%)	
CM (1500–3500, 100)	55	–	53	25	12	23	Thatcher et al. (1982)[20]
CEVA (4500, 600, 3, 80) + BMT, 2 courses	9	5	54	46	14	NR	Fahra et al. (1983)[21]
CAVE (1000, 50, 1.4, 125) Day 1 and 8 on courses 2 or 3	–	34	24	70	12	6 (DFS)	Brower et al. (1983)[22]
C (160–200 mg/kg) + BMT, 1 course	21	4	56	28	17	12 (DFS)	Souhami et al. (1983)[23]
CE (200 mg/kg, 400–600) + BMT, 2 courses	26	–	50	31	9.7	15 (DFS)	Souhami et al. (1985)[24]
CE (100 mg/kg, 1200) 2 courses	17	–	29	65	10	NR	Johnson et al. (1985)[25]
CE (1500–3500, 480) 3 courses	91	20	56	25	11	12	Thatcher et al. (1985)[26]
CE (2500, 489) 3 courses	55	15	54	21	11	11	Thatcher et al. (1985)[27]
CEP (100 mg/kg, 1200, 120) 1–2 courses	–	20	65	25	9.5	NR	Johnson et al. (1987)[28]
E (1200) 1–8 courses	–	21	–	24	5	NR	Luikart et al. (1987)[29]

A, doxorubicin; BMT, bone marrow transplantation; C, cyclophosphamide; CR, complete response; DFS, disease-free survival; E, etoposide; ES, extensive stage; LS, limited stage; M, methotrexate; NR, not recorded; P, cisplatin; PR, partial response; V, vincristine.

number of studies were undertaken which are summarized in Table 14.4.

To take an example, Spitzer et al. reported on patients with limited-stage SCLC who received conventional chemotherapy followed by high dose cylophosphamide and etoposide with or without vincristine and methotrexate, followed by autologous bone marrow transplantation (ABMT). Despite an improvement in complete response rate there was no obvious increase in response duration or survival compared with standard treatment.[37]

In a review of 178 patients from seven studies, 37% had a complete response after the late-intensification procedure but only 9.5% of patients were alive 1 year after therapy and 7.8% died during treatment, indicating no obvious survival advantage.[38]

Humblet et al.[44] conducted the only randomized study of high dose late intensification with

Table 14.3 Intensive induction for small cell lung cancer: randomized phase III trials

Regimen (mg/m²)	No. of patients		Response		Survival		Reference
	LS	ES	CR (%)	PR (%)	Median (months)	2 years (%)	
SD LMC (50, 10, 500)	1	8	0	45	5.0	0	Cohen et al.
HD LMC (100, 50, 1000)	4	19	30	66	10.5	13	(1977)[19]*
SD MeLVC (75, 2, 750)	8	6	38	25	10.8	NR	O'Donnell et al.
HD MeLVC (100, 2, 2000)	5	9	60	20	9.0	NR	(1985)[31]
SD CAV (1000, 50, 1)	18	33	22	39	NR	NR	Figuerdo et al.
HD CAV (1500–2250, 60, 1)	16	36	21	50	NR	NR	(1985)[32]
SD CAV (1000, 40, 1)	–	174	12	41	8.7	NR	Johnson et al.
HD CAV (1200, 70, 1) Courses 1–3	–	124	22	42	7.3	NR	(1987)[33]
SD CPAE (900, 80, 40, 75)	50	–	54	NR	NR	26	Arriagada et al.
HD CPAE (1200, 100, 40, 75) Course 1 only	55	–	67	NR	NR	43	(1993)[34]*
SD PE (80, 240)	–	46	22	61	10.7	NR	Ihde et al.
HD PE (135, 400) Courses 1 and 2	–	44	23	63	11.4	NR	(1994)[35]

A, doxorubicin; BMT, bone marrow transplantation; C, cyclophosphamide; CR, complete response; DFS, disease-free survival; E, etoposide; ES, extensive stage; HD, high dose; I, ifosfamide; L, CCNU; LS, limited stage; M, methotrexate; MeL, methylCCNU; NR, not recorded; P, cisplatin; PR, partial response; SD, standard dose; V, vincristine.
*Statistically significant.

autologous BMT (ABMT) compared with standard chemotherapy (Table 14.4). Patients with limited-stage disease who showed any response to standard induction chemotherapy and those with extensive-stage disease who achieved a complete response were randomized to either further conventional chemotherapy or to intensive chemotherapy with autologous bone marrow transplantation (ABMT). Although late intensification significantly extended relapse-free survival from 10 to 28 weeks ($P = 0.002$), median survival was not significantly different: 68 weeks for the intensified group and 55 weeks for the standard therapy group.[44]

Table 14.4 Late intensification: phase II studies

Induction regimen	LI regimen (mg/m²) unless otherwise stated	No. of patients	PR to CR†	Median survival (months)	Reference
PAE	P + A (120, 90–135) + E (720–1090) ± BMT	13	1	8.5	Klastersky et al. (1983)[39]
EAV	C (7000) ± BMT	36	5	11	Smith et al. (1985)[40]
ACEVM	C + E (180 mg/kg, 1000) + BMT	22	3	12 (LD) 7 (ES)	Banham et al. (1985)[41]
ACE ± P	C + E (100–200 mg/kg, 750–3500) ± BMT	6	5	12	Sculier et al. (1985)[42]
VIA or ECAV	C + E + V (4500, 600, 3) ± M (1500, 40–60) + BMT	32	9	14	Spitzer et al. (1986)[37]
CML–VVAP$_z$	C + E (120 mg/kg, 600) + BMT	29	1	5.5	Ihde et al. (1986)[43]
MVCA–PE	C + E + B (6000, 500, 300) + BMT	101	9	17 (13.8 no LI)	Humblett et al. (1987)[44]‡
PE–PEAV	C (150 mg/kg) no BMT	58	5	11.1	Goodman et al. (1991)[45]
Various	C + P + B (5625, 165, 480) + BMT	19	7	15	Elias et al. (1993)[46]

A, doxorubicin; B, carmustine; E, etoposide; ES, extensive stage; I, ifosfamide; L, lomustine; LI, late intensification; LS, limited stage; M, methotrexate; P, cisplatin; P$_z$, procarbazine; V, vincristine.
PR to CR, partial response with induction regimen converted to complete response with LI.
‡ Statistically significant.

There are inherent problems in late-intensification randomized trials, given that very large numbers of patients are required. Only about a third of patients in late-intensification programmes are actually suitable for the procedure because of toxicity during the induction regimen, lack of initial response or inability to withstand the side effects of late-intensification chemotherapy. The development of recombinant haemopoietic growth factors has allowed intensive accelerated chemotherapy to be given without the need for bone marrow transplantation.

ACCELERATED CHEMOTHERAPY

Weekly chemotherapy

Another way to try to increase dose intensity is by giving chemotherapy courses with as short an interval as possible between cycles. A number of studies of weekly chemotherapy were conducted in the early 1990s and a summary is presented in Table 14.5.

Originally the strategy was to alternate myelosuppressive with non-myelosuppressive chemotherapy. Overall response rates of 85%, with 44% complete response and a median survival of 12 months or more, were reported. These regimens were generally well tolerated.[38] A randomized trial from the London group alternated cisplatin and etoposide (PE) with ifosfamide and doxorubicin for 12 consecutive weeks. This accelerated regimen was compared with a standard 3-weekly treatment with alternating CAV/PE in good performance status-limited and extensive-stage patients.[51] The median survivals of 44 weeks versus 46 weeks and response rates were not significantly different. However, the received dose intensity was only 73% for the weekly group due to dose reductions and delays, and 92% on the standard 3-weekly regimen.[51] A similar study was conducted by the European Lung Cancer Working Party which also showed no survival advantage in patients treated with weekly multiple-drug chemotherapy as against standard combination treatment with CAE.[50] The National Cancer

Institute of Canada (NCIC) investigated weekly cisplatin administered for nine consecutive weeks with alternation of the other drugs in the CODE regimen (cisplatin, vincristine, doxorubicin, etoposide). Forty-eight patients with extensive stage had a median survival of 61 weeks and a 2-year survival of 30%; as a result of this an intergroup phase III trial was undertaken comparing the weekly CODE regimen with a standard alternating CAV/PE for extensive-stage SCLC.[49,52] Although response rate was higher, progression-free and overall survival were not significantly improved, with 10% of patients on both arms progression-free at 2 years and approximately 18% of patients on both arms alive at 2 years. However, overall treatment-related mortality was 0.9% on CAVE/PE versus 8.2% on CODE ($P = 0.04$) and the trial was stopped before the target accrual goal was met. This is the only randomized accelerated chemotherapy trial in which an increased dose intensity was achieved that did not lead to a survival benefit.

Accelerated chemotherapy with or without haemopoietic growth factors

Most chemotherapy regimens are dose limited by myelosuppression. It would be logical to use factors which can reduce the depth and duration of myelosuppression and thereby facilitate the use of more intensive chemotherapy regimens. Granulocyte colony stimulating factor (G-CSF) and granulocyte–macrophage colony stimulating factor (GM-CSF) are two of the factors which have been investigated most frequently in this context.

The earlier studies of G-CSF and later GM-CSF were not designed to test whether the interval between chemotherapy courses could be maintained or shortened, thereby leading to more dose-intensive therapy. The studies, summarized in Table 14.6, were more concerned with the effect of the CSF on haematological toxicity. Indeed, two studies actually showed greater toxicity with the haemopoietic growth factor when concurrent radiotherapy was given

Table 14.5 Trials of weekly chemotherapy

Regimen	No. of patients		CR (%)	PR (%)	Median survival (months)	Survival at 2 years (%)	DI† (%)	Reference
	LS	ES						
Phase II								
CA/MV/PE/V	34		47	35	16.6			Taylor et al. (1990)[47]
		42	38	43	11.4			
PE/IA	45		51	40	14.5			Miles et al. (1991)[48]
		25	48	44	10.5			
CVAE		48	40	54	15.2			Murray et al. (1991)[49]
Phase III								
ACE versus ACE/PVd/VM	48	60	21	37	10.8	8.5		Sculier et al. (1993)[50]
weekly	47	60	31	41	12.3	7.9	−14	
CAV/PE versus IA/PE	135	82	39	43	10.6	11.7		Souhami et al. (1994)[51]
weekly	141	80	37	44	10.8	11.8	−20	
CAV/PE versus CVAE	–	109	22	47	11.9			Murray et al. (1999)[52]
weekly	–	110	27	60	12.8	c.18	c.2x	

A, doxorubicin; C, cyclophosphamide; CR, complete response; E, etoposide; ES, extensive stage; I, ifosfamide; LS, limited stage; M, methotrexate; P, cisplatin; PR, partial response; V, vincristine; Vd, vindesine.
†DI, dose intensity, minus values indicate reduction in DI compared with standard chemotherapy.

Table 14.6 Phase III trials with and without G-CSF and GM-CSF

Regimen	No. of patients		Response		Survival		DI (%)	Reference
	LS	ES	CR (%)	PR (%)	Median (months)	2 years (%)		
ACE versus	29	75	19	61	12.2	NR	NR	Crawford et al.
ACE + G-CSF	27	68	30	42	11.4	NR	NR	(1991)[53]
ACE versus	25	39	87 (OR)†	13.1	13.1	9.1	88	Trillet et al. (1993,
ACE + G-CSF	22	43	79 (OR)†	11.5	11.5	13	96	1995)[54,55]
PE + RT versus	108	–	44	42	17	NR	86	Bunn et al.
PE + RT + GM-CSF	17	–	36	37	14	NR	75	(1995)[56]
C Ep EP × 4† versus	–	60	20	51	10.8	NR	84	Pujol et al.
C Ep EP + GMCSF × 6†	–	65	28	44	8.9	NR	76	(1997)[57]

A, doxorubicin; C, cyclophosphamide; CR, complete response; DI, dose intensity % of protocol dose; E, etoposide; Ep, epidoxorubicin; ES, extensive stage; G-CSF, granulocyte colony stimulating factor; GM-CSF, granulocyte–macrophage colony stimulating factor; LS, limited stage; MS, median survival; P, cisplatin; PR, partial response; RT, radiotherapy.
†OR, CR + PR.
‡Courses of chemotherapy.

with cisplatin[56] or when there was an attempt to increase the chemotherapy doses over the first four cycles.[57] In these early and some later randomized trials of chemotherapy with and without G-CSF and GM-CSF, no increase in received dose intensity could be obtained when cisplatin chemotherapy regimens were used (Tables 14.6 and 14.7), largely because non-haematological side effects such as renal toxicity and neurotoxicity. For example, in the trial of Miles et al.[58] the dose was 82% of that projected in the standard arm and 84% of that projected in patients receiving G-CSF. It is not surprising that there was no improvement in the patient outcome over the standard arm.[58] The major fault with the earlier studies was an attempt to intensify the dose of drugs where the main dose-limiting toxicity was non-haematological. However, when the more recent studies of regimens that did not include cisplatin are examined, the received dose intensity obtained with G-CSF or GM-CSF was increased and survival improved[60–63] (Table 14.7).

After studies that demonstrated the feasibility of accelerated chemotherapy,[64–66] a large randomized Medical Research Council trial of ACE (doxorubicin, cyclophosphamide, etoposide) was designed in which therapy was given every 3 weeks as standard or every 2 weeks with G-CSF in both limited- and extensive-stage patients with good performance status.[63] Rather surprisingly for this large pragmatic study, the increased dose intensity achieved was 33% (planned 50%) in the G-CSF group and there was modest survival improvement with no additional toxicity for the intensified group of patients.[63]

In another study by the Manchester group, G-CSF was used with the VICE regimen. Patients were randomized to receive G-CSF or no G-CSF; chemotherapy was given as soon as the blood count was satisfactory in both groups.

Table 14.7 Accelerated chemotherapy with and without G-CSF and GM-CSF

Regimen	No. of patients		Response		Survival		DI (%)	Reference
	LS	ES	CR (%)	PR (%)	Median (months)	2 years (%)		
PE/IA versus	12	5	71 (OR)†		NR	NR	82	Miles et al.
PE/IA + G-CSF	15	8	74 (OR)†		NR	NR	84	(1994)[58]
CVAE versus	–	31	23	61	8.0	6.5	72	Fukuoka et al.
CVAE + G-CSF	–	32	34	63	14.8	31	84	(1997)[59]*
VICE versus	28	3	58	36	16.3	15	118	Woll et al.
VICE + G-CSF	32	2	56	38	17.3	32	125	(1995)[60]
CAV/PE versus	–	113	15	61	10.9	8.5	82	Furuse et al.
CVAE + G-CSF	–	114	16	68	11.6	11.7	72	(1998)[61]
VICE 4 weekly versus	85	68	41	24	12.5	18	NR	Steward et al.
VICE 3 weekly ± GM-CSF	93	54	44	33	15.8	33	126	(1998)[62]*
ACE 3 weekly versus	151	51	28	50	11.8	8		Thatcher et al.
ACE + G-CSF 2 weekly	153	48	40	38	12.5	13	134	(2000)[63]*

A, doxorubicin; C, carboplatin; E, etoposide; I, ifosfamide; G-CSF, granulocyte colony stimulating factor; GM-CSF, granulocyte–macrophage colony stimulating factor; NR, not reported; P, cisplatin; V, vincristine.
*Statistically significant survival difference.

No dose reduction were performed over the six cycles of planned therapy. The G-CSF group received a significantly higher dose intensity than the control group (no G-CSF), with greatest dose intensity difference in the first three cycles (134% of the intensity of 4-weekly VICE versus 117%, $P = 0.01$). For all six cycles the dose intensity was 125% for G-CSF patients and 118% for controls. The median survival of 65 weeks for the controls and 69 weeks for G-CSF patients was not significantly different, but the proportion of patients alive at 2 years was 15% for the controls and 32% for the G-CSF higher dose intensity regimen.[60]

These studies indicate that when dose intensity is increased and cisplatin is avoided, treatment outcomes can be improved. The ICE or VICE regimens have the advantage that the dose-limiting toxicity is myelosuppression. Whilst an interval of 4–5 weeks is generally required to allow bone marrow recovery,[15,16] a large randomized trial established that a 26% dose intensification of the VICE regimen could be achieved with GM-CSF and this was associated with a significant improvement in the 2-year survival (33% versus 18%, $P = 0.0014$). Furthermore, extensive-stage patients who had good performance status also benefited from the accelerated intensified treatment.[62]

NEW APPROACHES

In addition to the growth factors discussed above, there are a number of other haemopoietic growth factors in development. The interleukins (IL) IL-3, IL-6 and IL-11 have all shown activity in the treatment of chemotherapy-induced thrombocytopaenia.[67–69] Erythropoietin is reported to be effective in the treatment and prevention of anaemia associated with chemotherapy and may have an effect on thrombocytopaenia.[70] However, to date, no studies have examined the role of these drugs in intensifying treatment. Treatment with combinations of growth factors is feasible and could be of future interest.[68]

The use of bone marrow transplantation for early and late intensification has already been discussed. More recently the use of peripheral blood progenitor cells has suggested new possibilities. Progenitor cells are mobilized from the bone marrow in significant numbers during normal recovery from myelosuppressive chemotherapy and additionally by the use of G-CSF and GM-CSF; IL-3 has also been used in such procedures.[71]

Unlike the situation in lymphomas and rare tumours, the logistic requirements and technical expertise needed for cell separation, cryopreservation and thawing, together with the necessary equipment, prevent the use of leukapheresis and cryopreserved peripheral blood progenitor cells to support high dose or dose-intensification therapy in common cancers. Recently the Manchester group has reported on the viability of harvested peripheral blood progenitor cells in whole blood compared with leukapheresis products stored for 48 h at 4°C. The viability of the cells was similar to that found after conventional cryopreservation and thawing and suggested that peripheral blood progenitor cells in the patient's whole blood could be stored for limited periods at 4°C and used to support multi-cyclic intensive chemotherapy.[72,73]

These observations led to the initiation of a cohort study with three groups of patients (Table 14.8). Haemopoietic progenitors were collected during each course and reinfused on day 3 of the next cycle. The first cohort was treated every 3 weeks with leukapheresis and cryopreservation every 2 weeks post-chemotherapy for six cycles. The second cohort was treated every 2 weeks with leukapheresis on day 1 of the chemotherapy cycle but with

---

Table 14.8 Accelerated ICE-type chemotherapy including peripheral blood progenitor cells (PBPC) support with whole blood

Regimen	Dose intensity increase, courses 1–4 (%)	Reference
No G-CSF	117	Woll et al. (1995)[60]
G-CSF no PBPC	134	Woll et al. (1995)[60]
3-weekly leukapheresis, cryopreservation	133	Pettengell et al. (1995)[73]
2-weekly leukapheresis, 4°C	200	Pettengell et al. (1995)[73]
2-weekly whole blood 4°C	190 (for all 6 cycles of therapy)	Pettengell et al. (1995)[73]

Abbreviation: G-CSF, granulocyte-colony-stimulating factor.

storage of the leukapheresis product at 4°C in a blood fridge and reinfusion after treatment. The third cohort was treated every 2 weeks and 500–750 ml of whole blood was drawn by venesection on day 1, immediately before the chemotherapy cycle, and stored at 4°C. The autologous whole blood was then reinfused the day after chemotherapy. The procedure was repeated for every cycle of chemotherapy. Results showed that the extremely myelosuppressive ICE regimen could be given every 2 weeks at full dose over six cycles using peripheral blood progenitor cell whole blood autotransfusions after each cycle. This technique achieved a 190–200% dose intensification.[73] Following this, a randomized phase II study was performed in which 50 patients with SCLC with good prognosis were allocated to receive standard 4-weekly ICE chemotherapy or 2-weekly treatment with peripheral progenitor cell autotransfusion support. There was a substantial increase in relative dose intensity of 180% in the autotransfusion arm compared with the standard regimen ($P = 0.0001$). Surprisingly, toxicity and the requirement for antibiotics, hospitalization etc. was less for patients receiving intensified treatment with autotransfusions.[74] A randomized phase III study is currently in progress to test whether this novel dose-intensification approach confers a survival benefit over standard treatment.

SUMMARY

A clear case for dose-intense therapy in small cell lung cancer has yet to be made. However, it is only recently that properly designed, well-executed studies have been performed to address this issue, and evidence is emerging for a survival advantage in selected patients.

REFERENCES

1. Skipper HE, Schabel Jr FM, Mellett LB et al. Implications of biochemical, cytokinetic, pharmacologic and toxicologic relationships in the design of optimal therapeutic schedules. Cancer Chemother Rep 1970;54:431–50.
2. Schabel Jr FM, Griswold Jr DP, Corbett TH, Laster WR. Increasing the therapeutic response rates to anticancer drugs by applying the basic principles of pharmacology. Cancer 1984; 54(suppl):1160–7.
3. DeVita VT. Principles of chemotherapy in cancer. In: DeVita VT, Hellman S, Rosenberg SA, editors. Principles and practice of oncology. Philadelphia: JB Lippincott, 1989:276–300.
4. Gurney H, Dodwell D, Thatcher N et al. Escalating drug delivery in cancer chemotherapy: a review of concepts and practice – part 1. Ann Oncol 1993;4:23–34.
5. DeVita VT. The influence of information on drug resistance on protocol design. Ann Oncol 1991;2:93–106.
6. Skipper HE. Dose intensity versus total dose of chemotherapy: an experimental basis. In: DeVita VT, Hellman S, Rosenberg SA, editors. Important advances in oncology. Philadelphia: JB Lippincott, 1990:43–64.
7. Coldman AJ, Goldie JH. Impact of dose-intense chemotherapy on the development of permanent drug resistance. Semin Oncol 1987;14(suppl 4): 29–33.
8. Klasa RJ, Murray N, Coldman AJ. Dose intensity meta-analysis of chemotherapy regimens in small cell carcinoma of the lung. J Clin Oncol 1991;9:499–508.
9. Sheehan RG, Balaban EP, Frenkel EP. The impact of dose intensity of standard chemotherapy regimens in extensive stage small cell lung cancer. Am J Clin Oncol 1993;16:250–5.
10. De Vathaire F, Arriagada R, De The H et al. Dose intensity of initial chemotherapy may have an impact on survival in limited small cell lung carcinoma. Lung Cancer 1993;8:301–8.
11. Gurney H, Dodwell D, Thatcher N et al. Escalating drug delivery in cancer chemotherapy: a review of concepts and practice – Part 2. Ann Oncol 1993;4:103–15.
12. Thatcher N, Lind M, Stout R et al. Carboplatin, ifosfamide and etoposide with mid-course vincristine and thoracic radiotherapy for 'limited' stage small cell carcinoma of the bronchus. Br J Cancer 1989;60:98–101.
13. Prendiville J, Radford J, Thatcher N et al. Intensive therapy for small-cell lung cancer using carboplatin alternating with cisplatin, ifosfamide, etoposide, mid-cycle vincristine and

radiotherapy. J Clin Oncol 1991;9:1446–52.

14. Prendiville J, Lorigan P, Hicks F et al. Therapy for small cell lung cancer using carboplatin, ifosfamide, etoposide (without dose reduction), mid-cycle vincristine with thoracic and cranial irradiation. Eur J Cancer 1994;30A:2085–90.

15. Thatcher N, Lorigan P, Burt P, Stout R. Intensive combined modality therapy in small cell lung cancer. Semin Oncol 1994;21(suppl 6):9–23.

16. Lorigan P, Ming Lee S, Betticher D et al. Chemotherapy with vincristine/ifosfamide/carboplatin/etoposide in small cell lung cancer. Semin Oncol 1995;22(suppl 7):32–41.

17. Smith IE, Perren TJ, Ashley SA et al. Carboplatin, etoposide and ifosfamide as intensive chemotherapy for small cell lung cancer. J Clin Oncol 1990;8:899–905.

18. Hatton MQF, Cassidy J, Bicknell S et al. Ifosfamide, carboplatin and etoposide for good prognosis small cell lung cancer. Are four courses adequate? Eur J Cancer 1995;31A:1022–3.

19. Cohen MH, Creaven PJ, Fossieck BE. Intensive chemotherapy of small cell bronchogenic carcinoma. Cancer Treat Rep 1977;61:349–54.

20. Thatcher N, Barber PV, Hunter RD et al. 11-week course of sequential methotrexate, thoracic irradiation, and moderate-dose cyclophosphamide for 'limited' stage small cell bronchogenic carcinoma. A study from the Manchester Lung Tumour Group. Lancet 1982;1:1040–3.

21. Farha P, Spitzer G, Valdivieso M et al. High-dose chemotherapy and autologous bone marrow transplantation for the treatment of small cell lung cancer. Cancer 1983;52:1351–5.

22. Brower M, Ihde DC, Johnston-Early A et al. Treatment of extensive stage small cell bronchogenic carcinoma. Am J Med 1983;75:993–1000.

23. Souhami RL, Harper PG, Linch D et al. High-dose cyclophosphamide with autologous marrow transplantation for small cell carcinoma of the bronchus. Cancer Chemother Pharmacol 1983;10:205–7.

24. Souhami RL, Finn G, Gregory WM et al. High-dose cyclophosphamide in small cell carcinoma of the lung. J Clin Oncol 1985;3:958–63.

25. Johnson DH, Wolff SN, Hainsworth JD et al. Extensive-stage small-cell bronchogenic carcinoma: intensive induction chemotherapy with high-dose cyclophosphamide plus high-dose etoposide. J Clin Oncol 1985;3:170–5.

26. Thatcher N, James RD, Steward WP et al. Three

months' treatment with cyclophosphamide, VP16-213 followed by methotrexate and thoracic radiotherapy for small-cell lung cancer. Cancer 1985;56:1332–6.

27. Thatcher N, Stout R, Smith DB et al. Three months' treatment with chemotherapy and radiotherapy for small-cell lung cancer. Br J Cancer 1985;52:327–32.

28. Johnson DH, Deleo MJ, Hande KR et al. High-dose induction chemotherapy with cyclophosphamide, etoposide and cisplatin for extensive-stage small-cell lung cancer. J Clin Oncol 1987;5:703–9.

29. Luikart SD, Propert KJ, Modeas CR et al. High-dose etoposide therapy for extensive small-cell lung cancer: a Cancer and Leukemia Group B study. Cancer Treat Rep 1987;71:533–4.

30. Souhami RL, Ruiz De Elvira MC. Chemotherapy dose intensity in small cell lung cancer. Lung Cancer 1994;10(suppl 1):175–85.

31. O'Donnell MR, Ruckdeschel JC, Baxter D et al. Intensive induction chemotherapy for small cell anaplastic carcinoma of the lung. Cancer Treat Rep 1985;69:571–5.

32. Figueredo AT, Hryniuk WM, Strautmanis I et al. Co-trimoxazole prophylaxis during high-dose chemotherapy of small cell lung cancer. J Clin Oncol 1985;3:54–64.

33. Johnson DH, Einhorn LH, Birch R et al. A randomized comparison of high-dose versus conventional-dose cyclophosphamide, doxorubicin, and vincristine for extensive-stage small-cell lung cancer: a phase III trial of the Southeastern Cancer Study Group. J Clin Oncol 1987;5:1731–8.

34. Arriagada R, Le Chevalier T, Pignon J-P et al. Initial chemotherapeutic doses and survival in patients with limited small cell lung cancer. N Engl J Med 1993;329:1848–52.

35. Ihde DC, Mulshine JL, Kramer BS et al. Prospective randomised comparison of high dose and standard dose etoposide and cisplatin chemotherapy in patients with extensive stage small cell lung cancer. J Clin Oncol 1994;12:2022–34.

36. Norton L, Simon R. Tumor size, sensitivity to therapy, and design of treatment schedules. Cancer Treat Rep 1977;61:1307–17.

37. Spitzer G, Farha P, Valdivieso M et al. High-dose intensification therapy with autologous bone marrow support for limited small-cell bronchogenic carcinoma. J Clin Oncol 1986;4:4–13.

38. Klastersky JA, Sculier J-P. Intensive chemo-

therapy of small cell lung cancer. Lung Cancer 1989;5:196–206.

39. Klastersky J, Nicaise C, Longeval E et al. Cisplatin, adriamycin and etoposide (CAV) for remission induction of small-cell bronchogenic carcinoma. Cancer 1982;50:652–8.

40. Smith IE, Evans BD, Harland SJ et al. High-dose cyclophosphamide with autologous bone-marrow rescue after conventional chemotherapy in the treatment of small-cell lung carcinoma. Cancer Chemother Pharmacol 1985;14:120–4.

41. Banham S, Dorward A, Hutcheon A et al. The role of VP16 in the treatment of small-cell lung cancer: studies of the West of Scotland Lung Cancer Group. Semin Oncol 1985;12(suppl 2): 2–6.

42. Sculier JP, Klastersky J, Stryckmans P et al. Late intensification in small-cell lung cancer: a phase I study of high doses of cyclophosphamide and etoposide with autologous bone marrow transplantation. J Clin Oncol 1985;3;184–91.

43. Ihde DC, Deisseroth AB, Lichter AS et al. Late intensive combined modality therapy followed by autologous bone marrow infusion in extensive-stage small-cell lung cancer. J Clin Oncol 1986;4:1443–54.

44. Humblet Y, Symann M, Bosly A et al. Late intensification chemotherapy with autologous bone marrow transplantation in selected small-cell carcinoma of the lung: a randomised study. J Clin Oncol 1987;5:1864–73.

45. Goodman GE, Crowley J, Livingston RB et al. Treatment of limited small-cell lung cancer with concurrent etoposide/cisplatin and radiotherapy followed by intensification with high-dose cyclophosphamide: a Southwest Oncology Group study. J Clin Oncol 1991;9:453–7.

46. Elias AD, Ayash L, Frei E et al. Intensive combined modality therapy for limited-stage small-cell lung cancer. J Natl Cancer Inst 1993; 85:559–66.

47. Taylor CW, Crowley J, Williamson SK et al. Treatment of small-cell lung cancer with an alternating chemotherapy regimen given at weekly intervals: a Southwest Oncology Group Pilot Study. J Clin Oncol 1990;8:1811–17.

48. Miles DW, Earl HM, Souhami RL et al. Intensive weekly chemotherapy for good-prognosis patients with small-cell lung cancer. J Clin Oncol 1991;9:280–5.

49. Murray N, Shah A, Osoba D et al. Intensive weekly chemotherapy for the treatment of exten-

sive-stage small-cell lung cancer. J Clin Oncol 1991;9:1632–8.

50. Sculier JP, Paesmans M, Bureau G et al. Multiple-drug weekly chemotherapy versus standard combination regimen in small-cell lung cancer: a Phase III randomized study conducted by the European Lung Cancer Working Party. J Clin Oncol 1993;11:1858–66.

51. Souhami RL, Rudd RM, Ruiz de Elvira MC et al. Randomised trial comparing weekly versus 3-weekly chemotherapy in small cell lung cancer: A Cancer Research Campaign Trial. J Clin Oncol 1994;12:1806–13.

52. Murray N, Livingston RB, Shepherd FA et al. Randomized study of CODE versus alternating CAV/EP for extensive-stage small-cell lung cancer: an Intergroup Study of the National Cancer Institute of Canada Clinical Trials Group and the Southwest Oncology Group. J Clin Oncol 1999;17:2300–8.

53. Crawford J, Ozer H, Stoller R et al. Reduction by granulocyte colony-stimulating factor of fever and neutropenia induced by chemotherapy in patients with small-cell lung cancer. N Engl J Med 1991;325:164–70.

54. Trillet-Lenoir V, Green J, Manegold C et al. Recombinant granulocyte colony stimulating factor reduces the infectious complications of cytotoxic chemotherapy. Eur J Cancer 1993;29A: 319–24.

55. Trillet-Lenoir V, Green JA, Manegold C et al. Recombinant granulocyte colony stimulating factor in the treatment of small cell lung cancer: a long-term follow-up. Eur J Cancer 1995;31A: 2115–16.

56. Bunn PA Jr, Crowley J, Kelly K et al. Chemoradiotherapy with or without granulocyte–macrophage colony-stimulating factor in the treatment of limited-stage small-cell lung cancer: a prospective phase III randomized study of the Southwest Oncology Group. J Clin Oncol 1995;13:1632–41.

57. Pujol J-L, Douillad J-Y, Riviere A et al. Dose-intensity of a four-drug chemotherapy regimen with or without recombinant human granulocyte–macrophage colony-stimulating factor in extensive stage small-cell lung cancer: a multi-center randomized phase III study. J Clin Oncol 1997;15:2082–9.

58. Miles DW, Fogarty MO, Ash CM et al. Received dose-intensity: a randomised trial of weekly chemotherapy with and without granulocyte

colony-stimulating factor in small-cell lung cancer. J Clin Oncol 1994;12:77–82.

59. Fukuoka M, Masuda N, Negoro S et al. CODE chemotherapy with and without granulocyte colony stimulating factor in small cell lung cancer. Br J Cancer 1997;75:306–9.

60. Woll PJ, Hodgetts J, Lomax L et al. Can cytotoxic dose intensity be increased by using granulocyte colony stimulating factor? A randomised controlled trial of lenograstim in small cell lung cancer. J Clin Oncol 1995;13:652–9.

61. Furuse K, Fukuoka M, Nishiwaki Y et al. Phase III study of intensive weekly chemotherapy with recombinant human granulocyte colony-stimulating factor versus standard chemotherapy in extensive-disease small-cell lung cancer. J Clin Oncol 1998;16:2126–32.

62. Steward WP, von Pawel J, Gatzemeier U et al. Effects of granulocyte macrophage colony stimulating factor and dose intensification of V-ICE chemotherapy in small cell lung cancer: a prospective randomised study of 300 patients. J Clin Oncol 1998;16:642–50.

63. Thatcher N, Girling D, Hopwood P et al. Improving survival without reducing quality of life in small cell lung cancer by increasing the dose-intensity of chemotherapy with G-CSF support: results of a British Medical Research Council Multi-center randomised trial. J Clin Oncol 2000;18:395–404.

64. Ardizzoni A, Sertoli MR, Corcione A et al. Accelerated chemotherapy with or without GM-CSF for small cell lung cancer: a non-randomised pilot study. Eur J Cancer 1990;26:937–41.

65. Thatcher N, Clark PI, Smith DB et al. Increasing and planned dose intensity of doxorubicin, cyclophosphamide and etoposide (ACE) by adding recombinant human methionyl granulocyte colony-stimulating factor (G-CSF; filgrastim) in the treatment of small cell lung cancer (SCLC). Clin Oncol 1995;7:293–9.

66. Thatcher N, Anderson H, Bleehen NM et al. The feasibility of using glycosylated recombinant human granulocyte colony-stimulating factor (G-CSF) to increase the planned dose intensity of doxorubicin, cyclophosphamide and etoposide (ACE) in the treatment of small cell lung cancer. Eur J Cancer 1995;31A:152–6.

67. Kudoh S, Sawa T, Kurihara N et al. Phase II study of recombinant human interleukin 3 administration following carboplatin and etoposide chemotherapy in small cell lung cancer patients. SDZ ILE 964 (IL-3) Study. Cancer Chemother Pharmacol 1996;38(suppl):89–95.

68. Crawford J, George M. The role of hemopoietic growth factors in support of ifosfamide/carboplatin, etoposide chemotherapy. Semin Oncol 1995;22(suppl 7):18–22.

69. Tepler I, Elias L, Smith JW et al. A randomized placebo-controlled trial of recombinant human interleukin-11 in cancer patients with severe thrombocytopenia due to chemotherapy. Blood 1996;87:3607–14.

70. De Campos E, Radford J, Steward W et al. Clinical and in vitro effects of recombinant human erythropoietin in patients receiving intensive chemotherapy for small cell lung cancer. J Clin Oncol 1995;13:1623–31.

71. Brugger W, Bross K, Frisch J et al. Mobilization of peripheral blood progenitor cells by sequential administration of interleukin-3 and granulocyte–macrophage colony-stimulating factor following polychemotherapy with etoposide, ifosfamide and cisplatin. Blood 1992;79(5): 1193–200.

72. Pettengell R, Woll PJ, O'Connor DA et al. Viability of haemopoietic progenitors from whole blood bone marrow and leukapheresis product: effect of storage media, temperature and time. Bone Marrow Transplant 1994;14: 703–9.

73. Pettengell R, Woll PJ, Thatcher N et al. Multicyclic, dose intensive chemotherapy supported by sequential reinfusion of haemopoietic progenitors in whole blood. J Clin Oncol 1995;13: 148–56.

74. Woll PJ, Lee SM, Lomax et al. Randomised phase II study of standard versus dose intensive ICE chemotherapy with reinfusion of haemopoietic progenitors in whole blood in small cell lung cancer. Proc ASCO 1996;15:333 (abstract 957).

15

High dose chemotherapy in germ cell tumours

Jonathan Shamash and R Timothy D Oliver

INTRODUCTION

This chapter examines the role of high dose chemotherapy in the management of germ cell tumours. Most of the work carried out in this area has been with male patients; germ cell tumours occurring in women are much rarer, although there is no evidence that the same principles of management should not apply.

STANDARD CHEMOTHERAPY OF GERM CELL TUMOURS

The standard management for patients with germ cell tumours who have metastatic disease is to use cisplatin-based combination chemotherapy. To date no treatment has been shown to be superior to PEB (cisplatin 100 mg/m², etoposide 500 mg/m² over 5 days in divided doses and bleomycin 30 000 units weekly).[1] Four cycles of the above treatment (often with omission of bleomycin on the fourth cycle) can be considered the therapy against which all new treatments should be compared. With such an approach, 80% of patients with

metastatic disease will achieve a durable remission. Following chemotherapy, many patients may have residual masses at previous sites of metastatic disease, but their persistence is not an indication for further chemotherapy treatment.[2-4] However, serious consideration should be given to resecting them: they may contain either necrotic tissue or mature teratoma, which has the potential for malignant transformation with time. Occasionally they will contain active carcinoma and if resection of all such masses is successful then such surgery may be curative in its own right. Surgically induced remissions may occur in 30–50% of such cases.[5-7]

'STANDARD SALVAGE CHEMOTHERAPY' FOR GERM CELL TUMOURS

Germ cell tumours are unusual in that following relapse a proportion of patients may be cured with further chemotherapy. Several approaches at this stage of the disease have been undertaken, the most common of which is to substitute ifosfamide for bleomycin and

Table 15.2 Prognostic variables for selection of patients for high dose chemotherapy[13]

	Risk score
Progressive disease before HDC	1
Mediastinal primary tumour	1
Refractory disease before HDC	1
Absolute refractory disease before HDC	2
β-hCG < 1000IU/l before HDC	2

Risk category score (summed)	Progression-free survival		Overall survival	
	At 1 year	2 years	1 year	2 years
0	56	51	73	61
1 or 2	28	27	50	34
>2	5	5	19	8

- progressive disease prior to HDC,
- β-hCG < 1000 IU/ml and
- mediastinal primary.

Thus a patient with a mediastinal primary who achieves a marker-positive partial remission to conventional cisplatin salvage and has a rising β-hCG prior to HDC which is still less than 1000 will score 2 and have an anticipated 2-year progression-free survival of 27%.

High dose chemotherapy has also been employed in patients with high tumour marker levels in whom the tumour markers failed to decline to half-life.[14] This is a much more controversial reason for intensifying treatment, as there is now clear evidence that a large proportion of patients with high β-hCG levels will normalize following the end of conventional treatment.[15] These patients, despite their tumour markers not declining to anticipated half-life, may be incorrectly considered as having resistant disease.

It is possible that patients whose tumour markers fail to decline to half-life [α-fetoprotein, (AFP) halving every 7 days or hCG halving every 48 h] in the absence of large masses being present, indicating possibly mature teratoma, are more likely to progress. Whether this is enough to justify intensification of treatment is arguable. To date there has been one randomized controlled trial assessing the role of HDC in patients with poor-prognosis disease; although the high dose regimen used may now be considered to be suboptimal, there was no evidence of any benefit of any immediate high dose consolidation in this study.[16]

DRUG COMPONENTS OF HIGH DOSE CHEMOTHERAPY PREPARATIVE REGIMENS

Platinum complexes

The initial attempt to intensify the dose of chemotherapy for relapsing germ cell tumours concentrated on dose escalation of alkylating agents, in particular cyclophosphamide. In the initial studies with non-platinum-based chemotherapy, partial responses were seen although they were short-lived.[17] As cisplatin has been responsible for fundamental improvement in the outcome of metastatic germ cell tumours, the inclusion of a platinum complex would appear necessary in any high dose regimen. Some studies have used intensified cisplatin; however, intensification can at best double the dose from the standard $100–200 \, mg/m^2$ before the onset of neurotoxicity or nephrotoxicity.[18,19] The analogue carboplatin, with its reduction in non-myeloid toxicity, is more suitable for dose intensification. The issue of how to dose carboplatin has followed the observation that its excretion is renal[20] and that within the conventional dose range the platelet nadir after carboplatin treatment correlated with the area under the curve achieved. This has meant that the best way to target a level of bone marrow suppression is to use the formula to achieve a specific area under the curve. Formally described by Calvert et al.,[20] it has gained widespread acceptance and there are some limited data to show that such a formula holds outside the normal dose range (AUC 5–8).[21,22] The maximum dose of carboplatin used as a single agent in high dose treatment is $2400 \, mg/m^2$ (when dosed on height and weight),[23] which corresponds to an AUC in a patient with normal renal function of approximately 35. Dose-limiting hepatotoxicity and gastrointestinal toxicity supervene, and neuropathy and ototoxicity begin to appear.

Evidence for a clear dose–response curve for carboplatin in teratoma is lacking. In the conventional dose range, carboplatin-based chemotherapy yields inferior results compared with similar cisplatin-based chemotherapy[24] and there is little evidence that in combination with etoposide, increasing the dose from a targeted AUC 20, or (if dose per square metre) $1500 \, mg/m^2$, leads to improved results.[25] When carboplatin has been combined with etoposide alone, common practice has been to use a dose of AUC 30, or $1500 \, mg/m^2$, and, if an oxazophosphorine is added, to reduce this dose to AUC 20, or $1200 \, mg/m^2$. The same doses have been used when tandem transplants have been performed, giving two doses of AUC 20 approximately a month apart.[14,26]

Etoposide

The introduction of etoposide in the treatment of germ cell tumours has been responsible for improving the cure rate, and etoposide is an ideal drug for dose intensification. The drug is frequently fractionated, and this has been shown to be superior to a single dose[27] within the conventional dose range. Studies have used doses ranging from $1 \, g/m^2$ in five divided doses to $2.4 \, g/m^2$ over 4 days. There is no evidence that increased doses of etoposide are responsible for adding to the nephrotoxicity of carboplatin[28] and there is no suggestion that those receiving the highest doses have improved survival. However, increasing mucositis occurs as doses are escalated, and hepatotoxicity is dose limiting.

Oxazophosphorines – cyclophosphamide and ifosfamide

The realization that cisplatin and ifosfamide regimens were able to salvage patients relapsing from PEB chemotherapy has led to the introduction of an oxazophosphorine in high dose regimens. Ifosfamide was used in many of the earlier studies. However, it is not easy to intensify the dose because, while $6 \, g/m^2$ forms the dose in standard VIP chemotherapy, the maximum safe dose appears to be $10 \, g/m^2$.[28] It appears that the ifosfamide has to be fractionated over 5 days. Despite this, significant nephrotoxicity can result and it appears to be related to the dose of carboplatin, with 8% of patients in one series requiring haemodialysis.[28] There is no evidence that nephrotoxicity delays haematological recovery. There appears to be a synergistic effect of ifosfamide on carboplatin-induced renal dysfunction,[28] and if ifosfamide is used the dose of carboplatin needs to be reduced to AUC 20, or $1200 \, mg/m^2$.

Fears about the contribution of ifosfamide to carboplatin-induced nephrotoxicity have led to the substitution of ifosfamide with cyclophosphamide. There is little convincing data to support the use of this drug in the conventional dose range, although it was included in some of the early protocols (VAB6 and POMB/ ACE).[29,30] Cyclophosphamide is more suitable than ifosfamide for dose intensification: up to 7 g/m^2 may be administered, which represents a three- to four-fold increase in intensity over the conventional dose range.[31] There is no evidence that cyclophosphamide significantly increases renal dysfunction, but haemorrhagic cystitis and cardiac dysfunction can occur.

Thiotepa

One study has incorporated thiotepa into the preparative regimen.[32] While this is well tolerated, the evidence that it contributes to improved results, compared with carboplatin or etoposide alone, is lacking. Mucositis is the main toxicity.

Taxanes

The taxanes represent a new group of agents which have been incorporated into therapy for refractory testicular cancers. Approximately 11% respond in the relapse setting and 4% of responses are complete.[33] The regimen TIP (cisplatin, paclitaxel and ifosfamide)[34] has been used for relapse/poor-risk patients with respectable results. However, when paclitaxel (210 mg/m^2 over 1 h) has been incorporated into HDC (with cyclophosphamide 6 g/m^2, etoposide 1500 mg/m^2 and carboplatin – AUC 20) toxicity has resulted from enterocolitis.[25] This may be due to an interaction between platinum and paclitaxel: when cyclophosphamide and paclitaxel have been used in high doses,[35] such effects have not been seen.

The failure to increase the dose of paclitaxel outside the standard range, the failure to demonstrate improved outcome over VIP[25] and the increase in toxicity mean that further investigation of paclitaxel is probably not warranted as part of carboplatin/etoposide-based preparative regimens.

Summary

High dose carboplatin and etoposide form the mainstay of cytotoxic drugs in the preparative regimen for testicular teratoma. When used together, a dose of carboplatin may be given either as a square metre dose, in which case 1500 mg/m^2 is often selected, or as an AUC calculated dose, in which case an AUC of 30 is selected. The addition of an oxazophosphorine is common: either ifosfamide at 10 g/m^2 (with the risk of nephrotoxicity) or cyclophosphamide at a dose of 6–7 g/m^2. The addition of cyclophosphamide or ifosfamide appears to allow a reduction in the dose of carboplatin to 1200 mg/m^2 or AUC 20. The role of other drugs remains uncertain, although thiotepa has been used.

ASSESSMENT OF PATIENTS PRIOR TO HIGH DOSE CHEMOTHERAPY

Collection of marrow or stem cells

The use of peripheral blood progenitor cells has led to more rapid engraftment compared with use of bone marrow cells and it is clear that although the absolute minimum number of CD34+ cells is 1×10^6/kg, a safer level is probably 3×10^6/kg. Reinfusion of stem cells following HDC usually leads to haemopoietic reconstitution, with neutrophils reaching 0.5×10^9/l by day 10 and an unsupported platelet count of 20×10^9/l by day 12. Stem cell mobilization may either follow chemotherapy or may be achieved by high dose growth factors alone. In patients who have been heavily pretreated, particularly if their peripheral blood count is low, cytogenetic analysis of the bone marrow may be considered because the presence of myelodysplasia is a contraindication to autologous transplantation.

Staging prior to high dose chemotherapy

Patients should have a computed tomography (CT) scan of chest, abdomen and pelvis as well as a magnetic resonance (MRI) or CT of the brain. The tumour marker level prior to chemotherapy has prognostic significance. Respiratory function is usually assessed because most patients would have received bleomycin prior to high dose chemotherapy and reductions in transfer factor are common. A substantially reduced K_{CO} (50% of normal or less) suggests that respiratory reserve is low and patients who develop septicaemia may be at significant risk because they are unable to meet their oxygen requirements. Assessment of renal function prior to HDC is mandatory; ideally this should be with an ethylenediaminetetra-acetic acid (EDTA) clearance and this may then be used to dose carboplatin.[20] High dose chemotherapy has been used in patients whose EDTA clearance is below 40 ml/min.[22] There is evidence that toxicity increases and, in addition, pre-HDC impaired renal function is itself a predictor for renal dysfunction following HDC.[25] Patients with clearance less than 60 ml/min should probably not have ifosfamide in their preparative regimen. The performance of audiographs prior to HDC is useful: patients who have significantly impaired hearing will be at higher risk of developing further damage from high dose carboplatin. Cardiac assessment using a multigated acquisition scan (MUGA) or echocardiogram in young patients who are asymptomatic is probably unnecessary, as patients are unlikely to have received cardiotoxic drugs prior to high dose treatment; however, it may be considered in those who are to receive high dose cyclophosphamide.

The descision on whether patients should have one or two high dose procedures depends partly on the ability to collect enough stem cells to rescue patients from two courses of HDC. Several series have reported tandem transplants;[14,26] the second transplant is usually not performed if the patient has not responded to the first. In the study by Margolin et al.,[14] patients who had persistent disease or relapse following conventional chemotherapy or had a high-risk presentation were given two cycles of carboplatin, ifosfamide and etoposide; 18 of the 20 patients received a second cycle, and 45% were progression-free. Overall, unfortunately it is unclear how refractory the patients were; three of the 20 patients who had high dose treatment were in complete remission. Nichols et al.[26] described two cycles of high dose carboplatin and etoposide administered with bone marrow rescue; all the patients had previous recurrent disease. Again, the second cycle of treatment was administered to those patients achieving a partial complete remission to the first. Fifty-eight per cent proceeded to the second high dose treatment. In the study by Lamp et al.,[21] 23 patients received one cycle of high dose carboplatin plus etoposide and 12 of these went on to receive a second cycle if they had not progressed. At present it is unclear what, if anything, a second high dose procedure adds to management.

Post high dose chemotherapy assessment and management

Following HDC the patient should be reassessed within 3 months; this would normally be with tumour markers and a repeat scan. Serious consideration should be given to resecting all residual disease if at all possible, although if masses have reduced considerably in size following high dose treatment, it clearly would be reasonable to watch these patients and re-scan them 1–2 months later, because further shrinkage within that time is more likely to suggest necrotic tissue.[3,36]

If patients have had brain metastases, serious consideration should be given to cranial irradiation following high dose therapy, if this has not been done before it.

Relapse following high dose chemotherapy

Most patients who relapse following high dose chemotherapy will do so within the year of the procedure and, if the sites are amenable to surgery, further consideration should be given to salvage surgery because a small proportion of patients will obtain durable remissions. Unfortunately, with the exception of this small group of patients, it is unlikely that relapse following HDC will be curable. In one report of those who relapse following HDC, only 4% were rendered progression-free by further management.[37] Several options have been pursued in this setting. In a review by Pont et al.,[38] both paclitaxel and oral etoposide were able to induce remissions although most of these were short-lived; oral etoposide has the advantage of ease of administration. More intensive therapy can be considered. A combination of actinomycin, high dose of methotrexate and etoposide has been used,[39] and a proportion (10%) will achieve a further remission with conventional BEP chemotherapy.

Of new agents under investigation, gemcitabine and the taxane derivatives have shown some promise. Gemcitabine appears to produce response rates in the region of 10–20%.[40]

In conclusion, relapse following HDC is frequently fatal. Consideration should be given to salvage surgery, fit patients may be candidates for innovative trials of further chemotherapy, and etoposide, gemcitabine or paclitaxel may produce responses in this group of patients. Table 15.3 shows a summary of single-group experiences of HDC in germ cell tumours.

FUTURE PROSPECTS

Chemotherapeutic approaches

New drugs and approaches which may be useful in the management of germ cell tumours are becoming available. The topoisomerase inhibitors topotecan and irinotecan appear to be synergistic with platinum complexes. Long-term remissions have been reported using cisplatin and irinotecan as first-line salvage. Topotecan is a drug which appears suitable for dose escalation because dose intensification above 10-fold is possible[46] and it is now being studied with etoposide and carboplatin.

Use of topoisomerase I inhibitor followed by topoisomerase II blockade (with etoposide) is a strategy which has shown synergy, and carboplatin, topotecan and etoposide may prove to be a useful high dose preparative regimen.

The diamine cyclohexane platinum II complex oxaliplatin appears to be as effective as cisplatin in germ cell lines and appears able to overcome acquired cisplatin resistance.[47] It is not nephrotoxic or ototoxic and this may make it a useful component of any salvage strategy. However dose-limiting peripheral neuropathy means that significant dose intensification is unlikely.

Gemcitabine plus cisplatin has proved a useful combination in a variety of tumours. Combinations with irinotecan may prove useful as salvage regimens in germ cell tumours.

It is clear from this review that HDC has an established role in patients who relapse after a response to cisplatin-based chemotherapy. However, its role in patients who are absolutely cisplatin refractory is more controversial because only 5% will derive long-term benefit; therefore there is an advantage to giving an induction treatment with conventional chemotherapy first, to test for platinum sensitivity. Patients with absolute refractory disease may then be identified for more radical approaches to treatment, such as the new non-myeloablative (mini-allograft) approaches that have recently given encouraging results in some adult solid cancers.

Molecular biotherapy approaches

In view of reports that absence of p53 mutation, overexpression of p53 and absent bcl-2 may be factors in the exquisite chemosensitivity of germ cell cancer as well as reports that patients with relapsed germ cell cancer have a high frequency of p53 mutation,[48] there is a role for further examination of gene therapy approaches using wild-type p53 and anti-sense bcl-2. None of these approaches has been tested in patients with germ cell tumours to date.

Table 15.3 Summary of single-group experiences of high dose chemotherapy in germ cell tumours

References	Regimen	No. of patients	Treatment-related deaths	Progression-free[a]	Refractory	Progression-free[b]	Comments
Motzer et al. (1996)[41]	Carboplatin 1500 mg/m² Etoposide 1200 mg/m² Cyclophosphamide 120 mg/kg +ABMT	38	5	12	23	6	Cyclophosphamide escalated from 60 to 150 mg/kg; 50% had 2 cycles
Barnett et al. (1993)[42]	Etoposide 3000 mg/m² Ifosfamide 6 g/m² Or cyclophosphamide 7.2 g/m² Carboplatin 800–1200 mg/m² +ABMT	21	2	14	4	0	
Shamash et al. (1999)[25]	Etoposide 1500 mg/m² Carboplatin 1200 mg/m² or AUC 20 Cyclophosphamide 6 g/m² or ifosfamide 9 g/m² +ABMT/ASCT	30	1	14	6	2	
Lampe et al. (1995)[21]	Carboplatin AUC 30 Etoposide 1200 mg/m² +ASCT	23	4	6	7	4	12 had tandem transplant
Nichols et al. (1992)[26]	Carboplatin 1500 mg/m² Etoposide 1200 mg/m² +ABMT	40	5	5	5	1	22 had tandem transplant
Margolin et al. (1996)[14]	Carboplatin 1200 mg/m² Etoposide 20 mg/kg Ifosfamide 6 g/m² +ABMT/ASCT	20	0	8	7	3	Tandem transplant 8 high-risk patients not proven refractory to first-line treatment
Motzer et al. (1997)[43]	Cyclophosphamide 150 mg/kg Carboplatin 1500 mg/m² Etoposide 1200 mg/m² +ASCT	30	0	15	NA	NA	First-line use: slow marker decline after VIP × 2 Single dose
Lyttelton et al. (1998)[22]	Carboplatin AUC 30 Etoposide 1800 mg/m²	31	1	11	22	5	Single dose
Siegert et al. (1994)[47]	Carboplatin 1500 mg/m² Etoposide 2400 mg/m² Ifosfamide 10 g/m² +ABMT	74	2	25	23	2	Dose escalator of carboplatin + ifosfamide and etoposide
Mandanas et al. (1998)[48]	Various mostly: Cyclophosphamide 120 mg/kg Etoposide 1200–2400 mg/m² Carboplatin 1600–2000 mg/m² +ABMT	21	2	11	9	2	Single high dose

ABMT, autologous bone marrow transplantation; ASCT, autologous stem cell transplantation; AUC, area under the curve; VIP, cisplatin, ifosfamide and etoposide.
[a]Total rendered progression free by the treatment.
[b]Number of refractory patients rendered progression free; these have a poorer outcome.

Amsterdam A, Vlamis V. High-dose carboplatin, etoposide, and cyclophosphamide for patients with refractory germ cell tumors: treatment results and prognostic factors for survival and toxicity. J Clin Oncol 1996;14(4):1098–105.

42. Barnett MJ, Coppin CM, Murray N et al. High-dose chemotherapy and autologous bone marrow transplantation for patients with poor prognosis nonseminomatous germ cell tumours. Br J Cancer 1993;68(3):594–8.

43. Motzer R, Mazumdar M, Bajorin D, Bosl G, Lyn P, Vlamis V. High-dose carboplatin, etoposide, and cyclophosphamide with autologous bone marrow transplantation in first line therapy for patients with poor risk germ cell tumours. J Clin Oncol 1997;15:2546–52.

44. Siegert W, Beyer J, Strochsheer I et al. High dose treatment with carboplatin, etoposide and ifosfamide followed by autologous stem-cell transplantation in relapsed or refractory germ cell cancer: a phase I/II study. J Clin Oncol 1994; 12(6):1223–31.

45. Mandanas R, Saez R, Epstein R, Confer D, Selby G. Long-term results of autologous marrow transplantation for relapsed or refractory male or female germ cell tumors. Bone Marrow Transplant 1998;21(6):569–76.

46. Sullivan D, Partyka J, Hernandez A et al. A phase I/II study of intensive-dose topotecan, ifosfamide (IFOS)/Mesna and etoposide (TIME) followed by autologous stem cell rescue in refractory malignancies. Proc ASCO 1999;18: (abstract 171).

47. Dunn TA, Schmoll HJ, Grunwald V, Bokemeyer C, Casper J. Comparative cytotoxicity of oxaliplatin and cisplatin in non-seminomatous germ cell cancer cell lines. Invest New Drugs 1997;15(2):109–14.

48. Nouri A, Oliver R. Tetraploid arrest with over expressed non-mutated p53 in germ cell cancers. Relevance to their chemosensitivity and possible application in non germ cell cancers. Int J Oncol 1997;11:1167–371.

Part 3

Supportive care and long-term complications

16

Blood products and supportive care

Mike Leach

CONTENTS Introduction • Special precautions • Red cell transfusion • Platelet transfusion • Granulocyte transfusion • Fresh frozen plasma and cryoprecipitate • Intravenous immunoglobulin • Plasma volume expanders • Albumin solutions • Summary

INTRODUCTION

Bone marrow toxicity is an almost universal consequence of high dose chemotherapy. Severe pancytopenia, with its inherent risk of bleeding and infection, carries a morbidity and mortality which has to be considered outside the prognostic parameters associated with the disease in question. Blood product support of the patient throughout this cytopenic phase is therefore of great importance and many high dose procedures would not be possible without this resource.

An ever-increasing array of blood product formulations are now available to the clinician and in this chapter I aim to outline an optimal practical approach to patient therapy with red cell, platelet, granulocyte and plasma products. Guidelines will be offered but I urge you to consider each clinical situation as unique. Cytopaenic patients need constant reassessment with regard to the extra risks imposed by the duration of neutropenia, concurrent drug therapy, the presence of fever, infection, splenomegaly, graft-versus-host disease and the effects of cardiopulmonary, hepatic or renal dysfunction.

The choice of product is of vital importance for the following reasons:

- to maximize the therapeutic/supportive potential to the patient,
- to minimize the complications of such therapy and
- to avoid unnecessary use of products, with its inherent cost implications and stretching of resources.

The measure of a guideline is not the elegance of its logic but by how much it improves patient care.[1]

SPECIAL PRECAUTIONS

Leukocyte-depleted products

With the advent of the theoretical risk of transmission of new variant Creutzfeldt–Jakob disease (CJD) by blood transfusion in the UK, a government decision was made to leukodeplete all cellular blood products routinely by the millennium. This decision inadvertently carries a number of benefits to the patient requiring blood product support during high dose therapy, as leukocyte contamination of red cell and platelet concentrates has been implicated in the following:[2]

- HLA and neutrophil-specific antigen alloimmunization,

- febrile transfusion reactions,
- refractoriness to platelet transfusion,
- transmission of cytomegalovirus infection and
- immune modulation, with possible implications for infection susceptibility and tumour recurrence.

A leukocyte-depleted red cell or platelet concentrate will contain less than 5×10^6 residual leukocytes when the product is filtered under validated conditions by the transfusion laboratory.

Gamma-irradiated blood components

Immunoreactive T lymphocytes can maintain their activity in cellular blood products during storage for some weeks. Following transfusion, such lymphocytes can be responsible for cell-mediated cytotoxicity in the recipient, with predominant damage to host cells in skin, gut, liver and bone marrow: the syndrome of transfusion-related graft-versus-host disease.[3] The risk associated with a transfusion depends on the number and viability of donor lymphocytes, the immune susceptibility of the patient and the degree of HLA disparity between the two. This condition, when established, responds poorly to treatment and is fatal in more than 90% of cases.[4] Prevention is therefore of utmost importance. Gamma irradiation of red cell and platelet concentrates prior to issue (minimum dose 25 Gy) will prevent this complication and has no deleterious effects on the product in question. The indications for the use of gamma-irradiated products in patients undergoing high dose therapy are therefore as follows:[5]

- all patients undergoing a stem cell transplant procedure,
- patients with Hodgkin's disease,
- patients with congenital cellular immunodeficiency,
- patients pretreated with purine analogues (e.g. fludarabine) and
- the use of blood components from relatives, who often share human leukocyte antigen (HLA) haplotypes with the patient, except in the case of donor lymphocyte infusions.

Cytomegalovirus-negative blood components

Cytomegalovirus (CMV)-negative blood components are normally recommended for CMV-negative recipients of autologous and allogeneic stem cell transplants. Acute CMV infection is responsible for fever, rash, hepatitis, pneumonitis and marrow failure in stem cell recipients.[6] It appears to increase the risk of other opportunistic infections and appears to precipitate or worsen acute graft-versus-host disease.[7] Transfusion-associated infection appears to be transmitted by viral genome inserted into leukocyte DNA, and the protective effect of intensive leukocyte depletion of products at source has been demonstrated.[8] Screening of donors for CMV may become less important as products are leukocyte depleted at source. Until a clear guideline on the risk of CMV transmission after leukodepletion becomes available, however, this policy should still be adhered to. In a patient whose CMV status is not known, products from seronegative donors should be selected until this is established.

Reactivation of CMV in a seropositive recipient may be responsible for inducing features identical to those of acute infection in those subjected to the immunosuppressive effects of high dose therapy. There appears to be little value in selecting CMV-negative products for these individuals as a means of reducing viral load, although, theoretically, acute infection is possible with a different viral strain.[9] There is no clinical evidence to date that this mechanism is important following stem cell transplant procedures.

RED CELL TRANSFUSION

Patients undergoing high dose therapy may be anaemic for a number of reasons:

- anaemia of chronic disorder, e.g. Hodgkin's disease,
- bone marrow infiltration,
- bleeding,
- haemolysis, e.g. cyclosporin-induced thrombotic thrombocytopenic purpura (TTP),
- nutritional or Septrin-induced folate deficiency or
- myelotoxicity of the therapy.

Although a reduction in red cell mass results in reduced oxygen-carrying capacity of the blood, compensatory mechanisms exist:[10]

- increased venous oxygen extraction and alveolar hyperventilation,
- a shift of the oxygen dissociation curve to the right,
- increased red cell 2,3-diphosphoglycerate (2,3-DPG) and
- increased cardiac output and blood tissue flow (aided by a fall in whole blood viscosity).

Indications

Despite these adaptations, the compensatory reserve of the patient is limited. The cardiovascular effects of age, coexistent fever and infection[11] and previous anthracycline therapy[12] need to be considered. Although there are no current UK guidelines with respect to red cell transfusion in this situation, it seems reasonable to aim to maintain a haemoglobin level greater than 8.0 g/dl. Below this level, a sharp increase in cardiac output is necessary in order to maintain tissue oxygenation and as levels fall to 0.5 g/dl a proportion of previously fit individuals will show evidence of myocardial ischaemia.[13] A randomized trial of a liberal versus a restrictive strategy for red cell transfusion in critically ill (non-haematology) patients showed a significantly lower mortality rate during hospitalization in the latter.[14] Clearly one should have a lower threshold for transfusion in a patient who is actively bleeding or haemolysing. The transfusion of red cells, with

improvement in the haematocrit and its effect on whole blood viscosity and platelet adhesion, may actually ameliorate the bleeding tendency in a given patient.[15] The clinician should anticipate the need for red cells in a patient who has been shown to have clinically significant alloantibodies, and crossmatching requests should ideally be made during working hours and early in the day, when screening for compatible donors will be necessary. For patients with unusual or complex combinations of antibodies, one should have compatible units available in the hospital blood bank to cover a serious and unexpected haemorrhage during their cytopaenic phase.

Red cell products

Red blood cells for transfusion are now almost universally available as concentrated cells (with or without optimal additive solution) with volume of 180 ml and haematocrit of 0.55–0.751/l. Such a preparation allows an increment in Hb of approximately 1 g/dl per unit and minimizes the risks of fluid overload but nevertheless can be infused rapidly should clinical circumstances dictate. Infusion rates not exceeding 1 ml/kg per hour are normally satisfactory. Patients at risk of, or with established, fluid overload may benefit from loop diuretic therapy given with each unit. This product has a shelf life of 35 days or longer, depending on the choice of anticoagulant. The use of red cells less than 5 days old, which have near normal oxygen affinity and 2,3-DPG levels, is theoretically attractive for use in patients undergoing high dose therapy but such use has not been evaluated in a clinical trial setting.

ABO-incompatible transplants

A number of sibling or unrelated donor allogeneic marrow/stem cell transplants will, despite full HLA matching, prove to be ABO incompatible. Major incompatibility exists when the donor cells possess an antigen that the recipient lacks, e.g. group A donor and group O recipient, whilst minor incompatibility exists when recipient cells possess an antigen the donor lacks, e.g. group O donor and group B recipient. Major and minor compatibility is a combination of the two, e.g. group A donor and group B recipient. This is important in three respects. Firstly, infusion of a marrow contaminated with red cells showing major incompatibility can cause a haemolytic transfusion reaction. This can be avoided by either red cell depleting the marrow on a cell separator or by giving 15 ml/kg of secretor plasma of donor group to the recipient prior to marrow infusion (so neutralizing natural anti-A or anti-B).[16] Secondly, haemolytic reactions can result from an incorrect choice of red cell donor group during the supportive phase before engraftment and before disappearance of recipient antibodies. For major ABO-incompatible marrow recipients, recipient-type red cells should be used until there are no detectable incompatible plasma antibodies. Plasma products should be donor type to prevent passive transfer of incompatible antibodies. For minor ABO-incompatible marrow recipients, red cells should be donor type and plasma products recipient type until recipient red cells have disappeared. If the transplant is minor and major ABO incompatible, group O red cell and group AB plasma should be used. Finally, ABO-incompatible transplants require greater red cell transfusion support during the cytopenic phase,[17] as natural antibodies normally persist beyond the time at which engraftment occurs, so suppressing red cell precursor activity.

Persistence of mixed chimaerism, i.e. presence of red cells of donor and recipient blood group, is not unusual following allogeneic transplantation resulting in mixed field reactions when blood grouping. This can cause confusion for the unwary: the corresponding natural antibody disappears from plasma. In fact, shifts in the relative proportions of donor- and recipient-derived red cells can be an indicator as to the health of the graft and of the persistence of recipient stem cells post-transplant.[18]

PLATELET TRANSFUSION

Severe thrombocytopenia due to impaired thrombopoiesis from bone marrow toxicity is an almost universal consequence of many high dose therapy regimens. The duration of thrombocytopenia will vary according to the nature of the disease being treated, the chemotherapy regimen and the type of transplant procedure being performed. A now well-recognized advantage of stem cells over bone marrow transplantation is that platelet recovery occurs some 7–10 days sooner.[19] Autologous bone marrow transplantation in patients treated for acute leukaemia is often associated with very slow platelet recovery and protracted haemorrhagic manifestations.

Although the myelosuppressive effect of therapy is most commonly the cause, severe thrombocytopenia may be worsened or prolonged by other coexistent pathologies as outlined below:

- infection, particularly when associated with disseminated intravascular coagulation,
- drug therapy, e.g. Septrin,
- folate deficiency,
- splenomegaly,
- cyclosporin-induced TTP,
- CMV infection and
- graft-versus-host disease.

As the response to platelet transfusion in thrombocytopenic patients is strongly influenced by the underlying cause, some careful thought should be given to the possible mechanisms operating. For example, platelet transfusion may be dangerous in the context of post-allogeneic transplant TTP and may precipitate further thrombotic sequelae. Furthermore, by identifying the cause, e.g. CMV infection or graft-versus-host disease, the clinician can address this directly, rather than assuming that the thrombocytopenia is merely due to delayed marrow recovery.

Indications for platelet transfusion

Therapeutic platelet transfusion is indicated in patients with severe thrombocytopenia who are actively bleeding. Prophylactic platelets should also be considered for those in whom spontaneous haemorrhage poses a substantial risk. The risk of haemorrhage correlates well with the absolute platelet count if platelet function and coagulation are normal. The following template should be used to help decide when platelet transfusion is indicated in patients who are thrombocytopenic post-chemotherapy.

Therapeutic platelet transfusion
This is recommended in patients who are actively bleeding with a platelet count $<50 \times 10^9/l$. Clearly, patients with haematomas developing close to vital structures, e.g. pharynx/larynx, orbit, central nervous system and major peripheral nerves, or those with life-threatening haemorrhage require more aggressive therapy. Spontaneous haemorrhage is unusual in those with a count of $>20 \times 10^9/l$. In this situation always consider coexistent platelet dysfunction (e.g. myelodysplasia, myeloid leukaemias, myeloma, uraemia, aspirin or nonsteroidal analgesic therapy) or coagulopathy due to infection and DIC.

Prophylactic platelet transfusion
This should be considered in the following situations:

- patients with platelet counts $<10 \times 10^9/l$;
- patients with platelet counts $<20 \times 10^9/l$ who are septic, require blood transfusion, bone marrow trephine or lumbar puncture, have a coagulopathy or show clinical signs of severe thrombocytopenia (new purpura, subconjunctival or retinal haemorrhage);
- patients requiring insertion of Hickman lines (or other invasive vascular devices) or minor surgery should be transfused to generate a platelet count of $>50 \times 10^9/l$ and
- patients requiring major surgery should be transfused to generate a starting platelet count of $>100 \times 10^9/l$.

As a general rule the threshold for transfusing prophylactic platelets should be lowered (consider transfusion when $<20 \times 10^9/l$) in the following situations where platelet turnover is accelerated:

- active infection
- fever
- coagulopathy and disseminated intravascular coagulation (DIC)
- hypersplenism and
- tissue trauma and active bleeding.

The debate continues regarding threshold platelet counts at which prophylactic platelet transfusion should be considered. Many consider counts above 20 to be safe,[20] though there is good evidence that the safe threshold for prophylactic platelets is lower,[21] i.e. platelets only transfused when the count fell below 10. The latter approach led to a 20% reduction in platelet usage in the study. The policy is likely to differ between institutions: the above schedule is put forward as a guide.

Platelet transfusion is not without adverse effect, particularly in patients who have been extensively pretreated. Repeated platelet exposures increase the risks of alloimmunization, transfusion refractoriness and the need for subsequent appropriate donor matching.

Platelet preparations

Random donor platelet concentrates are still the most frequently used product in clinical practice. These are produced from individual donor blood packs and are derived from prior prepared platelet-rich plasma or buffy coat preparations. The final concentrate has a nominal volume of 50–60 ml and contains 5.5×10^{10} to 7×10^{10} platelets. Normally, five packs of random platelet concentrate will constitute a treatment dose, i.e. 250–300 ml volume and 2.75×10^{11} to 3.5×10^{11} platelets. Single donor platelets are obtained by platelet pheresis using continuous-flow centrifugation procedures. They are attractive in that the product shows less red cell and leukocyte contamination, generates yields of 3×10^{11} to 6×10^{11} platelets and can be harvested with the needs of a particular patient, e.g. HLA matched or CMV negative, in mind. The procedure, however, is more involved and requires greater commitment by the donor. A single apheresis pack will normally constitute a treatment dose.

Platelets should, if possible, be ABO and Rhesus (Rh) D compatible. In emergencies and when platelet supplies are short, incompatible platelets can be administered. ABO antigens are weakly expressed on platelets but platelet increments do not appear adversely affected,[22] though this practice may increase the risks of HLA alloimmunization.[23] Haemolytic transfusion reactions have been documented following transfusion of group O platelets, with plasma containing high-titre anti-A or anti-B, to group A or B patients, respectively. Serum of potential platelet donors should be screened for such haemolysins.[24] Rhesus D positive platelets should be avoided in Rh D negative female patients of child-bearing age, as red cell contamination can induce the formation of anti-D, with implications for possible future haemolytic disease of the newborn. If Rh D positive platelets are inadvertently given in such a situation, the patient may be protected from immunization by 250 IU anti-D immunoglobulin (given subcutaneously) for each 5 units of platelets transfused.[24]

Platelets should be transfused through a standard 170-µm filter blood-giving set with an additional in-line leukocyte depletion filter if indicated. Platelets should not be transfused through a giving set which has been used for packed cells. The transfusion of a treatment dose of platelets should be complete within 30 min.

Platelet increments

Normally, around 65% of the transfused dose of platelets will be recovered in the recipient's circulation: 35% are lost due to splenic sequestration. The expected platelet increment with a standard transfusion dose can therefore be calculated as follows:

$$\text{Platelet increment } (\times 10^9/\text{l}) = \frac{\text{Dose transfused } (\times 10^9) \times 0.65}{\text{Blood volume (litres)}}$$

The expected increment, of 5 units of random donor platelets or of a single apheresis pack, following transfusion to an adult patient with a blood volume of 5 l will be around $50 \times 10^9/\text{l}$ (or $10 \times 10^9/\text{l}$ per random donor pack). The most meaningful increment is that taken at 1 h post-transfusion.

Patients who fail to achieve satisfactory increments should be investigated with respect to the following:

- HLA- or platelet-specific antigen alloimmunization and
- platelet consumption due to sepsis, coagulopathy, bleeding, hypersplenism or veno-occlusive disease.

It is important to recognize refractoriness due to alloimmunization, as it may be possible to identify compatible donors so that apheresis platelets can be harvested according to the needs of the patient. Most transfusion centres now have panels of HLA-typed donors, allowing selection for the needs of a particular patient on a local, regional or even national level. Clearly this needs close liaison between the clinician, serologist and transfusion service personnel, with anticipation of the likely needs of a patient according to the procedure being undertaken. In many cases excellent increments to such selected platelet products will again be documented with improved control of haemorrhagic complications. In female patients who have been previously alloimmunized in pregnancy, refractoriness to platelets may be seen earlier in the course of treatment. It should also be suspected where increments are good on some days but are disappointing on others. This is due to chance compatibility with certain donors of concentrates or apheresis platelets.

There is, however, a general trend towards worsening increments over time in those who are multiply transfused, even when all the above apparent causes are excluded.

Adverse reactions

With repeated exposure, adverse reactions to platelets are seen in virtually all patients. Febrile reactions with associated chills and rigors are frequently observed: a few patients develop itching and urticarial rashes. Both respond promptly to intravenous chlorpheniramine 10 mg and hydrocortisone 100 mg, and often reactions to subsequent transfusions can be prevented by premedication with the same. Such patients should be regularly monitored for the development of HLA- and platelet-specific HPA antigen alloimmunization because such reactions appear to parallel the development of such antibodies and associated platelet refractoriness. Often, HLA and/or HPA matching of subsequent platelet products can prevent or alleviate reactions in addition to improving increments.[25] Patients with an adverse reaction to their first transfusion of a blood product should be investigated for congenital IgA deficiency, particularly if they display anaphylactoid features. These individuals often have natural anti-IgA antibodies and react to small amounts of normal IgA in blood products. Subsequent transfusions should be from IgA-deficient donors registered with the transfusion centre.

A number of multitransfused patients will continue to experience such reactions, sometimes with associated bronchospasm, despite full investigation, HLA and HPA compatibility, premedication and leukocyte depletion of the platelet product. Such reactions are presumed to be cytokine mediated: platelet-derived interleukin-6, interleukin-8 and tumour necrosis factor α increase in plasma on storage and have been shown to be responsible for rigors and febrile reactions.[26] If blood products are leukocyte-depleted before storage then this cytokine accumulation is largely prevented[27] and such reactions are less frequently encountered. I have successfully used plasma-depleted platelet concentrates resuspended in platelet additive solution (Tsol, Baxter Healthcare) in this situation as a means of abolishing such reactions. Post-transfusion purpura (PTP) and transfusion-related acute lung injury (TRALI)[28] are both rare but well-recognized complications of platelet therapy. Their discussion, however, is outside the scope of this chapter.

GRANULOCYTE TRANSFUSION

The potential therapeutic benefits of administering normal donor granulocytes to neutropenic patients with established sepsis have long been attractive. The actual benefit, with regard to clearance of infection and improvement in patient survival, has not always been established, however, in the relatively few controlled trials addressing this issue. The introduction of peripheral blood stem cell transplantation and granulocyte colony stimulating factor therapy has led to a shortening of duration of neutropenia in many high dose therapy patients. Furthermore, there have been continued improvements in antibiotic regimens for patients with neutropenic sepsis, and the clinical scenarios where granulocyte transfusion might be indicated are less often encountered. Nevertheless, many clinicians believe that granulocyte transfusion still has a role in supportive therapy if all the following clinical criteria exist:

- the patient has prolonged severe neutropenia,
- the patient has established bacterial infection and
- the infection is refractory to antibiotic therapy or the organism shows in vitro multidrug resistance.

If these criteria are met and other therapeutic avenues are limited, then a course of granulocyte transfusions is an attractive option.

The role of granulocyte therapy in the treatment of refractory fungal infection in neutropenic patients is even more debatable, particularly because combined treatment with granulocytes and amphotericin appears synergistic in the development of serious pulmonary reactions.[29]

Granulocyte preparations

A therapeutic preparation should contain a minimum of 0.5×10^{10} to 1.0×10^{10} granulocytes. These should be administered on a daily basis for a minimum period of 4 days before response can be adequately assessed. The source of granulocytes is as follows.

- *Pooled buffy coats:* these are prepared from ABO and Rh D compatible buffy coat layers of fresh random donor packs. Ten pooled buffy coats will be required for a treatment dose and require crossmatching due to inevitable heavy red cell contamination.
- *Single-donor leukapheresis:* apheresis allows collection of 1.5×10^{10} to 2.0×10^{10} granulocytes during a 3–4-h donation procedure. Yields can be improved by prior administration of corticosteroids to mobilize marginating leukocytes and through the use of sedimenting agents to aid separation from red cells within the apheresis bowl. Apheresis also allows the selection of compatible donors for patients with pre-existing HLA or granulocyte-specific antibodies.

Granulocyte preparations should be CMV compatible and irradiated to prevent transfusion-related graft-versus-host disease; this treatment does not appear to impair subsequent granulocyte activity.[30] Transfused granulocytes have an in vivo half-life of a few hours. They should be administered as soon as possible after collection and preparation, as the optimal storage conditions have yet to be established.

Adverse effects

Once red cell, leukocyte and CMV compatibility is ensured and the preparation is irradiated, the main adverse effect appears to be due to cytokine-mediated fever and chills during or soon after administration. Such reactions usually respond to treatment with intravenous hydrocortisone and piriton: refractory cases may settle with intravenous pethidine 25 mg. The patient should be premedicated with the former prior to subsequent treatments once a febrile reaction has been documented. The most serious adverse reaction is that associated with dyspnoea and pulmonary infiltrates due to pulmonary capillary damage-induced granulocyte degranulation, proteolytic enzyme release and complement activation. As noted above, concomitant amphotericin therapy may increase the risk and, in this situation, these treatments should be given 12 h apart. Finally, recipients may develop HLA antibodies, particularly following pooled multi-donor granulocyte therapy. Clearly, such a development necessitates the use of apheresis granulocytes from HLA-compatible donors if adverse reactions are to be avoided and maximal therapeutic benefit maintained.

FRESH FROZEN PLASMA AND CRYOPRECIPITATE

Fresh frozen plasma (FFP) contains all the clotting factors necessary for normal haemostasis, though the levels of labile factors, factors V and VIII, may be low normal according to the time delay between donation of blood and freezing of plasma. The product has a volume of 200–250 ml, is stored at $-30°C$ and should be used within 2 h of thawing. The product should be ABO and Rh D compatible but does not require CMV testing, as it contains no viable leukocytes. A treatment dose of 10–15 ml/kg of FFP is necessary and may be indicated for certain complications of high dose therapy.

Cryoprecipitate is effectively a concentrate of fibrinogen, factor VIII and von Willebrand factor (VWF) which forms a pale fluffy precipitate when FFP is thawed slowly at 4°C. The supernatant plasma is removed and the cryoprecipitate with a volume of 20–25 ml is refrozen at $-30°C$. Cryoprecipitate should be ABO compatible and a treatment dose of 10 packs, when thawed, can be pooled for ease of administration. Both cryoprecipitate and FFP should be administered using a blood-giving set with integral 170 μm filter. Urticarial reactions should be managed as for platelet transfusion.

Disseminated intravascular coagulation may be seen as a complication of the underlying disease (particularly acute promyelocytic leukaemia, in which it is almost universal) or as a result of sepsis developing during the cytopaenic phase post-therapy. Treatment with FFP is indicated in patients with the laboratory features of DIC who are bleeding or require an invasive procedure. One should not be guided, in the former, by the response with respect to shortening or normalization of clotting times but by its haemostatic effect in the patient. In fact, normalization of clotting times is virtually impossible with FFP alone and the volumes required can lead to fluid overload. Cryoprecipitate can be used to maintain the serum fibrinogen level in such circumstances: one should aim to maintain a level of 1.5 g/l for a maximal haemostatic response. Treatment with platelet concentrates is also often necessary in such circumstances.

It is absolutely essential that the cause of acute DIC is identified and treated. Blood product therapy is of little or no benefit unless it is possible to address the underlying trigger.[31] All-*trans* retinoic acid (ATRA) is now recognized as a valuable adjunct to chemotherapy in the treatment of acute promyelocytic leukaemia and associated DIC.[32]

The disturbed coagulation and bleeding tendency associated with liver disease is multifactorial. Serious disturbance of liver function may be seen as a result of biliary obstruction, idiosyncratic drug reaction, sepsis or veno-occlusive disease in a patient being prepared for, or undergoing, high dose therapy. Treatment with FFP is indicated in patients who are bleeding or in those needing invasive procedures. In preparation for the latter, one should aim to reduce the prothrombin time to 1.6–1.8 times the control value.[33] The volumes of FFP necessary may limit its value in such circumstances, particularly if the patient is oedematous or oliguric before treatment. One should then consider the use of prothrombin complex concentrate (PCC), but the risks of inducing thrombosis or DIC are now well recognized.[33]

Plasma exchange with volume replacement using FFP is now the accepted treatment of TTP,[34] which may be seen as a complication of treatment with mitomycin or the use of cyclosporin during allogeneic bone marrow transplantation. Microangiopathic haemolysis often persists despite dose reduction or withdrawal of the drug, and plasma exchange may then be necessary. Daily 3-l exchange with FFP replacement is the treatment of choice and should be continued until an objective response is seen. There is evidence that refractory TTP may respond to continued exchange but with replacement using cryo-poor[35] or solvent/detergent-treated FFP.[36] Antibodies to a VWF cleaving protease have been identified in TTP;[37] these may allow the accumulation of high molecular weight VWF multimers which are at least partly responsible for the pathogenesis of the disease. Plasma exchange depletes these multimers and possibly the inhibitory antibody and cryo-poor or solvent/detergent-treated FFP replaces the missing enzyme without contributing more VWF to fuel the mechanism.

INTRAVENOUS IMMUNOGLOBULIN

Polyspecific pooled human intravenous immunoglobulin (i.v. Ig) therapy may be of some value to patients undergoing high dose therapy and haemopoietic stem cell transplantation. There is evidence that i.v. Ig may reduce the incidence of CMV reactivation and the severity of acute graft-versus-host disease[38] following allogeneic transplantation, though neither concept has been subject to analysis by randomized controlled clinical trial. Many patients are immunoparesed by their disease or prior treatment at the time of preparation for high dose therapy. One might expect that empirical treatment with i.v. Ig might at least be partially effective in reducing infective complications during the cytopenic phase, but again clinical trials are lacking. The treatment is expensive, may be capable of transmitting infection and can precipitate fluid overload and aseptic meningitis.

PLASMA VOLUME EXPANDERS

A variety of synthetic colloids are now available for the urgent restoration of intravascular volume. In the context of high dose therapy, they are most often indicated for the treatment of septicaemic shock. Fresh frozen plasma is of little or no value in restoring blood pressure; it is only indicated for treatment of coexistent coagulopathy due to DIC.

Gelatin solutions are derived from hydrolysed collagen, having a target molecular weight of 35 000; smaller molecules are often present in solution and, as they are filtered by the glomerulus, may encourage osmotic diuresis. Gelatin solutions are effective in restoring plasma volume and do not appear to interfere with haemostasis in vivo, though their calcium-yielding properties may induce clotting in venous blood taken into citrate. Hydroxyethyl starch consists of a solution of macromolecular polymers of starch (target MW range 200 000–450 000); smaller molecules are again present, and are filtered at the kidney. The oncotic properties of a 6% solution are similar to that of 5% albumin and they have the longest half-life of any synthetic material (approximately 15 h). Starch solutions have been implicated in the prolongation of clotting and bleeding times,[39] though the clinical significance of such is not clear at present.

Adverse reactions to synthetic plasma volume expanders are rare and usually self-limiting. These products are effective in restoring intravascular volume, are relatively inexpensive and do not transmit infection.

ALBUMIN SOLUTIONS

Human albumin solutions have been available for clinical use over many years. The clinical circumstances in which they are of maximal benefit are still not clearly defined: a recent meta-analysis of 30 studies looking at albumin in the treatment of hypovolaemia, burns and hypoalbuminaemia has actually suggested that albumin use was associated with an increased mortality.[40] There are no studies addressing the value of albumin solutions as a supportive treatment in patients receiving high dose chemotherapy. By extrapolating from consensus guidelines,[41] the use of albumin is justified in such patients in the following situations until well-controlled studies indicate otherwise:

- for plasma volume expansion where the plasma oncotic pressure is low, i.e. serum albumin <30 g/l and patients are malnourished,
- to initiate diuresis and control oedema and effusions in nephrotic syndrome,
- to maintain intravascular volume in patients with hypoalbuminaemia following removal of large volumes of ascites, e.g. >1.5 l and
- as a treatment of generalized oedema and hypoalbuminaemia in patients after surgery, where tissue oxygenation and wound healing might be compromised.

Human albumin is available in two forms. The iso-oncotic 4.5% solution (500 ml) is indicated for volume replacement on a background of hypoalbuminaemia. The hyper-oncotic 20% solution (100 ml) is indicated for treatment of hypoalbuminaemia where there has already been significant loss of fluid into the interstitium or into serous cavities. Hypoalbuminaemia in sick patients with malnutrition is better addressed by parenteral nutrition rather than through repeated use of albumin solutions.

When calculating the dose of albumin required it is important to remember that for a given dose only 60% will be recovered in the intravascular space. The actual increment in serum albumin level is subject to many influences. As a guide, 20 g of albumin (100 ml of 20% solution) will usually raise the serum albumin level by 4 g/l (60% recovery of 20 g in a patient with 3 l plasma volume).

Adverse reactions to albumin are rare. Cardiac failure can be precipitated by albumin infusions in susceptible patients. Albumin solutions may be capable of transmitting infection: there are particular concerns regarding new variant CJD and the non-lipid-enveloped viruses hepatitis A and parvovirus. As with any blood product, the decisions regarding their use have to be made after weighing potential clinical value against the risk of adverse events.

SUMMARY

An extensive range of blood products is now available to clinicians for the supportive treatment of patients undergoing high dose chemotherapy. I have put forward guidelines to assist in the choice of appropriate products in a variety of clinical circumstances. The topic is clearly complex and blood product formulations are changing all the time. I urge you to consider each clinical situation as unique and to devise a formula of supportive care according to the circumstances. Close liaison with transfusion services remains paramount, so that blood product requirement can be anticipated and preparations made available according to the needs of the patient.

REFERENCES

1. Clinical Resource and Audit Group. Clinical guidelines. Edinburgh: The Scottish Office, 1993.
2. Jennett B (Chairman). Consensus conference on leucocyte depletion of blood and blood components; 18–19 Mar 1993. Edinburgh: Royal College of Physicians of Edinburgh, 1993.
3. Anderson KC, Weinstein HJ. Transfusion-associated graft versus host disease. N Engl J Med 1990;323:315–21.
4. Sazama K, Holland PV. Transfusion induced graft-vs-host disease. In: Garratty G, editor. Immunobiology of transfusion medicine. New York: Marcel Dekker, 1993.
5. Voak D (Chairman) BCSH Blood Transfusion Task Force. Guidelines on gamma irradiation of blood components for the prevention of transfusion-associated graft-versus-host disease. Transfusion Med 1996;6:261–71.
6. Verdonck LF, van Heughten H, de Gast GC. Delay in platelet recovery after bone marrow transplantation: impact of cytomegalovirus infection. Blood 1985;66:921–5.
7. Meyers JD, Flournoy N, Thomas ED. Risk factors for cytomegalovirus infection after human marrow transplantation. J Infect Dis 1986;153:478–88.
8. De Graan-Hentzen YCE, Gratama JW, Mudde GC et al. Prevention of primary cytomegalovirus infection in patients with haematological malignancies by intensive white cell depletion of blood products. Transfusion 1989;29:757–60.
9. Chou S. Acquisition of donor strains of cytomegalovirus by renal transplant recipients. N Engl J Med 1986;314:1418–23.
10. Bellingham AJ. The red cell in adaptation to anaemic hypoxia. Clin Haematol 1974;3:577–94.
11. Lundsgaard-Hansen P. Treatment of acute blood loss. Vox Sang 1992;63:241–6.
12. Von Hoff DD, Layard MW, Basa P et al. Risk factors for doxorubicin induced congestive heart failure. Ann Intern Med 1979;91:710–17.
13. Boldt J, Kling D, Mark P, Hemplemann G. Influence of acute preoperative hemodilution on right ventricular function. J Cardiothorac Anesthesiol 1988;2:765–71.
14. Hebert PC, Wells G, Blajchman MA et al. A multicenter, randomised, controlled clinical trial of transfusion requirements in critical care. N Engl J Med 1999;340(6):409–17.
15. Hellem AJ, Borchgrevinck CF, Imes SB. The role of red cells in haemostasis: the relation between haematocrit, bleeding time and platelet adhesiveness. Br J Haematol 1961;7:42–50.
16. Hershko C, Gale RP, Ho W, Fitchen J. ABH antigens and bone marrow transplantation. Br J Haematol 1980;44:65–73.
17. Blacklock HA, Prentice HG, Evans JPM. ABO-incompatible marrow transplants: removal of red blood cells from donor marrow avoiding recipient antibody depletion. Lancet 1982;2:1061–4.
18. Hill RS, Peterson FB, Storb R. Mixed hematologic chimaerism after allogeneic marrow transplantation for severe aplastic anaemia is associated with a higher risk of graft rejection and a lessened incidence of acute graft-versus-host disease. Blood 1986;67:811–16.

19. To LB, Roberts MM, Haylock DN et al. Comparison of haematological recovery times and supportive care requirements of autologous recovery phase peripheral blood stem cell transplants, autologous bone marrow transplants and allogeneic bone marrow transplants. Bone Marrow Transplant 1992;9:277–84.

20. Beutler E. Platelet transfusion: the 20,000μL trigger. Blood 1993;81:1411–13.

21. Rebulla P, Finazzi G, Marangoni F et al. The threshold for prophylactic platelet transfusions in adults with acute myeloid leukaemia. N Engl J Med 1997;337(26):1870–5.

22. Lee EJ, Schiffer CA. ABO compatibility can influence the results of platelet transfusion. Results of a randomised trial. Transfusion 1989;29:384–9.

23. Carr R, Hutton JL, Jenkins JA, Lucas GF, Amphlett NW. Transfusion of ABO-mismatched platelets leads to early platelet refractoriness. Br J Haematol 1990;75:408–13.

24. Murphy MF (Convenor), Brozovic B, Murphy W, Ouwehand W, Waters AH. Guidelines for platelet transfusions. British Committee for Standards in Haematology. Working Party of the Blood Transfusion Task Force. Transfusion Med 1992;2:311–18.

25. Kekomaki S, Volin L, Koistinen P et al. Successful treatment of platelet transfusion refractoriness: the use of platelet transfusions matched for both human and leucocyte antigens (HLA) and platelet alloantigens (HPA) in alloimmunised patients with leukaemia. Eur J Haematol 1998;60:112–18.

26. Heddle NM, Klama L, Singer J. The role of the plasma from platelet concentrates in transfusion reactions. N Engl J Med 1994;331:625–8.

27. Nielsen HJ, Skov F, Dybkjaer E et al. Leucocyte and platelet derived bioactive substances in stored blood: effect of prestorage leucocyte filtration. Eur J Haematol 1997;58:273–8.

28. Leach M, Vora AJ, Jones DA, Lucas G. Transfusion-related acute lung injury (TRALI) following autologous stem cell transplant for relapsed acute myeloid leukaemia: a case report and review of the literature. Transfusion Med 1998;8:333–7.

29. Wright DG, Robichaud KJ, Pizzo PA et al. Lethal pulmonary reactions associated with the combined use of amphotericin B and leucocyte transfusions. N Engl J Med 1981;304:1185–9.

30. Eastlund DT, Charbonneau TT. Superoxide generation and cytotactic response of irradiated neutrophils. Transfusion 1988;28:368–70.

31. Mount MJ, King EG. Severe acute disseminated intravascular coagulation: A reappraisal of its pathophysiology, clinical significance and therapy based on 47 patients. Am J Med 1979;67:557–63.

32. Castaigne S, Chomienne C, Daniel MT et al. All-trans retinoic acid as a differentiation therapy for acute promyelocytic leukaemia. 1. Clinical results. Blood 1990;76:1704–9.

33. Contreras M (Convenor), Ala FA, Greaves M et al. Guidelines for the use of fresh frozen plasma. British Committee for Standards in Haematology, Working Party of the Blood Transfusion Task Force. Transfusion Med 1992;2:57–63.

34. Machin SJ. Thrombotic thrombocytopenic purpura. Br J Haematol 1984;56:191–7.

35. Rock G, Schumak KH, Sutton DMC, Buskard NA, Nair RC and the members of the Canadian Apheresis Group. Cryosupernatant as replacement fluid for plasma exchange in thrombotic thrombocytopenic purpura. Br J Haematol 1996;94:383–6.

36. Harrison CN, Lawrie AS, Iqbal A, Hunter A, Machin SJ. Plasma exchange with solvent/detergent-treated plasma of resistant thrombotic thrombocytopenic purpura. Br J Haematol 1996;94:756–8.

37. Tsai HM, Lian EC-Y. Antibodies to von Willebrand factor-cleaving protease in acute thrombotic thrombocytopenic purpura. N Engl J Med 1998;339(22):1585–94.

38. Guglielmo BJ, Wong-Beringer A, Linker CA. Immune globulin therapy in allogeneic bone marrow transplantation: a critical review. Bone Marrow Transplant 1994;13:499–510.

39. Strauss RG, Stansfield C, Henriksen RA, Villhauer PJ. Pentastarch may cause fewer effects on coagulation than hetastarch. Transfusion 1988;28:257–60.

40. Cochrane Injuries Group Albumin Reviewers. Human albumin administration in critically ill patients: systematic review of randomised controlled trials. BMJ 1998;317:235–40.

41. Durand-Zaleski I, Bonnet F, Rochant H, Bierling P, Lemaire F. Usefulness of consensus conferences: the case of albumin. Lancet 1992;340:1388–90.

17

Infections following high dose chemotherapy

Beryl A Oppenheim

CONTENTS   Introduction • Common infections following high dose therapy • An approach to the management of an infected patient following high dose therapy • Conclusions

INTRODUCTION

Infections are a major cause of morbidity and mortality in patients undergoing high dose therapy with stem cell rescue. Although there is a wealth of literature concerning the epidemiology, management and prevention of infections in the haematology/oncology setting in general, few studies have yet focused on the specific area of high dose therapy, so much of our current management is based on extrapolating best practice from other settings. Another problem relates to the fact that patients undergoing high dose therapy are not a homogeneous group and it is likely that underlying disease, co-morbidities, and type of high dose regimen will all significantly affect the type and severity of infections acquired following treatment.

This chapter will attempt to review the infections most commonly encountered in this setting, and will go on to discuss an approach to both managing and preventing such infections.

COMMON INFECTIONS FOLLOWING HIGH DOSE THERAPY

Bacterial infections

In common with other infections related to periods of neutropenia, the majority of proven early infections in patients undergoing high dose therapy are bacterial in nature and, from the limited data available, it would appear that these infections follow a similar pattern to those of other bacterial infections associated with neutropenia (Table 17.1).[1,2]

In recent years the predominant organisms causing bacteraemia and other infections in neutropenic patients have been gram-positive, most commonly the coagulase-negative staphylococci, the viridans streptococci, and, particularly in some centres, the enterococci. More typical 'pathogenic' bacteria such as *Staphylococcus aureus* and *Streptococcus pneumoniae* are relatively infrequently found in these patient groups. Typically, the gram-negatives make up less than one-third of all bacteraemic episodes and, where they are found, they are now often comprised mainly of environmental species such as *Strenotrophomonas maltophilia* and *Acinetobacter* spp., rather than organisms of enteric origin such as *Escherichia coli*.

The reasons for this rather surprising pattern

Table 17.1 Infections commonly encountered following high dose therapy	
Infection	**Major predisposing factors**
During neutropenic period	
Bacterial infections	
Coagulase-negative staphylococci	Neutropenia, central venous catheters
Viridans streptococci	Neutropenia, mucositis
Escherichia coli and other gram-negatives	Neutropenia, mucositis, central venous catheters
Clostridium difficile diarrhoea	Antibiotic and chemotherapeutic agents
Fungal infections	
Candida	Neutropenia, central venous catheters
Aspergillus	Prolonged neutropenia
Viral infections	
Herpes simplex	Neutropenia
Following engraftment	
Bacterial infections	
Bacterial pneumonia	
Fungal infections	
Aspergillus	Prolonged immunosuppression – may be associated with factors such as use of fludarabine, total body irradiation
Viral infections	
Varicella zoster	
Cytomegalovirus	
Other infections	
Pneumocystis	

of bacterial infection, which is very different from that seen in the 1970s and early 1980s when gram-negatives such as *E. coli*, *Klebsiella* sp., and *Pseudonomas aeruginosa* predominated, are not entirely clear.[3] The role of antibacterial prophylaxis is clearly important, but even centres that have never used prophylaxis report similar patterns of infection. The selective pressure exerted by antimicrobial treatment, both on individual patients and the hospital environment, is also likely to play a part. It is also possible that previously some of the above-mentioned bacteria were isolated from neutropenic patients but their significance was not realized and they were dismissed as contaminants.

In many series, both of neutropenic patients in general and of neutropenic bacteraemias following high dose chemotherapy, the coagulase-negative staphylococci are the most frequently isolated organisms. Despite this, our understanding of the pathogenesis, sources of infection and epidemiology remains poor.[4] Although the skin is an obvious source of coagulase-negative staphylococci, some studies have suggested that mucosal surfaces of the gastrointestinal and pulmonary systems may also be important. Regardless of the source or mechanism of entry of organisms, the presence of indwelling central venous catheters is a major contributory factor to infection. These catheters provide a surface to which bacteria can adhere, and the formation of biofilms may serve as sources of persistent septic foci. A particular problem with coagulase-negative staphylococcal infections in this setting is that many of the organisms are multiply antibiotic resistant. This means that the majority of infections will be treated using one of the two available glycopeptide antibiotics, vancomycin or teicoplanin, although there is continuing concern about the development of glycopeptide resistance in coagulase-negative staphylococci.

In many recent series, the viridans streptococci have been reported as either the first or second most frequently isolated organism causing neutropenic bacteraemias.[5] These bacteria are part of the normal flora of the mouth, oropharynx and intestinal tract, and the precise reasons for their sudden prominence in neutropenic infections are not fully understood. The association of neutropenia and oral mucositis does seem to be an important risk factor for the development of viridans streptococcal bacteraemia, while in some studies associations with specific chemotherapeutic agents (particularly high dose cytosine arabinoside) or antimicrobial agents used for prophylaxis have been noted. Although most patients with viridans streptococcal bacteraemia present with a fever that responds to antibiotics, a subgroup of these will develop a characteristic clinical picture with hypotension, a rash and, in some cases, onset of adult respiratory distress syndrome, with a high mortality rate.

Enterococci are becoming an increasingly common cause of hospital-acquired bacteraemia, being cited as the third commonest pathogen in some series. This finding has been paralleled in many centres treating neutropenic cancer patients, and a particular problem in some of these centres has been the acquisition of glycopeptide resistance, especially in *Enterococcus faecium*. When this occurs against a background of resistance to other antimicrobials such as beta-lactam and high-level aminoglycoside resistance, it is possible to be faced with a bacterium resistant to almost all available agents. The recent licensing in the UK of quinupristin–dalfopristin (Synercid) and linezolid (Zyvox) offers a new class of antimicrobial with activity against a number of problem gram positive bacteria, including glycopeptide resistant enterococci

As has already been noted, the incidence of gram-negative infections has dramatically decreased, both in centres using quinolone prophylaxis and in those where antibiotic prophylaxis is seldom used. However, gram-negative infections, particularly bacteraemias, still do occur and are considered to be associated with a higher mortality than most gram-positive infections. A particular problem which has recently emerged, particularly in some centres in Europe, has been the development of fluoroquinolone-resistant *E. coli* that causes bacteraemia in neutropenic patients.[6,7] If this finding becomes more widespread it may raise further questions about the risks and benefits of antibiotic prophylaxis in this setting. Another gram-negative which is now isolated far less frequently, but which still carries considerable morbidity and mortality, is *Ps. aeruginosa*. When this infection occurs it may be associated with necrotic spreading skin lesions, called ecthyma gangrenosum, and this may be particularly difficult to treat. Most authorities recommend combination therapy with two or three agents active against *Ps. aeruginosa*, given in high dosage. Because of the fears of severe *Ps. aeruginosa* infection during neutropenia, it is still recommended that any regimen used for empirical antibiotic therapy should retain anti-pseudomonal coverage.

Bacterial infections other than those causing bacteraemia or central venous catheter-related infections are rather uncommon. Urinary tract infections do occur, particularly if the patient has some underlying bladder or renal pathology, or urinary catheterization has been necessary. Although the respiratory tract is often the focus of infection following high dose chemotherapy, those infections which are microbiologically proven are often non-bacterial in nature.

A particular problem affecting neutropenic patients is the development of diarrhoea due to *Clostridium difficile*.[8] While this is often as a result of receiving antibiotic therapy, it is also recognized that cytotoxic agents themselves may predispose to this condition. Although some antibiotics such as clindamycin and the cephalosporins are associated with a particular risk of *Cl. difficile* infection, it is now known that this may occur following administration of almost any antibiotic. The diagnosis can be difficult to make because there are so many other possible causes of diarrhoea in an individual who has undergone high dose therapy. It is essential to submit faecal samples to the microbiology laboratory for toxin testing. Once a positive test is obtained, the management of *Cl. difficile* diarrhoea involves withdrawal of the offending antimicrobial (which may be very difficult in a critically ill patient) and the administration of either metronidazole or oral vancomycin. The use of oral vancomycin is generally discouraged because it is believed that it may contribute to the development of glycopeptide resistance in enterococci; metronidazole is now recommended as the first-line agent of choice. Recurrences of infection, which in many cases are known to be due to acquisition of different strains of *Cl. difficile*, can occur fairly commonly. More than one or two patients with *Cl. difficile* infections in a particular unit at the same time should alert clinicians to the need to review antibiotic policies and involve infection control teams because of the possibility of cross-infection problems.

Fungal infections

Fungal infections are a major cause of morbidity and mortality in neutropenic patients, as well as other immunosuppressed and critically ill individuals.[9] Although there are a number of risk factors for the development of an invasive fungal infection (IFI), such as use of steroids and previous antibiotics, it is well recognized that the most important of these is prolonged, profound neutropenia. Many of the regimens used for high dose treatments result in neutropenia which, although profound, may not persist for more than 14 days. It is therefore not surprising that invasive fungal infections are not commonly reported in analyses of infections following high dose chemotherapy, with rates of 1–2% being cited.[10] Despite this, however, because of the potentially disastrous consequences of an untreated fungal infection, it is essential to consider the possibility of IFI in all patients who fail to respond promptly to antibiotics. The two most common infecting organisms in this setting are *Candida* and *Aspergillus*, with *Candida* being more frequently noted in most series. However, a number of extremely rare, emerging fungal infections have been described, making cultural diagnosis particularly critical.

Candida is a yeast, and, in the setting of patients with haematological or other malignancies, may cause oropharyngeal candidiasis, fungaemias, central venous catheter-related infections or, more rarely, disseminated infection. Despite improved recognition and methods of treatment, published mortality still remains at around 40% for invasive candida infections, although mortality attributed only to the fungal infection itself may be lower.

Candida albicans is the most prevalent *Candida* species isolated from humans, and for many years was also the most common cause of invasive infections. However, in recent years there has been a dramatic shift in the patterns of candidal infections, particularly in oncology centres. A number of non-albicans *Candida* species are now causing significant numbers of infections. In many series the most frequent of these is *C. parapsilosis*, which may be associated with use of central venous catheters and/or parenteral nutrition. This species is of interest because the associated mortality appears to be lower than for other candidal infections and many patients respond promptly to central venous catheter removal and antifungal therapy. Mortality rates for most other candidal infections are similar to those for *C. albicans*. *Candida krusei* and *C. glabrata* are two species that appear to have emerged as a result of the widespread use of antifungal prophylaxis, and both are usually resistant to fluconazole. *Candida tropicalis* remains an unusual cause of infection but does appear to be more virulent and to be associated with a higher mortality rate.

The diagnosis of systemic candidal infection is usually made by isolation of the organism in blood cultures. The central venous catheter tip is often an important focus of infection. Acute dissemination to other organs can occur in association with a high mortality. A more unusual form of the infection is the chronic disseminated form also known as hepatosplenic candidiasis. This usually presents once neutrophil recovery has occurred, and the patient will have ongoing fevers and abnormalities in liver function tests. Radiological investigations are of particular importance in making the diagnosis of this condition, with CT and MRI scanning apparently offering significant advantages over ultrasound. Radiologically guided or laparoscopic biopsy may be essential to confirm the diagnosis.

Aspergillus is a filamentous fungus, and *A. fumigatus* is the most common species causing infection. Invasive aspergillus infections are a particular problem in cancer patients. Although typically associated with the prolonged neutropenia that is associated with induction therapy for acute leukaemia or allogeneic bone marrow transplantation, these infections have been described in patients after high dose treatment with stem cell rescue. The most common presentation of infection is invasive pulmonary aspergillosis, but skin lesions, sinusitis and disseminated infection may all occur. Infection can occur in all groups of individuals, but older age, male sex and underlying pulmonary disease appear to be risk factors. Clusters of infection have also been described in association with building work in hospitals and with malfunctioning ventilation systems. Invasive aspergillosis is associated with a high mortality. Early diagnosis and prompt institution of antifungal treatment appear to offer the best chance of a favourable outcome.

Viral infections

Viral infections often present later on in the course of follow-up of patients who have undergone high dose treatment and may need to be considered in an outpatient who presents with a variety of problems. The main viruses implicated in causing infections in this setting are the herpesviruses and, particularly during the winter months, the respiratory viruses.

The most common presentation of herpes simplex infection is oral ulcerative mucositis, although oesophagitis or infections in the genital or perianal areas may occur. The widespread use of acyclovir prophylaxis has significantly reduced these problems. Varicella zoster virus (VZV) reactivation is a significant problem following any kind of bone marrow transplantation (BMT), and appears to occur as frequently following high dose therapy as in the allogeneic or autologous BMT setting, although it may occur earlier in the course of treatment.[11] Acyclovir prophylaxis appears to delay the development of VZV infection, but the most appropriate duration of prophylaxis has not been defined.

Cytomegalovirus infection is a major problem following allogeneic BMT but appears to occur far less frequently in the high dose therapy setting. However, once disease has developed, mortality is high, with pneumonitis having a particularly poor prognosis.[12,13] Infection can occur either as a primary event or, more commonly, as reactivation in previously seropositive patients. In the allogeneic BMT setting, sensitive screening using quantitative polymerase chain reaction (PCR) followed by pre-emptive treatment for PCR-positive cases appears to be the most favoured approach to management and is now being fairly widely used routinely, but it is unlikely that this would prove cost-effective in the autologous setting. Future studies should focus on the value of screening particularly high-risk seropositive patients.[14]

Pneumocystis pneumonia

Pneumocystis carinii infection occurs in a wide variety of haematological malignancies, and following bone marrow and solid organ transplantation. Although its incidence following high dose therapy appears to be low, it is well documented[15] and the mortality is high. Prophylaxis is highly effective. Cotrimoxazole given three times weekly is widely used, with nebulized pentamidine as an alternative for patients unable to tolerate cotrimoxazole. Areas requiring further study are: whether prophylaxis is indicated in all patients undergoing high dose therapy (or only those in particular risk groups), and what is the optimal duration of prophylaxis.

AN APPROACH TO THE MANAGEMENT OF AN INFECTED PATIENT FOLLOWING HIGH DOSE THERAPY

Diagnosis of infection

History and physical examination
The majority of patients with infection following high dose therapy, particularly when they are neutropenic, present with a fever and few, if any, other signs of sepsis. Despite this, every attempt must be made to exclude a possible source of infection and to define the infecting agent.

The definition of a significant fever in this setting remains controversial, but many authorities recommend using a temperature of ⩾38.0°C. However, infection must still be con-

sidered in a very unwell patient who is apyrexial, or even hypothermic, particularly in association with hypotension.

Physical examination should focus on those areas most likely to provide a source for infection, such as the mouth and throat, the perianal area and the central vascular catheter exit site. Particular note should be taken of any skin lesions, as these may be pointers to infection with *Staph. aureus*, *Ps. aeruginosa* or fungi. Although the lungs are an important site of infection, auscultation may be normal; if there is any doubt, a chest radiograph should be performed.

Microbiological diagnosis
Specimens for culture should be taken prior to administration of antibiotics. Most are relatively simple to obtain and there is thus no need to delay the start of treatment.

Blood cultures are the mainstay of detecting infection in the neutropenic host and they can provide useful information in 30–50% of cases. At least two sets of cultures should be taken. If the patient has a central catheter, it is recommended that one set be taken from a peripheral vein and one set through each lumen of the catheter. There are a number of more specialized forms of culture that may be helpful in sorting out whether the catheter is the source of infection, such as differential quantitative blood cultures, but these are labour intensive and are not offered by all microbiology laboratories. Using modern blood culture detection systems, preliminary positive results can often be reported well within 24 h and these can play an important role in directing modification of antimicrobial treatment.

Other microbiological cultures are of more limited use. Throat and urine cultures are usually recommended. If the central venous catheter exit site is inflamed, this should be cultured. Stool should be examined for *Cl. difficile* and other enteric pathogens in patients who have diarrhoea. When skin lesions are present, skin scrapings should be submitted for microbiological staining and culture. Sputum is rarely produced in a neutropenic individual and, where a chest infection is suspected, a particularly valuable specimen is a bronchoalveolar lavage (BAL). Fibreoptic bronchoscopy is an extremely safe procedure in this setting and BAL fluid can be used to culture for bacteria and fungi as well as for some of the newer non-cultural methods described below. It is also the specimen of choice for the DEAFF test for cytomegalovirus (CMV), and respiratory viruses can be sought using both culture and rapid immunofluorescent staining, which can provide results within 1–2 h. The presence of *P. carinii* in BAL can also be investigated using immunofluorescent techniques.

The value of routine surveillance cultures is controversial. Although these specimens can be time-consuming and costly, some limited surveillance may be of benefit both to the individual patient and to the unit in general by directing antibiotic and infection control policies. Previous colonization with fungi, particularly *Aspergillus* spp., *Candida albicans* and *C. tropicalis*, has been associated with subsequent infection and may point towards early administration of an antifungal. Similarly, enteric carriage of *Ps. aeruginosa* can herald systemic infection, and colonization with this organism can be relatively simply eradicated using agents such as fluoroquinolones or colistin.

Non-cultural microbiological techniques

The development of non-cultural techniques is an exciting and fast-moving area which may, in the future, provide a far more accurate picture of the aetiology of infection in the neutropenic or post-transplant patient. To date, most developments have been in the areas of viral and fungal infections.

Modern methods of detection of CMV infection mainly revolve around the use of antigenaemia and quantitative PCR. It can be difficult to assess CMV antigenaemia in a neutropenic individual, and early results suggest quantitative PCR may be the investigation of choice. Although the rarity of CMV disease following high dose therapy indicates that routine screening for CMV post-treatment may not be cost-effective, CMV should be sought in any infected patient who has signs and symptoms that may be due to CMV, such as unexplained hepatic dysfunction, pneumonitis or unexplained pancytopaenia following engraftment, particularly if the patient has serological evidence of previous CMV infection.

Non-culture detection of fungi has mainly involved either detection of fungal antigens or PCR diagnosis in specimens such as blood, cerebrospinal fluid or BAL. Considerable interest has recently focused on the galactomannan ELISA for *Aspergillus* antigen, which is reported to be both sensitive and specific. For detection of fungal infection PCR is also showing promise, although at this stage a number of different approaches are being investigated, ranging from panfungal assays[16] to specific systems of detection for different fungi.

Imaging

Radiology has an important role to play in the detection of infection post-transplant. Although the chest radiograph is often normal until late on, even in the face of proven respiratory infection, it is an important baseline investigation in the febrile neutropenic patient and it should be repeated at regular intervals in patients who continue to show signs of infection.

High-resolution computed tomography (CT) scanning is now recognized as an extremely valuable investigation for invasive pulmonary infection. It is often positive when the chest radiograph is normal, and, in the hands of an experienced radiologist, features typical of invasive pulmonary aspergillosis such as the halo sign and the air-crescent sign can be detected.[17,18] As has been previously noted, CT and magnetic resonance imaging (MRI) are also valuable in the diagnosis of chronic disseminated candidiasis.

Approach to antimicrobial therapy

Initial antibiotic therapy

Any patient who has significant neutropenia and fever must be assumed to be infected, and prompt initiation of antimicrobial treatment in this setting can be potentially life-saving. This is one occasion when delaying treatment until microbiological results are available is unacceptable. For this reason, the concept of empirical treatment for neutropenic fevers has been established. A variety of appropriate empirical regimens have been described,[19] but for any individual unit it is recommended that standard protocols for empirical therapy be drawn up and strictly adhered to. Attempts to 'individualize' treatment to a specific patient's needs often result in misunderstandings and errors in providing the appropriate antimicrobial coverage. Protocols for empirical antimicrobials need to be based not only on published evidence, but also on an understanding of local patterns of infection.

Studies on the optimal use of empirical therapy have been ongoing since the 1970s – many co-ordinated by the European Organization for Research and Treatment of Cancer (EORTC) – and form the basis of our understanding of managing infection in neutropenic patients. However, most of the studies have included neutropenic patients with a wide variety of underlying diseases who have had a wide range of chemotherapeutic agents and procedures. It is only recently that it has been realized that empirical antibiotic therapy may be specifically tailored to the underlying disease and intervention, and reports of research in this area are now beginning to emerge.

For many years the literature supported the use of either an extended-spectrum penicillin (e.g. piperacillin) or anti-pseudomonal cephalosporin (e.g. ceftazidime) in combination with an aminoglycoside for empirical treatment. These combinations have the advantage of providing extremely broad-spectrum and potentially synergistic activity against some gram-negative bacilli. However, disadvantages include lack of activity against some gram-positive bacteria and toxicity of the aminoglycoside component which requires careful monitoring of serum levels. In an attempt to continue to use combination therapy but to avoid the toxicity of the aminoglycosides, double beta-lactam combina-

tions have been tried, but these have not generally found favour.

Although it is well recognized that treatment with an aminoglycoside alone is not acceptable because of the narrow window between therapeutic and toxic levels, it has been realized that this is not necessarily the case for all antibiotics, and single-drug or monotherapy using highly active beta-lactams or carbapenems have now been extensively investigated.[20] Ceftazidime, piperacillin/tazobactam, imipenem/cilastatin and meropenem are among the contenders for use as monotherapy for empirical treatment, and the EORTC has recently reported extremely favourable results comparing meropenem with their previous 'gold-standard' combination of ceftazidime and amikacin.[21]

Most of the studies of empirical antibiotic therapy have included patients with wide varieties of underlying diseases and periods of neutropenia, and these studies were designed to ensure appropriate management of those individuals at highest risk of mortality from neutropenic infection. It is now recognized that it may be possible to adopt a risk-management approach by which a subgroup of low-risk neutropenic patients may be considered for less intensive antimicrobial therapy. Such low-risk patients have generally included those with solid tumours in whom the duration of neutropenia is predicted to be short (<7 days) and in whom there are no significant co-morbidities.[22–24] A variety of regimens, such as outpatient intravenous antibiotic therapy, inpatient oral antibiotics and even outpatient oral antibiotics, have now been studied. The appropriateness of any of these approaches to certain groups of patients undergoing high dose therapies remains to be validated.

Modifications of empirical antibiotic regimens
Following initiation of empirical antimicrobial therapy, it is anticipated that the majority of patients will respond within 48–72 h. A continued fever beyond this time poses a dilemma for the clinician managing the patient (Fig. 17.1).

Clearly, if positive microbiological cultures have been obtained, treatment should be

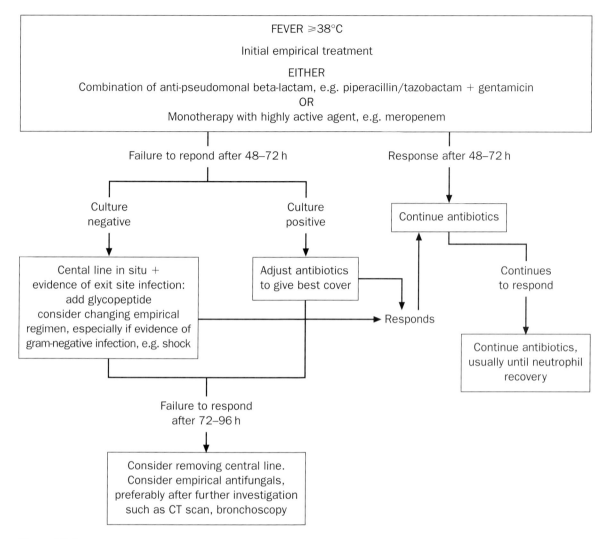

Figure 17.1
Approach to empirical antimicrobial therapy in neutropenic fevers.

adjusted to ensure best coverage of these organisms. Ironically, the most commonly isolated organisms causing bacteraemia, the coagulase-negative staphylococci, are often not covered by empirical regimens. The reason for this is that many of the coagulase-negative staphylococci are resistant to all beta-lactam antibiotics and would only be covered by the addition of one of the glycopeptide antibiotics, vancomycin or teicoplanin. A number of studies have investi-

gated the value of adding a glycopeptide to the initial antibiotic regimen, but this has generally not given any survival benefits and is usually discouraged because of toxicity, fears of the development of resistance and additional unnecessary cost.[25,26] For patients from whom a gram-positive organism resistant to the empirical regimen used is isolated, modification should involve the addition of either vancomycin or teicoplanin. Overall, both of these agents appear to give equivalent results in terms of efficacy, although teicoplanin may offer some advantages in ease of administration, non requirement of serum monitoring and fewer adverse events.[27]

In the consideration of fever which for more than 3 days fails to defervesce, in the absence of a positive culture or obvious source of infection, the following should be considered: bacterial infection resistant to the empirical choice, emergence of a new infection, non-bacterial causes of infection, inadequate levels of antimicrobials, drug fever, or a hidden source of infection such as catheters, abscesses or other deep infection. Consideration can be given to changing the initial empirical regimen, adding an aminoglycoside if this was not part of the initial choice, or adding a glycopeptide even in the absence of evidence of a gram-positive infection.

Empirical antifungal therapy
For those patients who continue with fever following 4–7 days of antibiotic treatment, the possibility of a fungal infection must be considered. While stem cell supported high dose therapy appears to carry a low risk of fungal infections, the possibility must be considered. The most appropriate timing for initiating antifungal therapy in a patient who has no signs or symptoms has not been established, although early treatment clearly is advantageous for those individuals who do have a systemic fungal infection. If there is evidence of a possible source of a fungal infection, particularly a pulmonary infiltrate, an early start to treatment is particularly important. In such cases every effort should be made to establish a diagnosis, using modalities such as CT scanning, BAL and, where available, non-cultural methods of diagnosis.

At present, amphotericin B remains the drug of choice for empirical antifungal treatment because of its broad spectrum.[28] However, reports are emerging that show that intravenous fluconazole or itraconazole can be used in this setting. These may prove particularly suitable in the somewhat lower risk setting of some types of high dose therapy. When used for empirical treatment, amphotericin B is usually recommended at a dosage of 1 mg/kg/day. Toxicity of amphotericin B is a problem. Acute toxic reactions such as chills and fever are common. Nephrotoxicity occurs in a high proportion of patients administered amphotericin B and can be potentiated by other nephrotoxic drugs such as aminoglycosides. In such cases, lipid-associated amphotericins can allow the ongoing administration of amphotericin with minimal if any renal problems.[29] Three lipid-based preparations are currently available and their formulation and licensed dosages are shown in Table 17.2.

Non-antimicrobial therapies
The management of individuals with severe infections who continue with prolonged profound neutropenia remains a problem, although it is unusual in the setting of stem cell supported high dose therapy. Granulocyte transfusions were widely used but fell into disfavour as improved antibiotic therapy allowed for the successful management of infections during neutropenia. However, the possibility of using granulocyte transfusions from granulocyte colony stimulating factor (G-CSF) stimulated donors has resulted in a resurgence of interest in this adjunctive therapy, particularly for patients with life-threatening fungal infections when there is no evidence of neutrophil recovery. The exact role of haemopoietic growth factors in either the prophylaxis or treatment of infections during neutropenia has not been fully defined. While G-CSF and granulocyte–macrophage (GM) CSF reduce the depth and duration of neutropenia and increase neutrophil number and quality, an overall benefit in terms of reducing mortality due to infection has not been shown. The greatest interest has been in the use of growth factors in severe fungal infections. Because of its stimulatory effects on monocyte and macrophage function, GM-CSF may be of particular use in this setting.

18

High dose chemotherapy and gonadal function

Simon J Howell and Stephen M Shalet

CONTENTS Introduction • Testicular function • Ovarian function • Summary

INTRODUCTION

High dose chemotherapy is being increasingly used in the treatment of a variety of malignancies. Its use is associated with significant morbidity in many patients, and alterations in gonadal function are among the most common long-term side effects of therapy. Germinal epithelial damage resulting in oligo- or azoospermia as a consequence of specific chemotherapeutic agents has long been recognized and there is also evidence of some degree of Leydig cell dysfunction following treatment. Testicular damage is drug specific and dose related.[1-4] The chance of recovery of spermatogenesis following cytotoxic insult and also the extent (normospermia or oligospermia) and speed of recovery are related to the agent used and the dose received.

Although the ovary is less vulnerable to the effects of cytotoxic chemotherapy than the testis, ovarian failure is not uncommon following these treatments. As with the testis, ovarian dysfunction is agent- and dose-dependent.[5-7] In addition, there is very clear evidence in women that age at the time of cytotoxic insult is important in determining the speed of onset and duration of amenorrhoea, and the chance of retaining normal ovarian function.[8-10] The course of ovarian function following chemotherapy is variable, and predicting the likely outcome in any individual patient can be difficult.

TESTICULAR FUNCTION

Many drugs, particularly alkylating agents, have been shown to be gonadotoxic, and the agents most commonly implicated are listed in Table 18.1. Data concerning the use of high dose chemotherapy are at present limited, but there is a large amount of information concerning the gonadal impact of standard cytotoxic chemotherapy. This is of importance not only because it helps to some extent to predict the impact of high dose treatment, but also because a proportion of patients undergoing high dose therapy will have previously received other chemotherapy regimens.

The impact on testicular function of chemotherapy used in the treatment of lymphomas, especially Hodgkin's disease, has been widely reported. Several studies have reported azoospermia with raised follicle stimulating hormone (FSH) levels in over 90% of men following cyclical chemotherapy with MVPP (mustine, vinblastine, procarbazine and prednisolone).[15,16] Testosterone levels are usually within the normal range but luteinizing

Table 18.1 Gonadotoxic drugs		
Group	**Definite gonadotoxicity**	**Reference**
Alkylating agents	Cyclophosphamide	Rivkees et al. (1988)[11]
	Chlorambucil	
	Mustine	
	Melphalan	
	Busulphan	Sanders et al. (1996)[12]
	Carmustine	Clayton et al. (1988)[13]
	Lomustine	Clayton et al. (1988)[13]
Antimetabolites	Cytarabine	
Vinca alkaloids	Vinblastine	Vilar et al. (1974)[14]
Others	Procarbazine	
	Cisplatin	Wallace et al. (1989)[7]

hormone (LH) levels are often near the upper limit of normal or frankly raised, suggesting a degree of Leydig cell impairment. Chemotherapy regimens used for the treatment of non-Hodgkin's lymphoma (NHL) are generally less gonadotoxic than those used for Hodgkin's disease. This is probably related to the absence of procarbazine in the standard regimens used for NHL,[6] although the reduction in the dose of alkylating agents may also be important. Azoospermia is also a common finding following the treatment of testicular cancers with either cisplatin- or carboplatin-based chemotherapy. However, this is usually temporary, with recovery of sperm counts in approximately 80% by 5 years.[17]

Many of the studies of testicular function following chemotherapy have demonstrated an effect of dose of the agents used in determining the extent of gonadal damage. Rivkees and Crawford[11] published an analysis of 30 studies which examined gonadal function after various chemotherapy regimens, which included a total of 116 males who had been treated with cyclophosphamide alone. Of the 116 patients, 52 (45%) had evidence of testicular dysfunction following treatment. The incidence of gonadal

dysfunction correlated with the total dose of cyclophosphamide; it occurred in approximately 50% of post-pubertal patients who received 200–300 mg/kg and over 80% of post-pubertal patients who received more than 300 mg/kg. The dose dependency of cytotoxic-induced gonadal damage has also been demonstrated in patients treated with MOPP/ABVD[18] and MOPP[3] for lymphoma. The higher doses of drug utilized in high dose regimens should therefore predict greater gonadal toxicity than that observed following conventional therapy. However, the gonadotoxicity of cytotoxic therapy is agent specific, and as the drugs used in high dose regimens often differ to some extent from those used in standard multiagent therapy, it is important to consider the available data concerning high dose treatment.

A number of studies have assessed testicular function after high dose chemotherapy. Most of these studies have included patients who also received total body irradiation (TBI), and as this is also gonadotoxic, it is difficult to assess the gonadal damage that is specifically a consequence of the chemotherapy. Howell et al.[19] studied a cohort of 68 men treated with one of four different high dose chemotherapy regimens; cyclophosphamide, BCNU and etoposide (CBV) ($n = 20$), busulphan and cyclophosphamide ($n = 23$), cyclophosphamide and TBI ($n = 15$) or high dose melphalan $\pm$ TBI ($n = 10$) for Hodgkin's disease, NHL, acute myeloid leukaemia (AML), acute lymphocytic leukaemia (ALL) and myeloma. In addition to TBI in 21 patients, most had received prior chemotherapy, 19 with MVPP or ChlVPP/EVA hybrid (chlorambucil, vinblastine, procarbazine, prednisolone, etoposide, vincristine and doxorubicin), which are known to result in gonadal damage in a high proportion of patients. A mean of 7.5 years after treatment, 60 of 68 patients (88%) had germinal epithelial damage, indicated by a raised FSH level, and in addition 33 patients (49%) had an LH level at or above the upper limit of normal, suggesting a degree of Leydig cell impairment. There were no significant differences in mean LH and FSH levels between the different treatment groups; the proportions of patients with raised FSH and LH levels are displayed in Fig. 18.1. The majority of men with normal FSH levels had received busulphan and cyclophosphamide (six of eight), suggesting that this regimen may be less toxic to the germinal epithelium. However, none of these patients had received TBI or procarbazine-containing chemotherapy, whilst all men in the CBV group had received prior treatment with either MVPP or ChlVPP/EVA hybrid, and the majority of the men in the other two groups had received TBI. It is probable that these differences in additional therapy account, at least in part, for the apparent difference in gonadotoxicity between the groups.

Sanders et al.[12] reported on a total of 155 men treated with cyclophosphamide (200 mg/kg) or busulphan and cyclophosphamide (busulphan 16 mg/day, cyclophosphamide 200 mg/kg) as preparation for bone marrow transplant (BMT). An average of 2–3 years post-transplant, 67 of the 109 who received cyclophosphamide (61%), but only 8 of 46 (17%) patients treated with busulphan and cyclophosphamide, had recovery of testicular function defined by normal LH, FSH and testosterone levels with evidence of

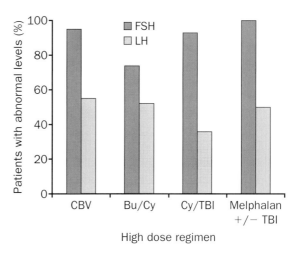

Figure 18.1
Proportion of patients with raised FSH and LH levels following high dose chemotherapy. Bu/Cy, Busulphan and cyclophosphamide; CBV, cyclophosphamide, BCNU and etoposide; Cy/TBI, cyclophosphamide and total body irradiation; FSH, follicle stimulating hormone; LH, luteinizing hormone; TBI, total body irradiation.

sperm production. The only prospective study to examine testicular function following high dose treatment reported on 13 men who received either BEAM (BCNU, etoposide, Ara-C and melphalan) ($n = 11$) or melphalan and single-fraction TBI ($n = 2$).[20] All had previously received multiagent chemotherapy and four had abnormal semen parameters before transplantation. All patients were azoospermic 2–3 months post-transplantation, associated with raised FSH levels. LH levels increased and testosterone levels decreased after transplantation, indicating that Leydig cell damage was apparent in addition to germ cell failure.

With regard to the treatment of boys before the onset of puberty, there are very few studies with a sufficiently long follow-up to enable reliable assessment of gonadal function to be made. Cyclophosphamide alone,[21] and combined with busulphan,[22] do not appear to prevent normal progress through puberty, although germinal epithelial dysfunction is affected in some, indicated by azoospermia or raised FSH levels. Following high dose cyclophosphamide in combination with TBI, testicular dysfunction is more common; 17 of 25 patients evaluated by Sanders et al.[21] had raised FSH levels and 10 of 25 had raised LH levels. Similar high rates of toxicity were also reported in a small group of boys treated with cyclophosphamide and TBI before puberty by Leiper et al:[23] there were raised LH levels in five out of six, and raised FSH in all six who had reached pubertal age.

There is thus no clear evidence that prepubertal boys are less susceptible to gonadal damage than adult men. Irrespective of age, cyclophosphamide alone at a dose of 200 mg/kg results in germinal epithelial failure in a little under half of individuals, but the addition of busulphan or TBI markedly increases the gonadotoxicity, with the vast majority of patients becoming azoospermic and mild Leydig cell dysfunction occurring in a proportion. Similar rates of gonadal dysfunction also occur following BEAM or melphalan and TBI.

Whilst the clinical impact of germinal epithelial damage and azoospermia is clear, there are fewer data concerning the impact of mild Leydig cell dysfunction, which occurs in a proportion of patients. A number of symptoms that occur in overt hypogonadism (fatigue, sexual dysfunction and altered mood) also occur more commonly in patients following cytotoxic chemotherapy. In addition, reduced bone mineral density (BMD), which is associated with testosterone deficiency, has also been demonstrated in cytotoxic-treated men, and bone density has been shown to correlate with testosterone levels in these patients.[24] A recent double blind placebo controlled trial of testosterone replacement in men with mild Leydig cell insufficiency following cytotoxic chemotherapy[25] did not, however, demonstrate any significant benefit of treatment. It was concluded,

therefore, that treatment should not be offered routinely to such patients.

In addition to impairment of steroidogenesis and sperm production, there has been concern that cytotoxic chemotherapy may also result in transmissible genetic damage. Animal studies have demonstrated untoward effects in offspring of animals treated with cytotoxic agents, but no clear evidence for this has been reported in humans. Increased aneuploid frequency has been observed in human sperm following chemotherapy for HD.[26,27] However, data on the outcome of pregnancies have not shown any increase in genetically mediated birth defects, altered sex ratios or birthweight effects in offspring of cancer survivors,[28] possibly as a result of selection bias against genetically abnormal sperm. On the evidence collected thus far, it is therefore reasonable to conclude that patients treated with high dose chemotherapy who remain fertile are not at increased risk of fathering children with genetic abnormalities.

Protection of testicular function

The deleterious effect of chemotherapy and radiotherapy on gonadal function has initiated a search for possible strategies to preserve fertility in patients undergoing therapy. Cryostorage of semen has become standard practice, and should be offered to all men before undergoing potentially sterilizing therapy. However, there are some limitations to this method of preserving fertility. Firstly, it is not a feasible option for prepubertal patients. Furthermore, testicular function in adult males with malignant disease is often impaired before treatment, resulting in poor sperm quality or difficulty in providing semen for storage. Thus, methods for protecting or enhancing the recovery of normal spermatogenesis following gonadotoxic therapy have been pursued.

The belief that prepubertal boys have a lower rate of permanent chemotherapy-induced gonadal damage,[11] due to the quiescent status of the germinal epithelium, has led many investigators to propose that suppression of testicular function in adult men may provide a degree of protection against cytotoxic therapy. Irrespective of the validity of the hypothesis, data derived from animal models have been encouraging, but there is at present no convincing evidence of similar success in humans. The most recent animal data suggest that hormonal treatment may enhance recovery of spermatogenesis from surviving stem cells rather than protect them from damage during cytotoxic insult.[29] Thus, suppression of gonadal function with a gonadotrophin releasing hormone (GnRH) agonist or testosterone for a fixed time after the completion of chemotherapy may prove more successful in reducing the impact of these treatments on fertility. The success of this will depend on whether any stem cells remain intact, and it is therefore likely to be of most benefit in those patients in whom the testicular insult is less severe, as it is these patients in whom there is significant preservation of A spermatogonia. Complete ablation of the germinal epithelium, as may occur in many men treated with high dose chemotherapy, will be irreversible.

Results from recent animal experiments have also indicated another possible method of preserving testicular function during gonadotoxic therapy. In 1994 Brinster et al.[30] demonstrated that spermatogonial stem cells isolated from a donor mouse could be injected into the seminiferous tubules of a sterile recipient mouse and result in the initiation of spermatogenesis. More recently, the same group have been able to demonstrate that spermatogenesis can be achieved in previously sterile mice following cryopreservation and then injection of donor stem cells into the testis. Potentially, therefore, stem cells could be harvested from the human testis before the start of sterilizing therapy, freeze-stored and reimplanted at a later date, with a subsequent return of spermatogenesis. A clinical trial testing this hypothesis is currently underway in adults: 11 men have had testicular tissue harvested shortly before commencing treatment with sterilizing chemotherapy for Hodgkin's disease or non-Hodgkin's lymphoma. In each case, a 0.5 cm cube of testicular tissue has been subjected to enzymatic digestion to produce a single-cell suspension which, following equilibration in cryoprotectant, has been stored in liquid nitrogen.[31] Five men have now successfully completed chemotherapy, and thawed testicular suspension has been reinjected into the donor testis. Results of follow-up semen analyses and hormonal evaluation are awaited with great interest.

OVARIAN FUNCTION

The gonadotoxic effects of chemotherapy in women were first reported by Louis et al.[32] in women treated with busulphan for CML. Since then a number of drugs have been implicated in the development of ovarian dysfunction.

The effects of cyclophosphamide, used in the treatment of breast cancer, renal disorders and rheumatological conditions, have been widely studied. Ovarian damage has been clearly shown to be dose- and age-dependent,[5,8] with progressively smaller doses required to induce permanent amenorrhoea with increasing age.[5] More recent data on the use of high dose cyclophosphamide as preparation for BMT are consistent with these findings.

Of 43 women treated with cyclophosphamide alone at a dose of 200 mg/kg, Sanders et al.[9] reported temporary amenorrhoea in all, but a return of normal menstrual cycles in 36 women between 3 and 42 months after transplantation. All patients less than 26 years of age at the time of transplant showed recovery of ovarian function, compared with only nine of 16 (56%) women aged 26 years or more. Of the 36 women in whom ovarian function recovered, however, five underwent an early menopause. In keeping with the age dependency of ovarian damage, women treated during childhood have a uniformly good prognosis in terms of ovarian function, following treatment with high dose cyclophosphamide alone.[21]

The addition of TBI to cyclophosphamide,

however, results in a much higher rate of permanent ovarian dysfunction.[9,12,33,34] In the study by Sanders et al.,[9] of 144 women who had been treated with cyclophosphamide (200 mg/kg) and TBI (12.0 or 15.75 Gy in six or seven divided doses), all had ovarian failure at 3 years, with recovery of ovarian function in only nine women between 3 and 7 years post-transplant. All of these nine women were less than 26 years old at the time of transplant. The likelihood of preservation of ovarian function is better in females treated before puberty, with normal spontaneous puberty reported in nine of 16 girls treated with cyclophosphamide (120 mg/kg) and hyperfractionated TBI (13.75–15.0 Gy).[35]

The combination of busulphan and cyclophosphamide is almost inevitably followed by ovarian failure. Of 73 adults treated with this regimen (busulphan 16 mg/kg and cyclophosphamide 200 mg/kg), only one recovered normal ovarian function after a median of 3 years of follow-up. The use of busulphan (14–16 mg/kg) during childhood is also associated with ovarian failure in the vast majority of patients.[36]

Data regarding other high dose regimens are limited. Following treatment with BEAM, all seven women studied by Chatterjee et al.[37] had ovarian failure indicated by amenorrhoea, raised gonadotrophin levels and low oestradiol levels. However, assessment of these women was carried out at 3–4 months after BMT, and recovery of ovarian function may have been observed later in a proportion of these women if they had been followed up for longer. Treatment with high dose melphalan (3 mg/kg), either alone or in combination with etoposide 1.6g/m², is associated with recovery of ovarian function in the majority of women.[38]

Longitudinal studies in patients treated with cytotoxic chemotherapy have demonstrated that the course of ovarian function after treatment can be varied (Fig. 18.2). A proportion of women with biochemical evidence of premature ovarian failure who are initially amenorrhoeic after treatment recover ovarian function, with a return of normal menses and fertility.[39] There is evidence of a reduction in ovarian follicle numbers after chemotherapy,[40] and the evolution of ovarian dysfunction with time is consistent with the destruction of a fixed number of oocytes. Older patients have a smaller pool of remaining oocytes before cytotoxic treatment and are therefore more likely to become permanently amenorrhoeic following therapy. Younger patients will often continue with normal ovarian function after cytotoxic insult, but they may undergo a premature menopause. Byrne et al.[41] took menstrual histories from over a thousand women who were still menstruating at the age of 21 after receiving treatment for malignancy during childhood. They found a much higher rate of premature menopause in these women compared with a control population; 42% of the treated women had reached the menopause by the age of 31 compared with only 5% of the controls.

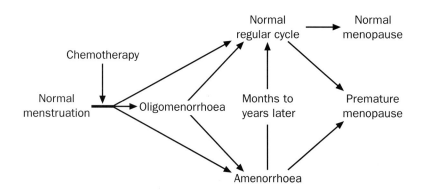

Figure 18.2
The course of ovarian function following cytotoxic chemotherapy.

In women who remain fertile following chemotherapy there is no evidence of an increase in birth defects during subsequent pregnancies. There is, however, some evidence for teratogenicity of several cytotoxic agents when they are administered during pregnancy.[42,43] Antimetabolites and, to a lesser extent, alkylating agents are associated with an increase in spontaneous abortions and congenital malformations following exposure during the first trimester. The risk of birth defects when chemotherapy is given during the second and third trimesters is probably no greater than the background rate. Women should therefore be advised to avoid conception during chemotherapy, and adequate contraception should probably be continued until the patient is in stable remission and is unlikely to require further cytotoxic therapy.

Whilst infertility is often the major concern for women undergoing potentially gonadotoxic therapy, the consequences of ovarian failure are not limited to the cessation of oocyte production but also include the loss of ovarian steroidogenesis. Symptoms of oestrogen deficiency, such as hot flushes, irritability and vaginal dryness, are not uncommon, and often necessitate treatment with hormone replacement therapy (HRT). The long-term effects of oestrogen deficiency have been well documented, with an increase in cardiovascular mortality, alterations in lipid profile and reduction in bone mineral density (BMD). Whilst some of these changes have been confirmed in women with chemotherapy-induced ovarian failure,[44] there is some evidence that ovarian dysfunction resulting from chemotherapy alone may not have exactly the same deleterious effects. Saarto et al.[45] have shown that high-density lipoprotein (HDL) cholesterol levels rise in women with cyclophosphamide-induced ovarian failure, in contrast to the fall in HDL cholesterol levels seen after natural and surgical menopause. This may in part negate the adverse effect of other changes in the lipid profile with respect to cardiovascular risk. In addition, although significant reductions in BMD have been reported in women with ovarian fail-

ure following gonadotoxic therapy,[44,46,47] the only cohorts studied in whom treatment was restricted to chemotherapy alone displayed only a small[46] or no significant reduction in BMD.[48]

The benefits of HRT in normal post-menopausal women have been well documented, with increases in BMD and a reduction in the risk of ischaemic heart disease; therefore HRT is usually recommended for women with premature ovarian failure. The BMD and lipid data suggest that HRT may be required less often in women with chemotherapy-induced premature ovarian failure. In addition, HRT has been shown to increase the risk of breast cancer in post-menopausal women and the incidence of breast tumours is also increased in women who have received radiotherapy to the chest. Thus, there is some concern about the additive risk associated with offering HRT under these circumstances. However, in the absence of solid evidence to the contrary, it seems likely that the benefits of HRT still outweigh the risks in the majority of younger women with cytotoxic-induced ovarian failure, particularly if they have symptoms of oestrogen deficiency. We would therefore recommend that most of these patients should receive sex steroid replacement therapy with a preparation containing oestrogen and progestogen.

Following high dose chemotherapy in women of premenopausal age, ovarian function should therefore be monitored regularly. Temporary amenorrhoea is very common but the absence of menses for more than 6 months following the completion of treatment warrants further investigation, with measurements of gonadotrophins and oestradiol. If these confirm ovarian failure, then HRT needs to be considered. The chance of ovarian recovery in a woman with clinical and biochemical evidence of ovarian failure will depend on her age and the chemotherapeutic agents used. If future pregnancies are desired and there is a possibility of ovarian recovery, it may be appropriate to defer HRT for a short time or to interrupt sex steroid therapy at intervals to reassess ovarian function. If normal ovarian function resumes following chemotherapy, patients should be warned about the possibility of an early menopause.

Prevention of ovarian failure

Because of the consequences of ovarian failure in young women, several strategies aimed at reducing the gonadotoxic effect of cancer treatment have been investigated. Animal models have intimated that suppression of the pituitary–gonadal axis with GnRH analogues may provide some protection against ovarian follicular depletion in rats[49] and monkeys[50] during treatment with chemotherapy. There are few published data in humans,[51,52] but one recent study claimed that GnRH agonists may partially protect against chemotherapy-induced ovarian damage.[51] However, there is no conclusive evidence of significant protection of the ovary from the toxic effects of radiotherapy or chemotherapy.

Whilst sperm banking may provide a means of preserving the reproductive capacity of some men, a similar approach in women is not feasible for several reasons. Firstly, whilst treatment can often be deferred for a few days to allow the collection of semen, the longer delay required to allow the harvesting of mature oocytes would often be unacceptable. Furthermore, only a handful of pregnancies have been established with cryopreserved oocytes and there is some concern that freezing may be associated with chromosomal abnormalities. Cryopreservation of embryos is much more successful but there is no guarantee of success, time restraints are still a problem, and the technique is of no use to a woman who has no permanent partner.

One approach, however, which may provide a method of preserving both the reproductive and steroidogenic capacity of the ovary is the cryopreservation of strips of ovarian tissue, which can be reimplanted at a later date. The method has been successfully tested in an animal model by Gosden et al,[53] who reported the restoration of fertility in a sheep by freeze-stored ovarian autografts. Recent work has shown that the majority of follicles are viable following thawing of cryopreserved human ovarian tissue,[54,55] and further work in women suggests that small pieces of ovarian tissue can be successfully transplanted to an ectopic site within the pelvic cavity (AJ Rutherford and RG Gosden, personal communication). Thus, harvesting strips of ovarian tissue, which can be frozen during gonadotoxic chemotherapy or radiotherapy and then reimplanted following the completion of treatment, may provide a realistic possibility of maintaining ovarian function in women who would otherwise have been rendered infertile. The recent report of the successful transplantation of cryopreserved autologous ovarian tissue into a previously oophorectomized woman with non-malignant disease[56] has provided evidence for the potential efficacy of this method. A clinical trial is currently underway at Christie Hospital, Manchester.[30] Twelve women with Hodgkin's disease, non-Hodgkin's lymphoma or ALL have undergone unilateral oophorectomy before potentially sterilizing chemotherapy. The cortex containing the primordial follicles has been stripped from the ovary, flattened, trimmed and then cut into strips which have then been stored in liquid nitrogen. One 36-year-old woman has undergone re-implantation of two cryopreserved ovarian strips 19 months after receiving high dose CBV for Hodgkin's disease.[57] Prior to re-implantation, oestradiol and gonadotrophin levels were in keeping with ovarian failure. Seven months later the patient reported resolution of her symptoms of oestrogen deficiency, associated with a detectable oestradiol level, suppression of LH and FSH and ultrasonographic evidence of endometrial hyperplasia. By 9 months, biochemical parameters had returned to pre-implantation levels, but the results suggested temporary function of the implanted ovarian tissue and are thus encouraging. There is a theoretical possibility of re-introducing tumour cells during the implantation of ovarian tissue; this will clearly limit the technique to conditions in which tumour involvement of the

---

Table 18.2 Summary of gonadal damage in high dose chemotherapy

Men

1. Testicular damage is drug- and dose-dependent but there is no reliable evidence of age dependency
2. High dose chemotherapy results in germinal epithelial damage in the vast majority of men
3. Mild Leydig cell dysfunction occurs in up to one-third of men, although this is not clinically significant in the majority of men
4. Sperm banking should be considered for all men before treatment
5. Hormonal manipulation following chemotherapy or cryopreservation of spermatogonial stem cells isolated from testicular biopsy may provide a method for maintaining fertility

Women

1. Ovarian damage is drug-, dose- and age-dependent
2. The course of ovarian function after chemotherapy is variable and late recovery (months to years after treatment) is not uncommon
3. High dose cyclophosphamide alone results in permanent amenorrhoea in only a small proportion of women
4. Addition of total body irradiation to a cyclophosphamide regimen results in a much higher rate of permanent ovarian dysfunction
5. Treatment with high dose busulphan almost inevitably results in permanent ovarian failure irrespective of age
6. Hormone replacement therapy should be considered in all women with cytotoxic-induced premature ovarian failure
7. Cryopreservation of ovarian tissue before treatment may provide a method of preserving ovarian function

---

ovaries is unlikely. Studies in severe combined immunodeficient (SCID) mice suggest that the risk of disease transmission by autotransplantation with lymphomas is low.[58]

SUMMARY

High dose chemotherapy is associated with significant gonadal damage (Table 18.2). The incidence of testicular and ovarian failure following treatment is drug-dependent and in women the impact on gonadal function is also significantly age-dependent. Prior chemotherapy and radiotherapy, and concomitant irradiation treatment, are also important factors in determining the likelihood of maintaining normal gonadal function following therapy. Several methods of preserving gonadal function during potentially sterilizing treatment have been considered. At present, sperm banking remains the only proven method in men, although hormonal manipulation to enhance recovery of spermatogenesis and cryopreservation of testicular germ cells are possibilities for the future. In women, the prospect of cryopreservation and reimplantation of ovarian tissue appears promising.

REFERENCES

1. Pryzant RM, Meistrich ML, Wilson G, Brown B, McLaughlin P. Long-term reduction in sperm count after chemotherapy with and without radiation therapy for non-Hodgkin's lymphomas [published erratum appears in J Clin Oncol 1993 May;11(5):1007]. J Clin Oncol 1993; 11(2):239–47.

2. Meistrich ML, Chawla SP, Da Cunha MF et al. Recovery of sperm production after chemotherapy for osteosarcoma. Cancer 1989;63(11): 2115–23.

3. da Cunha MF, Meistrich ML, Fuller LM et al. Recovery of spermatogenesis after treatment for Hodgkin's disease: limiting dose of MOPP chemotherapy. J Clin Oncol 1984;2(6):571–7.

4. Watson AR, Rance CP, Bain J. Long term effects of cyclophosphamide on testicular function. Br Med J Clin Res Ed 1985;291(6507):1457–60.

5. Koyama H, Wada T, Nishizawa Y, Iwanaga T, Aoki Y. Cyclophosphamide-induced ovarian failure and its therapeutic significance in patients with breast cancer. Cancer 1977;39(4): 1403–9.

6. Bokemeyer C, Schmoll HJ, van Rhee J, Kuczyk M, Schuppert F, Poliwoda H. Long-term gonadal toxicity after therapy for Hodgkin's and non-Hodgkin's lymphoma. Ann Hematol 1994;68(3):105–10.

7. Wallace WH, Shalet SM, Crowne EC, Morris Jones PH, Gattamaneni HR, Price DA. Gonadal dysfunction due to cis-platinum. Med Pediatr Oncol 1989;17(5):409–13.

8. Bines J, Oleske DM, Cobleigh MA. Ovarian function in premenopausal women treated with adjuvant chemotherapy for breast cancer. J Clin Oncol 1996;14(5):1718–29.

9. Sanders JE, Buckner CD, Amos D et al. Ovarian function following marrow transplantation for aplastic anemia or leukemia. J Clin Oncol 1988; 6(5):813–18.

10. Chapman RM, Sutcliffe SB, Malpas JS. Cytotoxic-induced ovarian failure in women with Hodgkin's disease. I. Hormone function. JAMA 1979;242(17):1877–81.

11. Rivkees SA, Crawford JD. The relationship of gonadal activity and chemotherapy-induced gonadal damage. JAMA 1988;259(14):2123–5.

12. Sanders JE, Hawley J, Levy W et al. Pregnancies following high-dose cyclophosphamide with or without high-dose busulfan or total-body irradi-ation and bone marrow transplantation. Blood 1996;87(7):3045–52.

13. Clayton PE, Shalet SM, Price DA, Campbell RH. Testicular damage after chemotherapy for childhood brain tumors. J Pediatr 1988;112(6): 922–6.

14. Vilar O. Effect of cytostatic drugs on human testicular function. In: Mancini RE, Martini L, editors. Male fertility and sterility, vol 5. London: Academic Press, 1974:423–40.

15. Chapman RM, Sutcliffe SB, Rees LH, Edwards CR, Malpas JS. Cyclical combination chemotherapy and gonadal function. Retrospective study in males. Lancet 1979;1(8111):285–9.

16. Whitehead E, Shalet SM, Blackledge G, Todd I, Crowther D, Beardwell CG. The effects of Hodgkin's disease and combination chemotherapy on gonadal function in the adult male. Cancer 1982;49(3):418–22.

17. Lampe H, Horwich A, Norman A, Nicholls J, Dearnaley DP. Fertility after chemotherapy for testicular germ cell cancers. J Clin Oncol 1997;15(1):239–45.

18. Viviani S, Ragni G, Santoro A et al. Testicular dysfunction in Hodgkin's disease before and after treatment. Eur J Cancer 1991;27(11): 1389–92.

19. Howell SJ, Radford JA, Shalet SM. Testicular function following cytotoxic chemotherapy – evidence of Leydig cell insufficiency. J Clin Oncol 1999;17(5):1493–8.

20. Chatterjee R, Mills W, Katz M, McGarrigle HH, Godstone AH. Germ cell failure and Leydig cell insufficiency in post-pubertal males after autologous bone marrow transplantation with BEAM for lymphoma. Bone Marrow Transplant 1994; 13(5):519–22.

21. Sanders JE, Buckner CD, Sullivan KM et al. Growth and development in children after bone marrow transplantation. Horm Res 1988; 30(2–3):92–7.

22. Michel G, Socie G, Gebhard F et al. Late effects of allogeneic bone marrow transplantation for children with acute myeloblastic leukemia in first complete remission: the impact of conditioning regimen without total-body irradiation – a report from the Societe Francaise de Greffe de Moelle. J Clin Oncol 1997;15(6): 2238–46.

23. Leiper AD, Stanhope R, Lau T et al. The effect of total body irradiation and bone marrow transplantation during childhood and adolescence on

growth and endocrine function. Br J Haematol 1987;67(4):419–26.

24. Holmes SJ, Whitehouse RW, Clark ST, Crowther DC, Adams JE, Shalet SM. Reduced bone mineral density in men following chemotherapy for Hodgkin's disease. Br J Cancer 1994;70(2):371–5.

25. Howell S, Radford J, Adams J et al. Randomised placebo controlled trial of testosterone replacement in men with mild Leydig cell insufficiency following cytotoxic chemotherapy. Clin Endocrinol 2001;55:315–24.

26. Monteil M, Rousseaux S, Chevret E, Pelletier R, Cozzi J, Sele B. Increased aneuploid frequency in spermatozoa from a Hodgkin's disease patient after chemotherapy and radiotherapy. Cytogenet Cell Genet 1997;76(3–4):134–8.

27. Robbins WA, Meistrich ML, Moore D et al. Chemotherapy induces transient sex chromosomal and autosomal aneuploidy in human sperm. Nature Genet 1997;16(1):74–8.

28. Robbins WA. Cytogenetic damage measured in human sperm following cancer chemotherapy. Mutat Res 1996;355(1–2):235–52.

29. Meistrich ML, Kangasniemi M. Hormone treatment after irradiation stimulates recovery of rat spermatogenesis from surviving spermatogonia. J Androl 1997;18(1):80–7.

30. Brinster RL, Zimmermann JW. Spermatogenesis following male germ-cell transplantation [see comments]. Proc Natl Acad Sci USA 1994;91(24):11298–302.

31. Radford JA, Shalet SM, Lieberman BA. Fertility after treatment for cancer. Br Med J 1999;319:935–6.

32. Loius J, Limarzi LR, Best WR. Treatment of chronic granulocytic leukaemia with Myerlan. Arch Intern Med 1956;97:299–308.

33. Keilholz U, Max R, Scheibenbogen C, Wuster C, Korbling M, Haas R. Endocrine function and bone metabolism 5 years after autologous bone marrow/blood-derived progenitor cell transplantation. Cancer 1997;79(8):1617–22.

34. Sanders JE. Endocrine problems in children after bone marrow transplant for hematologic malignancies. The Long-term Follow-up Team. Bone Marrow Transplant 1991;8(suppl 1):2–4.

35. Sarafoglou K, Boulad F, Gillio A, Sklar C. Gonadal function after bone marrow transplantation for acute leukemia during childhood [see comments]. J Pediatr 1997;130(2):210–16.

36. Teinturier C, Hartmann O, Valteau Couanet D, Benhamou E, Bougneres PF. Ovarian function after autologous bone marrow transplantation in childhood: high-dose busulfan is a major cause of ovarian failure. Bone Marrow Transplant 1998;22(10):989–94.

37. Chatterjee R, Mills W, Katz M, McGarrigle HH, Goldstone AH. Prospective study of pituitary–gonadal function to evaluate short-term effects of ablative chemotherapy or total body irradiation with autologous or allogenic marrow transplantation in post-menarcheal female patients. Bone Marrow Transplant 1994;13(5):511–17.

38. Jackson GH, Wood A, Taylor PR et al. Early high dose chemotherapy intensification with autologous bone marrow transplantation in lymphoma associated with retention of fertility and normal pregnancies in females. Scotland and Newcastle Lymphoma Group, UK. Leuk Lymphoma 1997;28(1–2):127–32.

39. Clark ST, Radford JA, Crowther D, Swindell R, Shalet SM. Gonadal function following chemotherapy for Hodgkin's disease: a comparative study of MVPP and a seven-drug hybrid regimen. J Clin Oncol 1995;13(1):134–9.

40. Nicosia SV, Matus Ridley M, Meadows AT. Gonadal effects of cancer therapy in girls. Cancer 1985;55(10):2364–72.

41. Byrne J, Fears TR, Gail MH et al. Early menopause in long-term survivors of cancer during adolescence. Am J Obstet Gynecol 1992;166(3):788–93.

42. Sorosky JI, Sood AK, Buekers TE. The use of chemotherapeutic agents during pregnancy. Obstet Gynecol Clin North Am 1997;24(3):591–9.

43. Barnicle MM. Chemotherapy and pregnancy. Semin Oncol Nurs 1992;8(2):124–32.

44. Bruning PF, Pit MJ, de Jong Bakker M, van den Ende A, Hart A, van Enk A. Bone mineral density after adjuvant chemotherapy for pre-menopausal breast cancer. Br J Cancer 1990;61(2):308–10.

45. Saarto T, Blomqvist C, Ehnholm C, Taskinen MR, Elomaa I. Effects of chemotherapy-induced castration on serum lipids and apoproteins in premenopausal women with node-positive breast cancer. J Clin Endocrinol Metab 1996;81(12):4453–7.

46. Ratcliffe MA, Lanham SA, Reid DM, Dawson AA. Bone mineral density (BMD) in patients with lymphoma: the effects of chemotherapy, intermittent corticosteroids and premature menopause. Hematol Oncol 1992;10(3–4):181–7.

47. Redman JR, Bajorunas DR, Wong G et al. Bone mineralization in women following successful treatment of Hodgkin's disease. Am J Med 1988;85(1):65–72.

48. Howell SJ, Berger G, Adams JE, Shalet SM. Bone mineral density in women with cytotoxic-induced ovarian failure. Clin Endocrinol Oxf 1998;49(3):397–402.

49. Bokser L, Szende B, Schally AV. Protective effects of D-Trp6-luteinising hormone-releasing hormone microcapsules against cyclophosphamide-induced gonadotoxicity in female rats. Br J Cancer 1990;61(6):861–5.

50. Ataya K, Rao LV, Lawrence E, Kimmel R. Luteinizing hormone-releasing hormone agonist inhibits cyclophosphamide-induced ovarian follicular depletion in rhesus monkeys. Biol Reprod 1995;52(2):365–72.

51. Blumenfeld Z, Avivi I, Linn S, Epelbaum R, Ben Shahar M, Haim N. Prevention of irreversible chemotherapy-induced ovarian damage in young women with lymphoma by a gonadotrophin-releasing hormone agonist in parallel to chemotherapy. Hum Reprod 1996;11(8):1620–6.

52. Waxman JH, Ahmed R, Smith D et al. Failure to preserve fertility in patients with Hodgkin's disease. Cancer Chemother Pharmacol 1987;19(2):159–62.

53. Gosden RG, Baird DT, Wade JC, Webb R. Restoration of fertility to oophorectomized sheep by ovarian autografts stored at −196 degrees C. Hum Reprod 1994;9(4):597–603.

54. Newton H, Aubard Y, Rutherford A, Sharma V, Gosden R. Low temperature storage and grafting of human ovarian tissue. Hum Reprod 1996;11(7):1487–91.

55. Hovatta O, Silye R, Krausz T et al. Cryopreservation of human ovarian tissue using dimethylsulphoxide and propanediol-sucrose as cryoprotectants. Hum Reprod 1996;11(6):1268–72.

56. Oktay K Karlikaya G. Ovarian function after transplantation of frozen banked autologous ovarian tissue. N Engl J Med 2000;342:1919.

57. Radford JA, Leiberman BA, Brison BR et al. Orthotopic reimplantation of cryopreserved ovarian cortical strips after high-dose chemotherapy for Hodgkin's lymphoma. Lancet 2001;357:1172–5.

58. Kim SS, Radford JA, Harris M et al. Ovarian tissue harvested from lymphoma patients to preserve fertility may be safe for autotransplantation. Human Reproduction 2001;16(10):2056–60.

19

Long-term complications after high dose chemotherapy and hematopoietic cell transplantation

H Joachim Deeg

CONTENTS   Introduction • Chronic GVHD • Infections • Airway and pulmonary disease • Autoimmunity • Neuroendocrine dysfunction • Cardiac disease • Ocular problems • Musculoskeletal problems • Dental problems • Genitourinary dysfunction • Gastrointestinal and hepatic complications • Post-transplant malignancies • Neurological complications • Psychosocial effects and rehabilitation

INTRODUCTION

Myelosuppression is frequently the dose-limiting factor of cytotoxic anti-cancer therapy. Rescue from marrow failure by hematopoietic stem cell transplantation (HSCT), in principle, allows one to disregard this side effect and to escalate chemotherapeutic dose intensity to levels at which toxicity in the next most susceptible organ(s) is approached. Such high dose therapy, however, also carries the risk of delayed complications related to the intensity of therapy, the effects of stem cell rescue/transplantation, or both. In the USA more than 35 000 patients annually receive high dose therapy and autologous or allogeneic stem cell transplantation. Because the success rate also has risen for several indications of this treatment modality, a rapidly growing population of survivors is at risk of developing late complications.

Most patients undergoing HSCT who survive the acute post-transplant period and who do not experience a recurrence of their underlying disease within 1–2 years of transplantation, lead active and productive lives. Some patients, however, develop chronic or delayed complications (Table 19.1).[1–3] Certain complications, such as chronic graft-versus-host disease (GVHD) and prolonged immunodeficiency, occur only in patients given an allogeneic HSCT and are directly related to genetic differences between donor cells and patient tissues. Other problems, such as infertility or cataracts, are due to the intensity of the treatment regimen and occur in both allogeneic and autologous transplant patients. Others (chronic pulmonary disease, secondary malignancies and others) are multifactorial in etiology. To what extent therapy given before HSCT impacts on delayed complications after HSCT is difficult or impossible to distinguish.

The focus of this overview will be the pathophysiology and the clinical spectrum of delayed complications (Table 19.1).

Table 19.1 Delayed complications
Chronic graft-versus-host disease
Immunodeficiency and infections
Airway and pulmonary disease
Autoimmune disorders
Neuroendocrine dysfunction
Impairment of growth and development
Infertility
Cardiac disease
Ocular problems
Musculoskeletal disease
Dental problems
Dysfunction of the genitourinary tract
Gastrointestinal and hepatic complications
Post-transplant malignancies
Central and peripheral nervous system impairment
Psychosocial effects

CHRONIC GVHD

Chronic GVHD is the most frequent delayed complication in allogeneic HSCT recipients, affecting as many as 40–60% of patients. Chronic GVHD may develop as early as 2 months and as late as 18 months after HSCT.[4] It may have a progressive onset (i.e. progression from acute GVHD to a chronic form), may occur after successful treatment of acute GVHD and a quiescent phase, or may be de novo in patients who never experienced acute GVHD.[5] The prognosis is worst with progressive and best with de novo onset. A limited form of chronic GVHD (involving the skin ± liver) may not require systemic therapy. Extensive chronic GVHD is generally treated with glucocorticoids, cyclosporine, FK506, phototherapy with PUVA and other modalities, either alone or in combination. Two-thirds of patients with standard-risk chronic GVHD will respond to primary therapy, e.g. with steroids plus cyclosporine. Because of the underlying characteristics of chronic GVHD and the immunosuppressive effects of its therapy, potentially fatal infections are a major complication. Depending upon risk factors present, the mortality from chronic GVHD ranges from 10% to almost 40%. For a detailed discussion of chronic GVHD, the reader is referred to recent comprehensive reviews.[4]

INFECTIONS

Frequently, infections occur early after HSCT when anatomical barriers have been damaged by high dose therapy, pancytopenia is present and patients are severely immunodeficient. Late infections are observed particularly in patients with chronic GVHD. The spectrum includes bacterial and fungal septicemias and pneumonias, otitis media and meningitis, and late activation of varicella zoster virus (VZV) or cytomegalovirus (CMV) in patients given antiviral prophylaxis.[6] Hepatitis B and C virus may result in chronic hepatitis and cirrhosis.[7,8] The types of infection observed after high dose therapy and autologous or allogeneic HSCT are similar; however, the frequency is higher, and the time interval at risk is longer, after allogeneic transplantation. This is true, in particular, in recipients of HSCT from unrelated volunteer donors; about 20% of recipients require immunosuppressive therapy for several years. A detailed description of infections and their management is given elsewhere.[6]

AIRWAY AND PULMONARY DISEASE

Airways and lungs are sensitive to cytotoxic chemotherapy and irradiation, but are also prominent targets of viral, bacterial and fungal infections.[6] Mucositis in the early post-transplant period interferes with mucociliary clearance, leading to mucous retention in the lower airways, inflammatory alterations and tissue repair. Inflammation can be aggravated by sinus drainage associated with post-nasal drip.

The possible responses of the lung to injury

are limited; they are most prominent in the interstitium. The repair process leads to scarring, which in turn will interfere with gas exchange and respiratory dynamics and kinetics. The bronchial tree may also be involved by GVHD.[9] In particular, severe structural and functional damage as seen with bronchiolitis obliterans appears to be related to chronic GVHD.[4] As a sequel to various insults, chronic pulmonary complications affect at least 15–20% of patients after allogeneic and 5–10% of patients after autologous HSCT.[10–12] This is of significance since pulmonary dysfunction is an important indicator for long-term outcome.[13]

Interstitial pneumonitis

Late-onset interstitial pneumonitis, sometimes with marked interstitial fibrosis, is seen almost exclusively in patients with chronic GVHD.[14] These patients usually fail to respond to bronchodilators but improve on immunosuppressive therapy, generally required anyway because of other typical clinical and pathological findings of chronic GVHD. Occasionally, late-onset interstitial pneumonitis may be caused by infectious organisms. The use of prolonged prophylaxis with ganciclovir, while successful in preventing CMV disease early post-transplant, has led to an increased frequency in late CMV infections, including pneumonitis, which are observed in 10–15% of patients 1 year or later after HSCT.[15]

Restrictive disease

Patients who have abnormal pre-transplant pulmonary function test results (PFTs), in particular decreased diffusing capacity ($D_{CO_{sb}}$ and increased oxygen gradient ($P_{(A-a)O_2}$), have a higher mortality after transplantation than patients whose tests are normal.[16] Excess mortality is only in part due to respiratory failure, however. Post-transplant PFTs similarly have predictive value.[13] A decline in total lung capacity (TLC) and D_{CO} is frequent by 3 months after HSCT; restrictive defects (<80% of predicted values) are present in one-third of all patients studied. In one study, such a defect (or a loss of $\geq$15% of TLC) was associated with a two-fold increase in non-relapse mortality related to respiratory failure (not significantly associated with chronic GVHD). The effect was most pronounced more than 1 year post-transplant.

Restrictive changes are not correlated with the type of high dose therapy given or with the presence of chronic GVHD; generally, they do not result in severe symptoms. However, because restrictive disease is associated with increased long-term mortality, sequential evaluation of lung function is warranted since aggressive bronchial hygiene and prompt therapy of infection may be useful in slowing disease progression.[17]

Obstructive disease

Obstructive pulmonary changes might represent sequelae to extensive restrictive changes in the small airways, or, with obstructive bronchiolitis, may be related to small airway destruction.[18] Recurrent aspirations secondary to esophageal dysfunction (e.g. associated with GVHD) or post-nasal drip contribute to airway inflammation and obstructive lung disease. Obstructive defects as defined by FEV_1/FVC of <80% of predicted are present in 25% of patients by 3 months post-transplant. Patients with chronic GVHD also may have low immunoglobulin G (IgG) and IgA levels which further contribute to the susceptibility to infections. Obstructive pulmonary disease in this setting usually does not respond to bronchodilator treatment; about 30–40% of patients improve on immunosuppressive therapy with glucocorticoids and cyclosporine (CSP). Some patients with end stage pulmonary disease have been treated successfully with pulmonary transplants.[19]

Bronchiolitis obliterans

In the past, progressive bronchiolitis obliterans was observed as early as 3 months and as late as 2 years after HSCT in 10% of all patients with active chronic GVHD.[20,21] The findings of bronchiolitis obliterans after HSCT are similar to those after lung or heart–lung transplants.[22] Pulmonary function tests show a reduction in forced mid-expiratory flow to 10% or 20% of predicted values and a reduction in the forced vital capacity. The diffusion capacity is usually normal. Pulmonary ventilation scans show decreased activity patterns corresponding to areas of obliteration of bronchiolar walls along with atelectatic areas. It is thought that the histological changes are due to a graft-versus-host reaction, possibly aggravated by infection.

The clinical course of bronchiolitis varies from mild, with slow deterioration, to diffuse necrotizing and rapidly fatal bronchiolitis of the small airways. Combination therapy with glucocorticoids and CSP is indicated; some investigators add azathioprine.

The incidence of bronchiolitis obliterans appears to be falling, possibly due to changes in prophylaxis and treatment of infection.[23]

AUTOIMMUNITY

All high dose therapy regimens currently in use are associated with profound immunosuppression. Even after the reinfusion of autologous stem cells, there is an interval of several months of slow immunological recovery.[24]

With an allogeneic stem cell source, donor-derived cells recognize recipient antigens as non-self (alloreactivity), a process which forms the basis for the development of GVHD.[25] However, once donor-derived cells are established in the recipient, these cells, by generating the new immune system of the recipient, have to be considered as expressing 'autoreactivity' if they exhibit humoral or cellular reactivity against host tissue. In addition, the presence of thymic damage, due to high dose therapy (and, in allogeneic recipients, acute GVHD), would

be expected to interfere with the negative selection of autoreactive cells and, thus, facilitate the development of cellular and, indirectly, humoral autoreactivity.[26,27]

Autoantibodies are observed frequently after HSCT, particularly in patients with chronic GVHD. However, a correlation between these antibodies and GVHD activity has not been shown.[28] Generally patients are asymptomatic and no therapy is indicated. Some patients may develop myasthenia gravis, typically 1–2 years after HSCT.[29] The anti-acetylcholine receptor antibodies are donor-derived, as shown by immunoglobulin allotyping.[30] Treatment is identical to that of non-transplant patients with myasthenia gravis.

The pattern of immunoglobulin recovery after HSCT follows the sequence observed in onotogeny: IgM, IgG1 followed by IgG3 with IgG2, IgG4 and IgA lagging behind.[24] Antibodies observed early after HSCT are to a large extent mono- or oligoclonal and, with the exception of autoreactivity, have irrelevant specificities. With lengthening of the post-transplant interval, there is a rise of specific titers to infectious antigens. Patterns of abnormal immune reactivity of the donor, e.g. atopic asthma, psoriasis and food allergies,[31,32] are also transferred to the recipients.[24]

At the interphase between donor-derived immunity and GVHD-associated autoimmunity, may be situated immune reactions against infectious agents. There is evidence that donor immunity to both herpesviruses and CMV may be mechanistically involved in the subsequent development of chronic GVHD.[33–36] Prophylactic antiviral therapy may reduce the risk of chronic GVHD.

Numerous hematological problems have been observed after transplantation.[37–39] Marrow can be a target of GVHD, and persistent thrombocytopenia has been identified as a poor prognostic factor for chronic GVHD.[40] However, immune-mediated thrombocytopenia has also been observed after high dose therapy followed by syngeneic and autologous transplants, and in these instances, should be treated like idiopathic thrombocytopenic purpura (ITP).[43] High dose i.v. Ig has been successful in some patients.[41] Immune-mediated neutropenia is less frequent; if spontaneous recovery does not occur, therapy with steroids is warranted. Patients transplanted from an ABO incompatible donor may experience hemolysis and severe anemia for months or even years after transplantation due to persisting host isoagglutinins until long-lived host cells have been eliminated.[42] Occasionally, patients developing classical pure red cell aplasia have been treated successfully with immunosuppressive therapy.[43]

NEUROENDOCRINE DYSFUNCTION

As cytotoxic therapy and gamma irradiation damage endocrine glands,[44] high-dose regimens followed by HSCT are expected to affect endocrine function.

Thyroid

Overt or compensated hypothyroidism and the 'euthyroid sick syndrome' (ETS) are the most common abnormalities. After total body irradiation (TBI), incidences of thyroid dysfunction as high as 57% at 3 months and 29% at 14 months (suggesting some recovery) have been reported in adult patients.[45] In patients given high dose chemotherapy, the incidence was only 14% both at 3 and 14 months. In one study, ETS was associated with a significantly lower survival (34% versus 96% in controls; $P < 0.0001$).[46] Among pediatric patients given TBI, thyroid dysfunction has been observed in 85%.[47] The risk of thyroid dysfunction is further enhanced in patients who also received cranial irradiation or irradiation to the neck.[48] Hypothyroidism may not become manifest until years after transplantation.[49] The incidence is highest in children and lower in the adult population.

Patients are also at an increased risk of developing benign or malignant thyroid tumors, related directly to radiation exposure and to increased thyroid stimulating hormone (TSH) levels.[50,51] All patients who have received irradiation (including TBI) to the thyroid should be followed for life with annual physical evaluation and thyroid function studies as indicated.[48] Patients with hypothyroidism should receive replacement therapy; however, because some patients show spontaneous recovery, intermittent trials off therapy may be indicated.

Adrenal glands

Many recipients of high dose therapy and HSCT receive glucocorticoids in the pre-, peri- or post-transplant period and as a consequence may show the classic side effects of steroid therapy and experience iatrogenic suppression of endogenous cortisol production.

Only limited data on adrenal function are available in patients who no longer receive immunosuppression. One study showed 24% of patients to have subnormal 11-deoxycortisol levels at 1–8 years post-transplant; however, no patient was symptomatic.[49] Subnormal stimulated cortisol levels are also observed in patients given central nervous system irradiation, and a central (primary) effect may play a role in patients post-transplant.[52]

Hypothalamic–pituitary axis

Cranial irradiation, accentuated by TBI, may have profound effects on the pituitary gland.[52–54] Thyrotropin releasing hormone (TRH) may be low early after high dose therapy, and TRH-induced TSH responses may be subnormal and delayed.[52] Release of gonadotropin in response to luteinizing hormone releasing hormone (LHRH) may be elevated.[52] Leydig cell function is usually normal, as is prolactin secretion and the pituitary–adrenal axis. Growth hormone levels are decreased after cranial irradiation (±TBI), and deficiency becomes apparent earlier with younger age at transplant.[53]

Gonadal function, puberty and fertility

Several reviews have been published recently[55–58] and this is dealt with in Chapter 18.

CARDIAC DISEASE

Cardiac insufficiency and coronary artery disease have been recognized as consequences of intensive cytotoxic therapy, in particular high dose anthracycline, and mediastinal irradiation given for Hodgkin's disease.[59] Cardiomyopathies also occur post-transplant, albeit infrequently.[60] Early cardiac insufficiency may be seen in patients treated with cyclophosphamide 200 mg/kg, sometimes before treatment is completed. Pretransplant determination of the ejection fraction has not been a reliable tool in predicting this complication. It has been suggested that cardiac toxicity is avoided if cyclophosphamide is administered as a dose per square metre rather than per kilogram.[60]

Some cases of myocardial infarction have occurred at various time intervals after high dose therapy and transplantation,[61] but a cause–effect relationship has not been proven.

OCULAR PROBLEMS

Cataracts are frequent in the population at large, and the incidence increases with age. Various physicochemical insults to the eye are cataractogenic or enhance cataract formation in a lens with pre-existing damage. Patients who receive high dose therapy and HSCT have already previously received chemotherapeutic agents, and are frequently exposed to glucocorticoids and gamma irradiation, both of which are known to cause cataracts.

In patients who are given TBI, posterior capsular cataracts develop, beginning approximately 1 year after transplant.[62] With single-dose TBI (usually 920–1000 cGy), the incidence may be 80% at 5–6 years. With fractionated TBI, the incidence is approximately 50% at cumulative doses greater than 1200 cGy,

and 30–35% at doses of 1200 cGy or less. The incidence of cataracts is also correlated with an increase in the radiation exposure rate.[63,64] Among patients who are not exposed to TBI or cranial irradiation, cataracts occur in about 20%, almost exclusively related to the use of steroids.

Approaches to cataract prevention in the setting of high dose therapy and HSCT are experimental. Treatment of cataracts with contact lenses may be difficult in patients with chronic GVHD and insufficient tear production (sicca syndrome). The treatment of choice is lens extraction and implantation of an artificial lens. With the improved quality of modern lenses, they are now implanted routinely even in children.[65]

Other ocular complications are generally related to immunosuppressive therapy, chronic GVHD and associated infections.[65] Infections and GVHD may also cause scar formation (e.g. in the tarsus) and lead to synechiae, ectropion, corneal damage and potentially perforation if not treated meticulously and aggressively. Long-term antibiotic coverage and the use of artificial tears can prevent some infections and scarring. Late-onset keratoconjunctivitis sicca has also been described in patients without chronic GVHD, although the possibility that it represents an abortive form of GVHD cannot be excluded.[2,66] Obstruction of the nasolacrimal duct, related either to GVHD or conditioning-induced fibrosis, has been observed,[67] but is infrequent.

MUSCULOSKELETAL PROBLEMS

Myopathy and myositis

The most common complication that involves the musculoskeletal system is steroid-induced myopathy. Because patients frequently lack energy and initiative, muscle weakness further adds to inactivity and loss of muscle and bone mass. It is important, therefore, to maintain and gradually increase the level of physical activity to counter a progressive decline in physical function.

Occasionally, patients with chronic GVHD have involvement of muscle, fascia and serous membranes, including the synovia, although joint effusions may occur in patients without any other sign of GVHD.

Osteoporosis

The development of osteoporosis is related to several factors, including irradiation, glucocorticoid therapy, inactivity and, in women, iatrogenic hypogonadism.[68] Osteopenia or osteoporosis occurs in 20–50% of patients undergoing HSCT. The bone alkaline phosphatase may be elevated, particularly in women, as may the C-terminal propeptide. There may also be increased hydroxyproline excretion. An excellent method to evaluate osteopenia/osteoporosis is dual energy X-ray absorptiometry, which, in one study of women after high dose therapy and transplantation (using WHO criteria), revealed osteopenia in 33% and osteoporosis in 18% of patients.[68] In women, hormone supplementation with estrogens and medroxyprogesterone increases bone mass.[69] Bisphosphonates may be useful for patients of either gender. Whenever possible, glucocorticoids should be discontinued and a carefully planned exercise program should be instituted.

Avascular necrosis of the bone

Avascular necrosis is a classic side effect of glucocorticoid therapy. It may occur with a long delay even after short courses of high dose therapy for GVHD.[70] Several reports suggest an incidence of 4–8% at 5 years.[71,72] Symptoms develop at approximately 1 year. The hip joint is involved most frequently (65–80% of cases), followed by the humerus; in most patients more than one joint is affected. In addition to glucocorticoid therapy (for acute or chronic GVHD), male gender and age may increase the risk. In addition, irradiation-based therapy, type of GVHD prophylaxis, and acute or chronic GVHD may be associated with an increased risk of avascular necrosis.[70] Once avascular necrosis has developed, the only definitive treatment is joint replacement, particularly in weight-bearing joints such as the hip.

DENTAL PROBLEMS

Oral and pharyngeal mucosa is frequently involved with acute and chronic GVHD.[73] An oral sicca syndrome may also be due to high dose conditioning and may result in poor oral hygiene with recurrent infection and periodontitis. Dental decay occurs because of a lack of cleansing by saliva, which is of altered consistency and reduced volume.[74] As the mouth may be painful, patients are hesitant to brush their teeth and to take care of teeth and mucosa. One study[75] found that the incidence of dental decay was comparable in children given chemotherapy alone and in patients given high dose therapy and HSCT.[76] Treatment includes diligent hygiene, fluoride treatment, artificial saliva and other supportive measures.

In very young children, irradiation interferes with dental and facial development.[77] There may be poor calcification, micrognathia, mandibular hypoplasia, root blunting and apical closure.[75] The changes are most severe in children less than 7 years of age at the time of transplantation. While chemotherapy mostly results in qualitative disturbances of dentine and enamel, irradiation induces both quantitative and qualitative alterations.[78] No effective prophylactic measures are currently available; careful planning (and where possible, timing) of high dose therapy may minimize these side effects.

GENITOURINARY DYSFUNCTION

Bladder

Cystitis with microscopic or macroscopic hematuria occurs in 10–15% of patients after high dose therapy.[79] While cystitis is usually an acute problem, some patients will have protracted hematuria, and scarring of the bladder wall with volume loss may present a chronic problem manifested by urinary frequency. Treatment early on consists of bladder irrigation, cystoscopic fulguration and, in extreme cases, in cystectomy with the construction of an artificial bladder from a bowel loop. In patients with severe scarring, anti-spasmodic treatment may be beneficial. Viruria with adenovirus, polyomavirus, or other viruses may also be responsible for hematuria.

Patients receiving immunosuppressive therapy for chronic GVHD, particularly women with GVHD of the vagina, are at risk for recurrent urinary tract infections which require prompt antibiotic therapy.

Kidneys

Renal failure related to antibiotic therapy, CSP or chemotherapy given before HSCT is a frequent occurrence in the early post-transplant period.[80] Late renal function impairment, in contrast to observations in solid organ transplant recipients, is less frequent. However, in patients previously treated aggressively with nephrotoxic chemotherapy (e.g. with platinum compounds), renal insufficiency has been observed in as many as 20–25% by 2 years after high dose therapy and transplantation.[81] The term 'marrow transplant nephropathy' has been coined for this syndrome of azotemia, hypertension and a disproportionate degree of anemia.[81] There may also be features of a hemolytic uremic syndrome. Total body irradiation may also lead to long-term renal damage, as determined by creatinine levels, blood urea nitrogen,[51] Cr-EDTA residual activity, proteinuria or hematocrit changes.[82] Renal shielding for TBI doses >1200 cGy may have a protective effect and the use of angiotensin converting enzyme inhibitors may have a preventive effect.[83] Once nephropathy has developed, control of hypertension is the mainstay of therapy.

Renal failure associated with hemolytic uremic syndrome or microangiopathic hemolytic anemia also occurs in patients who are not heavily pretreated and are not treated with TBI. Plasmapheresis and the use of glucocorticoids are therapeutic options. In some patients the disease stabilizes upon blood pressure control.

Genital organs

Complications related to chronic GVHD may also involve the genital organs, in particular the glans penis and vagina. Vaginitis can be severe and cause considerable distress and dyspareunia. Prolonged treatment, topically with estrogens and systemically, for example with glucocorticoids, is indicated to prevent the development of atrophic vaginitis and adhesions.

GASTROINTESTINAL AND HEPATIC COMPLICATIONS

Gastrointestinal tract

The gastrointestinal (GI) tract is a frequent target of acute transplant-related complications; chronic problems generally are related to GVHD. Involvement of the esophagus by chronic GVHD may lead to strictures and web formation.[84] Chronic GVHD of the small bowel may result in malabsorption.

Pneumatosis cystoides intestinalis occurs in patients after high dose therapy, generally while receiving glucocorticoid therapy.[85] The diagnosis is usually made within 2–3 months. No specific therapy is available and it usually resolves spontaneously.

A potential problem is the late occurrence of viral disease. Because viral infections are being controlled very successfully with acyclovir and ganciclovir prophylaxis in the early post-transplant period, as many as 15% of patients experience late-onset (12–18 months) CMV esophagitis or enteritis.[15]

Liver

Liver function abnormalities related to high dose therapy and GVHD or infections, in particular viral infections, are frequent in the early post-transplant period.[86] At 3 or more months after transplant, the most frequent cause of enzyme or bilirubin elevations is chronic GVHD. However, viral hepatitis has to be considered at any time after HSCT. In the absence of cutaneous manifestations, VZV may cause hepatitis. Prompt therapy with acklovir is indicated.[87]

Of considerable concern are the late sequelae of hepatitis, i.e. cirrhosis and hepatoma. Numerous cases of post-transplant cirrhosis have been recognized, most probably secondary to hepatitis C virus.[88] Several hepatic malignancies, including unusual fibrous histiocytomas, have been observed.[89]

Anecdotal cases of hemosiderosis of the liver have occurred post-transplant, and are thought to be related to altered iron absorption.[90]

POST-TRANSPLANT MALIGNANCIES

Conditions under which malignancies develop at a significantly higher frequency than in the population at large include chromosomal instability (e.g. ataxia telangiectasia or Fanconi's anemia), immunosuppression or chronic antigenic stimulation (both resulting in disruption of normal regulatory mechanisms), and infection with viruses, such as Epstein–Barr virus (EBV). Some or all of these factors are present in recipients of high dose therapy and HSCT.[1,2,91] In addition, the therapeutic agents may be mutagenic.

Secondary cancers occur in patients treated with conventional dose chemotherapy, radiation, or both, for Hodgkin disease, non-Hodgkin lymphoma, leukemia, or solid tumors.[92] An increased incidence of malignant tumors has also been reported in patients receiving immunosuppressive treatment after renal transplantation,[93] and the high incidence of neoplasms in individuals exposed to ionizing

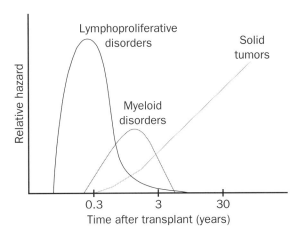

Figure 19.1
Schematic representation of the time course and relative frequency of post-transplant malignancies.

irradiation, be it for medical reasons or accidentally, is well documented.[94]

Experimental models of allogeneic transplantation have shown that lymphomas arising post-allogenic transplant are virus induced[94] and that there is a five- to six-fold increase in the incidence of solid tumors.[95] It was not surprising, therefore, that new malignancies were also recognized as a complication in human HSCT recipients. These malignancies are basically composed of lymphoproliferative disorders, hematopoietic disorders and solid tumors (Fig. 19.1).[92]

Post-transplant lymphoproliferative disorders

Post-transplant lymphoproliferative disorders (PTLD) occur after HSCT and are the most thoroughly studied of all post-transplant malignancies.[96] B cell PTLD consists of an uncontrolled proliferation of B lymphocytes, presumably due to suppressed immunity, antigenic stimulation and an intrinsic capacity of EBV to transform cells. One of the EBV-encoded proteins, LMP-1, induces *bcl*-2 and thereby opposes cell death. Most of the cases occur in donor-derived B lymphocytes. The most frequent presentation of PTLD is with fever, and lymphadenopathy; spleen, liver, bowel and other organs are often involved. The diagnosis can now be supported and the effect of therapy be monitored by semiquantitative polymerase chain reaction of the EBV DNA.

The overall incidence of PTLD at 5 years after transplantation is in the range of 1.0–1.6%.[96,97] Factors associated with increased risk include T cell depletion of the stem cell inoculum, HLA non-identity or transplant from an unrelated donor, the use of anti-thymocyte globulin or anti-CD3 monoclonal antibody (MAB) for acute GVHD prophylaxis or in the preparative regimen, and an underlying diagnosis of primary immunodeficiency. The majority of cases occur during the first few months after transplantation; late cases can occur but are generally not EBV associated.[97]

In early studies PTLDs were generally rapidly fatal. More recently, complete responses have been achieved with interferon-α, intravenous immunoglobulin and monoclonal antibodies directed at B cell antigens CD21 and CD24.[98] Currently, the best approach may be cellular therapy with donor lymphocytes.[99–101]

One recent analysis suggests that there is also an increased incidence of Hodgkin's disease after HSCT. The mechanism is currently not clear; an association with antigenic stimulation has been suggested.[102]

Solid tumors

Solid tumors occur not only after allogeneic but also after syngeneic and autologous HSCT. These tumors arise in host cells. Unlike PTLD, the lag time for solid tumors is several years and if a solid tumor is observed within 6–12 months of HSCT it is likely that the tumor was already present pretransplant. It is possible that a patient's post-transplant immunocompromise may allow for accelerated tumor growth.[103]

In one recent survey of 2150 patients, 15 developed a solid tumor (eight of 1400 after allo- and seven of 750 after autotransplant) for

a cumulative probability of 5.6% at 13 years.[96] Use of TBI in the treatment regimen was the major risk factor (relative risk = 6). A 3.7% incidence of solid tumors after autologous HSCT for Hodgkin's disease was reported in another survey.[91] Among autologous transplant recipients at the Fred Hutchinson Cancer Research Center, 625 survived at least 3 years and 205 at least 5 years. Among these 625 patients, 14 developed a new malignancy (see Table 19.2); 10 had received high dose TBI, and four had been treated with chemotherapy.

An analysis of approximately 20 000 patients transplanted from an allogeneic donor in Seattle or reported to the International Bone Marrow Transplant Registry indicates a risk of solid tumors of 6.7% at 15 years post-transplant; head and neck cancer, squamous cell carcinomas and melanomas of the skin, liver, brain, thyroid, bone and connective tissue were common sites.[88] There was a positive correlation of the dose of TBI and the risk of malignancy. Chronic GVHD and male gender were strongly linked with squamous cell carcinoma of the buccal cavity. The overall risk was highest in young patients transplanted for acute leukemia and declined with increasing age at HSCT.

These results suggest that prevention of chronic GVHD, and whenever possible omission of irradiation, are important prophylactic measures. The results in patients with Fanconi's anemia also indicate that transplantation of normal hematopoietic stem cells corrects hematopoiesis but does not prevent the development of malignancies in other tissues and organs.

The mechanism or mechanisms leading to solid tumor development after HSCT are not well delineated, but the etiology appears to be multifactorial. It is remarkable that there has not been a significant increase in the incidence of otherwise common cancers such as lung and breast carcinoma. Conversely, the relatively high incidence of melanomas, squamous cell carcinomas of skin or mucous membranes, and liver tumors is of note. Only limited studies on oncogene mutations and chromosomal instabil-

Table 19.2 Secondary malignancies after autologous transplantation

Secondary malignancy (no. of cases)	Original disease (no. of patients)	Interval since transplant (months)
Adenocarcinoma (6)	NHL (5); AML (1)	38, 47, 49, 50, 65, 116
Squamous cell carcinoma (2)	NHL; HD	24, 26
MDS/AML (3)	ALL; HD; MM	28, 56, 70
Malignant melanoma (1)	ALL	35
Glioblastoma (1)	NHL	10
Basal cell carcinoma (4)	AML (2); NHL; breast carcinoma	4, 13, 88, 106
ALL (1)	Neuroblastoma	11
Myxoid chondrosarcoma (1)	ALL	56
Thyroid carcinoma (1)	NHL	111

ALL, Acute lymphoblastic leukemia; AML, acute myeloid leukemia; HD, Hodgkin's disease; MDS, myelodysplastic syndrome; MM, multiple myeloma; NHL, non-Hodgkin's lymphoma.

ity have been carried out. Occasional *ras* mutations have been observed and unpublished data suggest a high incidence of p53 mutations.[104]

Hematological malignancies

Leukemia developing after high dose therapy and HSCT may represent disease relapse or a true secondary leukemia, either a morphologically distinct leukemia developing in host cells or new leukemia developing in donor cells.[90,105]

In recent years the development of myelodysplastic syndrome (MDS) and leukemia after high dose chemotherapy and autologous HSCT has attracted considerable attention. In reports from four centers, 1254 patients who received an autologous HSCT shared an estimated incidence of MDS at 3–5 years of 4–18%, with time to diagnosis of 2.5–8.5 years.[106,107] An increased incidence of MDS has also been reported after autologous HSCT for solid tumors, in particular for breast cancer.[108] In a recent update of results at the University of Minnesota, the estimated probability of MDS in patients transplanted for Hodgkin's disease or non-Hodgkin's lymphoma was 13.5% at 6 years. In multivariate analysis, the use of peripheral blood rather than marrow stem cells (relative risk = 5.8) and age over 35 years at HSCT (relative risk = 3.5) were significant risk factors. Since MDS has been observed predominantly after autologous HSCT, a central question is whether MDS is truly related to the transplant procedure or, rather, to therapy given before cells for HSCT are being harvested. A recent report on patients with multiple myeloma suggests that the major factor contributing to the development of MDS or leukemia is the extent of therapy given before HSCT.[109]

Treatment of post-transplant MDS includes chemotherapy (which often is not well tolerated) and allogeneic HSCT. Transplantation is potentially curative but the success rate has been low, maybe 15%.[110]

NEUROLOGICAL COMPLICATIONS

Treatment-related chronic or delayed neurological complications are well recognized after conventional chemoradiotherapy. The high dose conditioning regimens used in preparation for HSCT and the immunocompromised state in the post-transplant period are expected to further accentuate those problems.

A severe syndrome, observed mostly in the early era of transplantation, is leukoencephalopathy.[111] The damage to the white matter of the brain is related to extensive intrathecal administration of methotrexate alone or combined with cranial irradiation (1800–2400 cGy or even higher doses) and the use of TBI. Recovery is uncommon. Leukoencephalopathy has been diagnosed infrequently in recent years.

In addition, there are reports on multifocal cerebral demyelination, inflammatory demyelinating polyneuropathy, immune-mediated myelopathy and encephalopathy.[112,113] The possibility of CNS involvement by GVHD has been debated but has generally been rejected. However, HSCT results in patients with Hurler's disease show that the patient's microglia is being replaced by donor cells and, hence, donor–host interactions might take place in the CNS.[114] Several clearly documented cases of peripheral neuropathy with reduced nerve conduction velocity related to chronic GVHD have been reported.[115,116]

Infections of the CNS usually occur during the first few weeks after high dose therapy and HSCT. However, infections with *Toxoplasma gondii* have been diagnosed 6–8 months after transplantation.[117] Patients with chronic GVHD are particularly prone to develop septicemia and meningitis caused by encapsulated organisms.[6] Patients with chronic GVHD who receive immunosuppressive therapy should, therefore, also be given prophylactic antibiotics.

Patients may also have impaired memory, shortened attention span and defects in verbal fluency.[118] Children, particularly those who also received cranial irradiation, are likely to score lower than controls in visual–motor processing tasks and various IQ tests.[119]

PSYCHOSOCIAL EFFECTS AND REHABILITATION

Research on issues of survivorship in cancer patients in general and HSCT patients in particular is a young discipline.[120,121] However, it is clear from recent studies that long-term adjustments and rehabilitation after HSCT depend strongly on pretransplant conditions and events along the way.

Several studies have compared the quality of life of patients who received a transplant with the quality of life of patients who had comparable diagnoses but were given maintenance chemotherapy.[122] With regard to symptoms of depression, multifocal psychiatric symptomatology and scores according to several quality-of-life instruments, no significant differences between the two groups were found. However, in at least in one study, 20% of transplant recipients had failed to return to full-time employment 40 months after transplantation;[122] another group reported that only 9% of 4-year survivors had failed to return to full-time occupation.[123]

Reduced attention span, short-term memory deficit, depression, inability to attain sexual satisfaction, and low self-esteem because of reduced physical functioning all contribute to psychosocial morbidity.[122,124,125]

A recent analysis of long-term results in 212 patients with aplastic anemia who had survived at least 2 years after transplantation and who had been followed for up to 26 years shows that chronic GVHD is the major risk factor for long-term complications and outcome. Survival at 20 years was 89% for patients without and 69% for patients with chronic GVHD. Chronic skin problems, cataracts, chronic pulmonary disease, musculoskeletal problems and depression all were more frequent in patients with chronic GVHD,[8] but problems arise even after autologous transplantation.[126] Changes in body image due to skin disfigurement, weight loss and weakness, in addition to medications, especially glucocorticoids or CSP, and their side effects, weigh heavily on some patients. Patients with joint contractures or pulmonary disease may be crippled for years. Realistic and open pretransplant communication about potential long-term complications, and pretransplant identification of patients at high risk for post-transplant physical and psychosocial morbidity, will help to deal successfully with these problems as they arise.

In pediatric and adolescent patients, the desire to be equal to their peers may cause considerable problems with compliance, and problems with self-esteem, body image and sexuality may be particularly severe. A multidisciplinary approach involving adolescent medicine physicians and endocrinologists along with group therapy appears most promising. Rehabilitation must begin at the time of diagnosis and should involve a long-term treatment plan.

REFERENCES

1. Deeg HJ. Delayed complications and long-term effects after bone marrow transplantation. Hematol Oncol Clin North Am 1990;4:641–57.
2. Duell T, Van Lint MT, Ljungman P et al. Health and functional status of long-term survivors of bone marrow transplantation. EBMT Working Party on Late Effects and EULEP Study Group on Late Effects. European Group for Blood and Marrow Transplantation. Ann Intern Med 1997;126:184–92.
3. Socie G, Stone JV, Wingard JR et al. Long-term survival and late deaths after allogeneic bone marrow transplantation. Late Effects Working Committee of the International Bone Marrow Transplant Registry. N Engl J Med 1999;341: 14–21.
4. Sullivan KM. Graft-versus-host-disease. In: Thomas ED, Blume KG, Forman SJ, editors. Hematopoietic cell transplantation, 2nd edn. Boston: Blackwell Science, 1999:515–36.
5. Sullivan KM, Shulman HM, Storb R et al. Chronic graft-versus-host disease in 52 patients: adverse natural course and successful treatment with combination immunosuppression. Blood 1981;57:267–76.
6. Bowden RA, Ljungman P, Paya CV, editors. Transplant infections. Philadelphia: Lippincott-Raven Publishers, 1998.
7. Strasser SI, Sullivan KM, Myerson D. Cirrhosis of the liver in long-term marrow transplant survivors. Blood 1999;93:3259–66.
8. Deeg HJ, Leisenring W, Storb R et al. Long-term outcome after marrow transplantation for severe aplastic anemia. Blood 1998;91:3637–45.
9. Madtes DK, Crawford SW. Lung injuries associated with graft-versus-host reactions. In: Ferrara JLM, Deeg HJ, Burakoff SJ, editors. Graft-vs-host disease, 2nd edn. New York: Marcel Dekker, 1997:425–46.
10. Palmas A, Tefferi A, Myers JL et al. Late-onset noninfectious pulmonary complications after allogeneic bone marrow transplantation. Br J Haematol 1998;100:680–7.
11. Tirona MR, Gordon DS, Crocker I et al. High dose cyclophosphamide, fractionated total body irradiation with involved field irradiation and autologous bone marrow transplantation in malignant lymphoma. Leuk Lymphoma 1996;20:249–57.
12. Jules-Elysee K, Stover DE, Yahalom J, White DA, Gulati SC. Pulmonary complications in lymphoma patients treated with high-dose therapy autologous bone marrow transplantation. Am Rev Respir Dis 1992;146:485–91.
13. Crawford SW, Pepe M, Lin D, Benedetti F, Deeg HJ. Abnormalities of pulmonary function tests after marrow transplantation predict nonrelapse mortality. Am J Respir Crit Care Med 1995;152:690–5.
14. Kantrow SP, Hackman RC, Boeckh M, Myerson D, Crawford SW. Idiopathic pneumonia syndrome: changing spectrum of lung injury after marrow transplantation. Transplantation 1997; 63:1079–86.
15. Boeckh M, Riddell SR, Cunningham T, Myerson D, Flowers M, Bowden RA. Increased risk of late CMV infection and disease in allogeneic marrow transplant recipients after ganciclovir prophylaxis is due to a lack of CMV-specific T cell responses. Blood 1996;88:302 (abstract 1195).
16. Crawford SW, Fisher L. Predictive value of pulmonary function tests before marrow transplantation. Chest 1992;101:1257–64.
17. Crawford SW. Respiratory infections following organ transplantation. Curr Opin Pulmonary Med 1995;1:209–15.
18. Clark JG, Schwartz DA, Flournoy N, Sullivan KM, Crawford SW, Thomas ED. Risk factors for airflow obstruction in recipients of bone marrow transplants. Ann Intern Med 1987;107: 648–56.

19. Boas SR, Noyes BE, Kurland G, Armitage J, Orenstein D. Pediatric lung transplantation for graft-versus-host disease following bone marrow transplantation. Chest 1994;105:1584–6.

20. Sullivan KM, Mori M, Sanders J et al. Late complications of allogeneic and autologous marrow transplantation [Review]. Bone Marrow Transplant 1992;10:127–34.

21. Philit F, Wiesendanger T, Archimbaud E, Mornex JF, Brune J, Cordier JF. Post-transplant obstructive lung disease ('bronchiolitis obliterans'): a clinical comparative study of bone marrow and lung transplant patients. Eur Respir J 1995;8:551–8.

22. Sharples LD, Tamm M, McNeil K, Higenbottam TW, Stewart S, Wallwork J. Development of bronchiolitis obliterans syndrome in recipients of heart–lung transplantation – early risk factors. Transplantation 1996;61:560–6.

23. Sullivan KM, Storek J, Kopecky KJ et al. A controlled trial of long-term administration of intravenous immunoglobulin to prevent late infection and chronic graft-vs.-host disease after marrow transplantation: clinical outcome and effect on subsequent immune recovery. Biol Blood Marrow Transplant 1996;2:44–53.

24. Storek J, Witherspoon RP. Immunological reconstitution after hemopoietic stem cell transplantation. In: Atkinson K, editor. Clinical bone marrow and blood stem cell transplantation: a reference textbook. Cambridge University Press, 2000:11.

25. Billingham RE. The biology of graft-versus-host reactions. The Harvey Lectures. New York: Academic Press, 1966:21–78.

26. Hakim FT, Mackall CL. The immune system: effector and target of graft-versus-host disease. In: Ferrara JLM, Deeg HJ, Burakoff SJ, editors. Graft-vs.-host disease, 2nd edn. New York: Marcel Dekker, 1997:257–90.

27. Hess AD. The immunobiology of syngeneic/ autologous graft-versus-host disease. In: Ferrara JLM, Deeg HJ, Burakoff SJ, editors. Graft-vs.-host disease, 2nd edn. New York: Marcel Dekker, 1997:561–86.

28. Rouquette-Gally AM, Boyeldieu D, Prost AC, Gluckman E. Autoimmunity after allogeneic bone marrow transplantation. Transplantation 1988;46:238–40.

29. Mackey JR, Desai S, Larratt L, Cwik V, Nabholtz JM. Myasthenia gravis in association with allogeneic bone marrow transplantation: clinical observations, therapeutic implications and review of literature. Bone Marrow Transplant 1997;19:939–42.

30. Smith CIE, Aarli JA, Biberfeld P et al. Myasthenia gravis after bone-marrow transplantation. Evidence for a donor origin. N Engl J Med 1983;309:1565–8.

31. Bellou A, Kanny G, Fremont S, Moneret-Vautrin DA. Transfer of atopy following bone marrow transplantation. Ann Allergy Asthma Immunol 1997;78:513–16.

32. Snowden JA, Heaton DC. Development of psoriasis after syngeneic bone marrow transplant from psoriatic donor: further evidence for adoptive autoimmunity. Br J Dermatol 1997; 137:130–2.

33. Hebart H, Einsele H, Klein R et al. CMV infection after allogeneic bone marrow transplantation is associated with the occurrence of various autoantibodies and monoclonal gammopathies. Br J Haematol 1996;95:138–44.

34. Soderberg C, Larsson S, Rozell BL, Sumitran-Karuppan S, Ljungman P, Moller E. Cytomegalovirus-induced CD13-specific autoimmunity – a possible cause of chronic graft-vs-host disease. Transplantation 1996;61:600–9.

35. Jacobsen N, Lönnqvist B, Ringdén O et al. Graft-versus-leukaemia activity associated with cytomegalovirus seropositive bone marrow donors but separated from graft-versus-host disease in allograft recipients with AML. Eur J Haematol 1987;38:350–5.

36. Naucler CS, Larsson S, Moller E. A novel mechanism for virus-induced autoimmunity in humans [Review]. Immunol Rev 1996;152: 175–92.

37. Klumpp TR. Immunohematologic complications of bone marrow transplantation [Review]. Bone Marrow Transplant 1991;8:159–70.

38. Sivakumaran M, Hutchinson RM, Pringle H et al. Thrombocytopenia following autologous bone marrow transplantation: evidence for autoimmune aetiology and B cell clonal involvement. Bone Marrow Transplant 1995; 15:531–6.

39. De Lord C, Marsh JC, Smith JG, Singer CR, Gordon-Smith EC. Fatal autoimmune pancytopenia following bone marrow transplantation for aplastic anaemia. Bone Marrow Transplant 1996;18:237–9.

40. Wingard JR, Piantadosi S, Vogelsang GB et al. Predictors of death from chronic graft versus

host disease after bone marrow transplantation. Blood 1989;74:1428–35.

41. Lee SJ, Churchill WH, Konugres A, Gilliland DG, Antin JH. Idiopathic thrombocytopenic purpura following allogeneic bone marrow transplantation – treatment with anti-D immunoglobulin. Bone Marrow Transplant 1997;19:173–4.

42. Sniecinski IJ, Oien L, Petz LD, Blume KG. Immunohematologic consequences of major ABO-mismatched bone marrow transplantation. Transplantation 1988;45:530–4.

43. Roychowdhury DF, Linker CA. Pure red cell aplasia complicating an ABO-compatible allogeneic bone marrow transplantation, treated successfully with antithymocyte globulin. Bone Marrow Transplant 1995;16:471–2.

44. Locatelli F, Giorgiani G, Pession A, Bozzola M. Late effects in children after bone marrow transplantation: a review. Haematologica 1993; 78:319–28.

45. Toubert ME, Socié G, Gluckman E et al. Short- and long-term follow up of thyroid dysfunction after allogeneic bone marrow transplantation without the use of preparative total body irradiation. Br J Haematol 1997;98:453–7.

46. Vexiau P, Perez-Castiglioni P, Socié G et al. The 'euthyroid sick syndrome': incidence, risk factors and prognostic value soon after allogeneic bone marrow transplantation. Br J Haematol 1993;85:778–82.

47. Borgstrom B, Bolme P. Thyroid function in children after allogeneic bone marrow transplantation. Bone Marrow Transplant 1994;13:59–64.

48. Neglia JP, Nesbit ME, Jr. Care and treatment of long-term survivors of childhood cancer [Review]. Cancer 1993;71:3386–91.

49. Sanders JE and the Long-Term Follow-Up Team. Endocrine problems in children after bone marrow transplant for hematologic malignancies. Bone Marrow Transplant 1991;8:2–4.

50. Uderzo C, Van Lint MT, Rovelli A et al. Papillary thyroid carcinoma after total body irradiation. Arch Dis Child 1994;71:256–8.

51. Lupoli G, Cascone E, Vitale G et al. Risk factors and prevention of thyroid carcinoma [Review]. Minerva Endocrinol 1996;21:93–100.

52. Kubota C, Shinohara O, Hinohara T et al. Changes in hypothalamic-pituitary function following bone marrow transplantation in children. Acta Paediatr Jpn 1994;36:37–43.

53. Brauner R, Adan L, Souberbielle JC et al. Contribution of growth hormone deficiency to the growth failure that follows bone marrow transplantation. J Pediatr 1997;130:785–92.

54. Clement-De-Boers A, Oostdijk W, Van Weel-Sipman MH, Van den Broeck J, Wit JM, Vossen JM. Final height and hormonal function after bone marrow transplantation in children. J Pediatr 1996;129:544–50.

55. Sanders JE. Growth and development after hematopoietic cell transplantation. In: Thomas ED, Blume KG, Forman SJ, editors. Hematopoietic cell transplantation, 2nd edn. Boston: Blackwell Science, 1999:764–75.

56. Mayer EI, Dopfer RE, Klingebiel T, Scheel-Walter H, Ranke MB, Niethammer D. Longitudinal gonadal function after bone marrow transplantation for acute lymphoblastic leukemia during childhood. Pediatr Transplant 1999;3:38–44.

57. Sanders JE, Hawley J, Levy W et al. Pregnancies following high-dose cyclophosphamide with or without high-dose busulfan or total-body irradiation and bone marrow transplantation. Blood 1996;87:3045–52.

58. Chatterjee R, Mills W, Katz M, McGarrigle HH, Goldstone AH. Germ cell failure and Leydig cell insufficiency in post-pubertal males after autologous bone marrow transplantation with BEAM for lymphoma. Bone Marrow Transplant 1994;13:519–22.

59. Yahalom J. Re-visiting the role of radiation therapy in Hodgkin's disease [Review]. Isr J Med Sci 1995;31:137–43.

60. Braverman AC, Antin JH, Plappert MT, Cook EF, Lee RT. Cyclophosphamide cardiotoxicity in bone marrow transplantation: a prospective evaluation of new dosing regimens. J Clin Oncol 1991;9:1215–23.

61. Hochster H, Wasserheit C, Speyer J. Cardiotoxicity and cardioprotection during chemotherapy [Review]. Curr Opin Oncol 1995; 7:304–9.

62. Benyunes MC, Sullivan KM, Deeg HJ et al. Cataracts after bone marrow transplantation: long-term follow-up of adults treated with fractionated total body irradiation. Int J Radiat Oncol Biol Phys 1995;32:661–70.

63. Belkacemi Y, Ozsahin M, Pene F et al. Cataractogenesis after total body irradiation. Int J Radiat Oncol Biol Phys 1996;35:53–60.

64. Fife K, Milan S, Westbrook K, Powles R, Tait D. Risk factors for requiring cataract surgery

following total body irradiation. Radiother Oncol 1994;33:93–8.

65. Tichelli A. Late ocular complications after bone marrow transplantation [Review]. Nouv Rev Fr Hematol 1994;36(suppl 1):79–82.

66. Tichelli A, Duell T, Weiss M et al. Late-onset keratoconjunctivitis sicca syndrome after bone marrow transplantation: incidence and risk factors. European Group of Blood and Marrow Transplantation (EBMT) Working Party on Late Effects. Bone Marrow Transplant 1996;17: 1105–11.

67. Hanada R, Ueoka Y. Obstruction of nasolacrimal ducts closely related to graft-versus-host disease after bone marrow transplantation. Bone Marrow Transplant 1989;4:125–6.

68. Castaneda S, Carmona L, Carvajal I, Arranz R, Diaz A, Garcia-Vadillo A. Reduction of bone mass in women after bone marrow transplantation. Calcif Tissue Int 1997;60:343–7.

69. Castelo-Branco C, Rovira M, Pons F et al. The effect of hormone replacement therapy on bone mass in patients with ovarian failure due to bone marrow transplantation. Maturitas 1996; 23:307–12.

70. Fink JC, Leisenring WM, Sullivan KM, Sherrard DJ, Weiss NS. Avascular necrosis following bone marrow transplantation: a case–control study. Bone 1998;22:67–71.

71. Fletcher BD, Crom DB, Krance KA, Kun LE. Radiation-induced bone abnormalities after bone marrow transplantation for childhood leukemia. Radiology 1994;191:231–5.

72. Socié G, Cahn JY, Carmelo J et al. Avascular necrosis of bone after allogeneic bone marrow transplantation: analysis of risk factors for 4388 patients by the Societe Francaise de Greffe de Moelle (SFGM). Br J Haematol 1997;97: 865–70.

73. Schubert MM, Williams BE, Lloid ME, Donaldson G, Chapko MK. Clinical assessment scale for the rating of oral mucosal changes associated with bone marrow transplantation. Cancer 1992;69:2469–77.

74. Izutsu KT, Sullivan KM, Schubert MM et al. Disordered salivary immunoglobulin secretion and sodium transport in human chronic graft-versus-host disease. Transplantation 1983;35: 441–6.

75. Nasman M, Bjork O, Soderhall S, Ringden O, Dahllof G. Disturbances in the oral cavity in pediatric long-term survivors after different forms of antineoplastic therapy. Pediatr Dent 1994;16:217–23.

76. Pajari U, Ollila P, Lanning M. Incidence of dental caries in children with acute lymphoblastic leukemia is related to the therapy used. ASDC J Dent Child 1995;62:349–52.

77. Dahllöf G, Barr M, Bolme P et al. Disturbances in dental development after total body irradiation in bone marrow transplant recipients. Oral Surg Oral Med Oral Pathol 1988;65:41–4.

78. Dahllöf G, Rozell B, Forsberg CM, Borgstrom B. Histologic changes in dental morphology induced by high dose chemotherapy and total body irradiation. Oral Surg Oral Med Oral Pathol 1994;77:56–60.

79. Yang CC, Hurd DD, Case LD, Assimos DG. Hemorrhagic cystitis in bone marrow transplantation. Urology 1994;44:322–8.

80. Zager RA. Acute renal failure in the setting of bone marrow transplantation. Kidney Int 1994; 46:1443–58.

81. Cohen EP, Lawton CA, Moulder JE. Bone marrow transplant nephropathy: radiation nephritis revisited [Review]. Neph 1995;70:217–22.

82. Niemer-Tucker MM, Sluysmans MM, Bakker B, Davelaar J, Zurcher C, Broerse JJ. Long-term consequences of high-dose total-body irradiation on hepatic and renal function in primates. Int J Radiat Biol 1995;68:83–96.

83. Cohen EP, Moulder JE, Fish BL, Hill P. Prophylaxis of experimental bone marrow transplant nephropathy. J Lab Clin Med 1994; 124:371–80.

84. Strasser SI, McDonald GB. Gastrointestinal and hepatic complications. In: Thomas ED, Blume KG, Forman SJ, editors. Hematopoietic cell transplantation, 2nd edn. Boston: Blackwell Science, 1999:627–58.

85. Navari RM, Sharma P, Deeg HJ, McDonald GB, Thomas ED. Pneumatosis cystoides intestinalis following allogeneic marrow transplantation. Transplant Proc 1983;15:1720–4.

86. Strasser SI, McDonald GB. Hepatobiliary complications of hematopoietic cell transplantation. In: Schiff ER, Sorrell MF, Maddrey WC, editors. Schiff's diseases of the liver, 8th edn. Philadelphia: Lippincott-Raven, 1999:1617–41.

87. Han CS, Miller W, Haake R, Weisdorf D. Varicella zoster infection after bone marrow transplantation: incidence, risk factors and complications. Bone Marrow Transplant 1994;13: 277–83.

88. Ljungman P, Johansson N, Aschan J et al. Long-term effects of hepatitis C virus infection in allogeneic bone marrow transplant recipients. Blood 1995;86:1614–18.

89. Curtis RE, Rowlings PA, Deeg HJ et al. Solid cancers after bone marrow transplantation. N Engl J Med 1997;336:897–904.

90. Mahendra P, Hood IM, Bass G, Patterson P, Marcus RE. Severe hemosiderosis post allogenic bone marrow transplantation. Hematol Oncol 1996;14:33–5.

91. Socié G. Secondary malignancies. Curr Opin Hematol 1996;3:468–70.

92. Deeg HJ, Socié G. Malignancies after hematopoietic stem cell transplantation: many questions, some answers. Blood 1998;91:1833–44.

93. The Committee for the Compilation of Materials on Damage Caused by the Atomic Bombs in Hiroshima and Nagasaki. Hiroshima and Nagasaki: the physical, medical, and social effects of the atomic bombings. New York: Basic Books, 1981.

94. Schwartz RS, Beldotti L. Malignant lymphomas following allogeneic disease: Transition from an immunological to a neoplastic disorder. Science 1965;149:1511–14.

95. Deeg HJ, Storb R, Prentice R et al. Increased cancer risk in canine radiation chimeras. Blood 1980;55:233–9.

96. Cohen JI. Epstein–Barr virus lymphoproliferative disease associated with acquired immunodeficiency [Review]. Medicine 1991;70:137–60.

97. Bhatia S, Ramsay NK, Steinbuch M et al. Malignant neoplasms following bone marrow transplantation. Blood 1996;87:3633–9.

98. Curtis RE, Travis LB, Rowlings PA et al. Risk of lymphoproliferative disorders following bone marrow transplantation: a multi-institutional study. Blood 1999;94:2208–16.

99. Benkerrou M, Durandy A, Fischer A. Therapy for transplant-related lymphoproliferative diseases [Review]. Hematol Oncol Clin North Am 1993;7:467–75.

100. Papadopoulos EB, Ladanyi M, Emanuel D et al. Infusions of donor leukocytes to treat Epstein–Barr virus-associated lymphoproliferative disorders after allogeneic bone marrow transplantation. N Engl J Med 1994;330:1185–91.

101. Rooney CM, Smith CA, Ng CY et al. Use of gene-modified virus-specific T lymphocytes to control Epstein–Bar-virus-related lymphoproliferation. Lancet 1995;345:9–13.

102. Heslop HE, Ng CY, Li C et al. Long-term restoration of immunity against Epstein–Barr virus infection by adoptive transfer of gene-modified virus-specific T lymphocytes. Nature Med 1996;2:551–5.

103. Rowlings PA, Curtis RE, Passweg JR et al. Increased incidence of hodgkin disease following allogeneic bone marrow transplantation. J Clin Oncol 1999;17:3122–7.

104. Wodzig KW, Beijleveld LJ, Damoiseaux JG, Arends JW, van Breda Vriesman PJ. Malignant neoplasms in cyclosporin A-induced autoimmunity (CyA-AI). Int J Cancer 1997;72:530–5.

105. Socié G, Scieux C, Gluckman E et al. Squamous cell carcinomas after allogeneic bone marrow transplantation for aplastic anemia: further evidence of a multistep process. Transplantation 1998;66:667–70.

106. Thomas ED, Bryant JI, Buckner CD et al. Leukaemic transformation of engrafted human marrow cells in vivo. Lancet 1972;i:1310–13.

107. Darrington DL, Vose JM, Anderson JR et al. Incidence and characterization of secondary myelodysplastic syndrome and acute myelogenous leukemia following high-dose chemoradiotherapy and autologous stem-cell transplantation for lymphoid malignancies. J Clin Oncol 1994;12:2527–34.

108. Traweek ST, Slovak ML, Nademanee AP, Brynes RK, Niland JC, Forman SJ. Myelodysplasia and acute myeloid leukemia occurring after autologous bone marrow transplantation for lymphoma [Review]. Leuk Lymphoma 1996;20:365–72.

109. Roman-Unfer S, Bitran JD, Hanauer S et al. Acute myeloid leukemia and myelodysplasia following intensive chemotherapy for breast cancer. Bone Marrow Transplant 1995;16:163–8.

110. Govindarajan R, Jagannath S, Flick JT et al. Preceding standard therapy is the likely cause of MDS after autotransplants for multiple myeloma. Br J Haematol 1996;95:349–53.

111. Anderson JE, Gooley TA, Schoch G et al. Stem cell transplantation for secondary acute myeloid leukemia: evaluation of transplantation as initial therapy or following induction chemotherapy. Blood 1997;89:2578–85.

112. Thompson CB, Sanders JE, Flournoy N, Buckner CD, Thomas ED. The risks of central nervous system relapse and leukoencephalopathy in patients receiving marrow transplants for acute leukemia. Blood 1986;67:195–9.

113. Griggs JJ, Commichau CS, Rapoport AP, Griggs RC. Chronic inflammatory demyelinating polyneuropathy in non-Hodgkin's lymphoma. Am J Hematol 1997;54:332–4.

114. Openshaw H, Slatkin NE, Parker PM, Forman SJ. Immune-mediated myelopathy after allogeneic marrow transplantation. Bone Marrow Transplant 1995;15:633–6.

115. Unger ER, Sung JH, Manivel JC, Chenggis ML, Blazar BR, Krivit W. Male donor-derived cells in the brains of female sex-mismatched bone marrow transplant recipients; a Y-chromosome specific in situ hybridization study. J Neuropathol Exp Neurol 1993;52(5):460–70.

116. Amato AA, Barohn RJ, Sahenk Z, Tutschka PJ, Mendell JR. Polyneuropathy complicating bone marrow and solid organ transplantation [Review]. Neurology 1993;43:1513–18.

117. Greenspan A, Deeg HJ, Cottler-Fox M, Sirdofski M, Spitzer TR, Kattah J. Incapacitating peripheral neuropathy as a manifestation of chronic graft-versus-host disease. Bone Marrow Transplant 1990;5:349–52.

118. Slavin MA, Meyers JD, Remington JS, Hackman RC. *Toxoplasma gondii* infection in marrow transplant recipients: a 20 year experience. Bone Marrow Transplant 1994;13:549–57.

119. Sanders J, Flowers M, Siadak M, McGuire T. Negative impact of prior central nervous system (CNS) irradiation on growth and neuropsychological function (NPsF) after total body irradiation (TBI) and bone marrow transplant (BMT). Blood 1994;84:250 (abstract).

120. Chou RH, Wong GB, Kramer JH et al. Toxicities of total-body irradiation for pediatric bone marrow transplantation. Int J Radiat Oncol Biol Phys 1996;34:843–51.

121. Meyers CA, Weitzner M, Byrne K, Valentine A, Champlin RE, Przepiorka D. Evaluation of the neurobehavioral functioning of patients before, during, and after bone marrow transplantation. J Clin Oncol 1994;12:820–6.

122. Molassiotis A. Late psychosocial effects of conditioning for BMT. Br J Nurs 1996;5:1296–302.

123. Molassiotis A, van den Akker OBA, Milligan DW et al. Quality of life in long-term survivors of marrow transplantation: comparison with a matched group receiving maintenance chemotherapy. Bone Marrow Transplant 1992;17:249–58.

124. Syrjala KL, Chapko MK, Vitaliano PP, Cummings C, Sullivan KM. Recovery after allogeneic marrow transplantation: prospective study of predictors of long-term physical and psychosocial functioning. Bone Marrow Transplant 1993;11:319–27.

125. Leigh S, Wilson KC, Burns R, Clark RE. Psychosocial morbidity in bone marrow transplant recipients: a prospective study. Bone Marrow Transplant 1995;16:635–40.

126. Baker F, Wingard JR, Curbow B et al. Quality of life of bone marrow transplant long-term survivors. Bone Marrow Transplant 1994;13:589–96.

127. Deeg HJ, Witherspoon RP, Sullivan KM, Flowers M. Long-term observations following hematopoietic cell transplantation. In: Dicke KA, Keating A, editors. Autologous blood and marrow transplantation. Charlottesville: Carden Jennings Publishing, 1999:507–9.

20

Overview of allogeneic procedures: immune modulation and non-myeloablative allogeneic hematopoietic stem cell transplantation

George E Georges and Rainer F Storb

CONTENTS   Introduction • Principles of conventional allogeneic HSCT • Toxicity limits the clinical use of conventional allogeneic HSCT • Results of myeloablative allogeneic HSCT in elderly patients • Immune modulation of allografting: graft-versus-leukemia effect • Mixed chimerism after allogeneic hematopoietic stem cell transplantation • Evidence that host-versus-graft and graft-versus-host reactions are mediated by T cells • Immune modulation: allografts with non-myeloablative pre- and post-transplant immunosuppression • Future directions • Conclusions

INTRODUCTION

The curative potential of allogeneic hematopoietic stem cell transplantation (HSCT) represents a major therapeutic advance for the treatment of malignant and non-malignant hematologic diseases. The basis of conventional allogeneic HSCT involves the use of a myeloablative high dose chemo/radiotherapy conditioning regimen followed by infusion of histocompatible donor marrow or peripheral blood stem cells (PBSC) to rescue hematopoiesis. Significant progress has been made over the past 30 years, with improved survival of patients treated with this approach. For a variety of hematologic malignancies, allogeneic HSCT is now considered a standard of care for patients under the age of 50 years who have a human leukocyte antigen (HLA) matched donor. One of the major limitations of conventional allogeneic HSCT is that the toxicity associated with high dose chemoradiotherapy is high, particularly in older patients or in patients previously treated with extensive chemo- or radiotherapy. This chapter will focus on recent developments in allogeneic HSCT in which an improved understanding and control of immune modulation has led to non-myeloablative conditioning regimens which have been developed for clinical use. These new approaches may significantly change how allogeneic HSCT will be conducted in the future.

PRINCIPLES OF CONVENTIONAL ALLOGENEIC HSCT

Allogeneic HSCT developed from the initial observation by Jacobsen et al.[1] in 1949 that mice could be protected from marrow lethal effects of ionizing radiation by shielding their spleens with lead. This finding led to experiments in the 1950s which showed that transplantation of donor marrow or splenocytes after lethal irradiation conferred radioprotection.[2-4] From these experiments, the current conventional treatment schema was developed for patients with various hematopoietic diseases such as leukemia.[5]

Conventional allogeneic transplantation relies upon high dose, myeloablative chemoradiotherapy to (1) eradicate underlying disease, (2) create marrow space and (3) suppress the recipient's immune system in preparation for the allograft so that rejection of the donor stem cell graft does not occur. The intensity and the lack of specificity of the myeloablative regimen result in obliteration of all elements of the host normal hematopoietic system. The host sustains an acute and profound pancytopenia. Infusion of the donor stem cell graft is critical in order to rescue hematopoiesis and reconstitute the recipients' immune system following the otherwise lethal marrow toxicity of the conditioning regimen. Importantly, the allograft is critical to eliminate residual disease via a graft-versus-host (GVH) reaction. Following infusion of the donor graft, immune suppression is necessary to prevent graft-versus-host disease (GVHD) and establish long-term graft–host tolerance (Table 20.1).

TOXICITY LIMITS THE CLINICAL USE OF CONVENTIONAL ALLOGENEIC HSCT

While this approach has led to long-term cures of otherwise incurable diseases, widespread application of allogeneic HSCT has been limited by toxicity associated with the myeloablative conditioning regimens. In an attempt to achieve maximal tumor eradication, conditioning regimens have been intensified to a point where organ toxicities are common, resulting in morbidity and mortality (Table 20.2).[5] In addition, the pancytopenia induced by the high dose regimens increase the risk for serious and even lethal infections, despite the use of prophylactic broad-spectrum antibiotics. In addition, the regimen-related toxicity, particularly to the liver and kidney, frequently restricts the ability to give optimal post-grafting immunosuppression, which is necessary to avoid GVHD. Because of the toxicities associated with myeloablative regimens, over the past 30 years allogeneic grafts have been conducted in the setting of highly specialized intensive care hospital wards.

Patients with extensive prior chemotherapy, prior irradiation of chest or abdomen, previous marrow transplants, and pre-existing damage to lungs, kidneys and heart are at particularly high risk for life-threatening regimen-related toxicities, in particular veno-occlusive disease of the liver (VOD) and idiopathic interstitial pneumonia (IP). At most transplant centers, the severity of the complications from myeloablative chemotherapy and allotransplants has limited its use to relatively young patients or patients less than 55 years of age. Effective strategies to reduce the toxicity of transplant regimens are necessary to improve overall survival, reduce delayed side effects, and improve quality of life of long-term survivors.

RESULTS OF MYELOABLATIVE ALLOGENEIC HSCT IN ELDERLY PATIENTS

Ringden performed a retrospective analysis of 2180 HLA-identical sibling bone marrow transplants in adults (>30 years) with leukemia from the European Bone Marrow Transplant Registry to assess risk of age on transplant outcome.[6] Patients over 45 years of age with advanced leukemia had a significantly higher risk of treatment-related mortality, and the 45- to 50-year-old cohort had a higher risk of interstitial pneumonia. Hansen et al.[7] reported that patients greater than 50 years of age undergoing unrelated HLA-matched HSCT for chronic

Table 20.1 Outline for conventional myeloablative allografting

Time course	Therapy	Function	Effect
Pretransplant	Myeloablative chemo/radiotherapy conditioning	(1) Control HVG reaction (2) Eradicate underlying disease (3) Create marrow space	(1) Requires hospitalization (2) Risk of severe toxicity: VOD, IP (see Table 20.2) (3) Pancytopenia (4) Increased risk of infection
Transplant	Bone marrow or PBSC allograft	Rescue hematopoiesis	(1) Engraftment at 10 to 25+ days after transplant: ANC rises >500 cells/μl (2) Introduce complete donor hematopoietic chimerism
Post-transplant	Immunosuppression (CSP + MTX) or, alternatively, T cell depletion of marrow at time of transplant	Prevent GVHD	(1) Reconstitute immunity (2) Decrease incidence of GVHD (3) Induction of donor–host tolerance (4) GVL effect (5) Cure of underlying disease

ANC, Absolute neutrophil count; CSP, cyclosporine; GVHD, graft-versus-host disease; GVL, graft-versus-leukemia; HVG, host-versus-graft; IP, idiopathic pneumonia; MTX, methotrexate; PBSC, peripheral blood stem cells; VOD, veno-occlusive disease of the liver.

myeloid leukemia (CML) had a higher risk of death than patients who were 21–50 years of age (relative risk 3.4). Clift et al.[8] reported that increasing age was an independent risk factor predictive of poorer survival after HLA-identical allotransplant for CML in chronic phase. Although results of these studies suggest that the toxicity of conventional allotransplants in elderly patients is not uniformly prohibitive, assessment of outcome from HSCT using high dose regimens must be evaluated with respect to the confounding problem of rigorous patient selection.

Of the more than 1600 allogeneic transplants performed for the treatment of CML at the Fred Hutchinson Cancer Research Center (FHCRC),

Table 20.2 Toxicity of high dose conditioning regimens used for conventional allografting	
Acute side effects	**Delayed side effects**
Alopecia	Cataracts
Nausea and vomiting	Infertility
Oral pharyngeal mucositis	Hypothyroidism
Diarrhea	Radiation nephritis
Pancytopenia	Restrictive lung disease
Veno-occlusive disease of the liver	Secondary malignancies
Interstitial pneumonitis	Impaired growth and development in children
Infection due to neutropenia	Reduced IQ in children or psychosocial problems
Gastrointestinal hemorrhage	Osteoporosis
Hemorrhagic cystitis	
Cardiomyopathy	
Dermatitis	
Peripheral neuropathy	
Acute renal failure	
Parotitis	

including more than 900 from HLA-identical siblings, we have transplanted only 68 patients aged 50–62 years and three patients age greater than 62 years. These statistics suggest that physicians and patients are reluctant to consider allografting at a more advanced age. The few patients above age 50 who have been referred for allogeneic HSCT are subject to rigorous selection and are unlikely to be representative of the general patient population. This may explain why results in the 50- to 60-year-old group are not significantly different than in the 40- to 50-year-old group.

Long-term patient survivals for allografting for non-Hodgkin's lymphoma (NHL), multiple myeloma (MM), and chronic lymphocytic leukemia (CLL) have been much lower than for patients with CML in chronic phase. This was due in part to significantly higher transplant-related mortality experienced by patients with NHL, MM and CLL. Several factors contributed to this, including adverse effects of prior

chemotherapy, radiation, infections and, in some cases, the disease on organ function, for example renal dysfunction in multiple myeloma. In particular, patients greater than 50 years with NHL, MM or CLL tolerated conventional allogeneic HSCT poorly, and transplant-related mortality exceeded 50%. Although patients had incurable disease using conventional dose therapy, there was no evidence of disease progression among those patients who died early after allografting. The small number of allografts performed in patients greater than 50 years of age reflects the reluctance of physicians at our center to recommend allografts for these patients. This reluctance, in turn, results from the knowledge that fatal toxicities are frequently seen in these patients with conventional myeloablative regimens.

With the exception of acute lymphoblastic leukemia (ALL) and Hodgkin's disease (HD), however, the incidence of hematologic malignancies in the population increases in patients older than 55 years of age. There is substantial discrepancy between the median age of patients who have undergone allogeneic HSCT for hematologic malignancies and the median age at time of diagnosis.

Figure 20.1 shows the age distribution of patients who received an allogeneic HSCT at FHCRC between 1980 and 1998 and the age distribution of all patients at time of disease diagnosis, based on data presented by the National Cancer Institute Surveillance, Epidemiology and End Results (SEER) Cancer Statistics, 1986.[9]

Thus, using conventional allogeneic HSCT, the majority of patients are not generally con-

sidered eligible for the potentially curative treatment offered by allografting. These data strongly support the efforts in developing safe and effective allografting protocols that can be applied to older or previously heavily treated patients.

IMMUNE MODULATION OF ALLOGRAFTING: GRAFT-VERSUS-LEUKEMIA EFFECT

Over time, two important observations related to HSCT have emerged. First, some hematologic malignancies cannot be cured, despite the

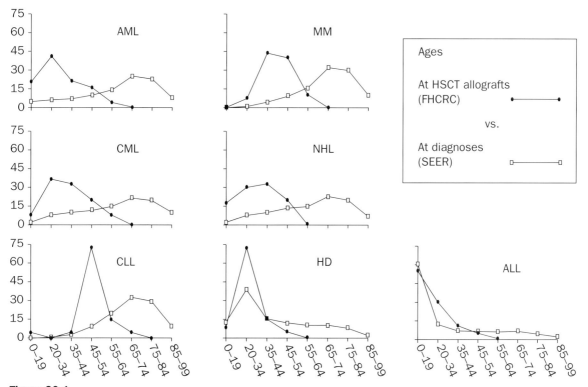

Figure 20.1
Age distribution curves of patients with various hematologic diseases undergoing allogeneic hematopoeitic stem cell transplantation (HSCT) at the Fred Hutchinson Cancer Research Center (solid circle). These are compared with the National Cancer Institute Surveillance, Epidemiology and End Results Cancer Statistics database distribution of patients with respect to age at diagnosis (open square). With the exception of Hodgkin's disease (HD) and acute lymphoblastic leukemia (ALL), note the discrepancy between ages at diagnoses and ages at the times of conventional allogeneic HSCT. AML, acute myeloid leukemia; MM, multiple myeloma; CML, chronic myeloid leukemia; NHL, non-Hodgkin's lymphoma; CLL, chronic lymphocytic leukemia. Adapted from Molina AJ, Storb R. Hematopoietic stem cell transplants in older adults. In: Rowe J et al., editors. Handbook of Bone Marrow Transplantation. London: Martin Dunitz, 2000.

most intensive conditioning regimens.[5] This observation was predicted in murine experiments in the 1960s that showed that mouse leukemia could only be eradicated by several thousand centiGray (cGy) of total body irradiation (TBI).[10] This level of TBI translates to a dose that is an order of magnitude greater than what is maximally tolerated in humans. Second, allogeneic HSC grafts serve not only to rescue hematopoiesis in a myeloablated patient, but provide a graft-versus-leukemia (GVL) effect that is responsible for many of the observed cures. The allogeneic effect was first predicted by Barnes et al.[11] in murine studies in 1956. In 1965, Mathe et al.[12] termed this effect 'adoptive immunotherapy'. In 1979 and 1981, Weiden et al.[13,14] published the first articles that clearly showed the GVL benefit provided by the allograft by demonstrating that patients after allogeneic HSCT with acute or chronic GVHD had a significantly decreased risk of relapse. These observations were confirmed by other investigators.[15–19] It had been observed that donor buffy coat infusion enhanced engraftment and increased the risk of GVHD.[20] Donor buffy coat infusions were then given to patients to increase the GVL effect of marrow allografts.[21] More recently, donor lymphocyte infusions (DLI) were given as therapy for patients whose leukemia had relapsed after allogeneic transplantation.[22–27]

Attempts to treat relapse with high dose regimens followed by second allografts have been associated with a high incidence of transplant-related mortality.[28–33] At relapse, T lymphocytes are usually still of donor origin and, therefore, immunologically tolerant of host tissues, including the malignant cells. Following relapse after T-cell-depleted marrow transplant, patients are frequently mixed T cell chimeras.[27] Given these findings, Kolb et al. reasoned that donor lymphocytes infused into the recipient would not be rejected and might exert a GVH/GVL effect.[22] There are now many reports on the use of DLI to treat relapse of hematological malignancy after allografting. The largest experience and greatest success have been in patients with CML; complete

responses were seen in 50–80% of patients.[22–27] Patients with complete cytogenetic responses after DLI usually become negative by polymerase chain reaction (PCR) for *bcr-abl* transcripts and experience sustained disease control.[24]

Although fewer patients have been treated, complete remissions have been reported after DLI for relapsed MM, NHL and CLL, as well as acute myeloid leukemia (AML), myelodysplastic syndrome (MDS) and ALL.[34,35] Most data have been reported for MM. In a collation of several small reports, 19 of 25 patients with MM had partial or complete responses to DLI, with sustained complete responses of between 8 and 24 months in four patients.[36–40]

Despite the success of DLI, a mortality of 10–20% has been reported as a result of acute and chronic GVHD. Acute or chronic GVHD occurs in approximately 50% of patients and severe myelosuppression in 15–20% of patients.[24]

Myelosuppression, predominantly seen in patients with CML, was usually reversible as donor marrow cells repopulated the marrow space. The presence of predominantly donor myeloid cells[41] or donor CD34+[42] cells may be protective from aplasia as the donor myeloid elements are not destroyed by the GVH reaction of the donor T cells. Disease response, myelosuppression, and GVHD have usually occurred by 2 months after DLI, but may occur more slowly and be T cell dose dependent.[27] Attempts to reduce the toxicity of DLI have included the use of peripheral blood mononuclear cells (PBMC) administered in a dose escalation scheme based on T cell numbers, selectively removing CD8+ T cells thought to be primarily responsible for GVHD[25,40] and infusing T cells transduced with the suicide gene herpes simplex virus thymidine kinase (*HSV*-TK).[43]

Correlations between the development of GVHD and/or myelosuppression, dose of T cells given and disease response to DLI have been made.[24,26,27] In the setting of a dose escalation study of DLI recipients with relapsed CML and mixed T-cell chimerism, McKinnon et al.[27]

reported that disease response and GVHD were correlated with the dose of T cells (CD3+) infused. Seven of 21 patients treated had complete responses after infusion of relatively low doses of T cells (1×10^7/kg) without the development of GVHD, suggesting that a GVL effect can occur after DLI in the absence of clinical GVHD. At CD3+ cell doses of less than 1×10^7/kg, anti-tumor responses were not observed.

MIXED CHIMERISM AFTER ALLOGENEIC HEMATOPOIETIC STEM CELL TRANSPLANTATION

Relapse after allogeneic HSCT for hematologic malignancy typically presents as a state of mixed hematopoietic chimerism: tolerant donor T cells coexist with malignant host cells. Only in such mixed chimeras is DLI successful; the presence of donor T cells prevents the rejection of infused donor lymphocytes. Disease remission is achieved with conversion to complete donor chimerism and elimination of host malignant cells. Sporadic cases of stable mixed hematopoietic chimerism have also been observed in patients after myeloablative allogeneic transplant. Although the number of cases are few, in patients with non-malignant diseases such as thalassemia major and sickle cell disease stable mixed chimerism has been sufficient to cure phenotypic expression of the inherited hematologic disease.[44,45] Given the success of DLI in converting mixed chimeras to complete donor chimerism, we reasoned that an allotransplant approach intentionally aimed to achieve mixed chimerism could be developed. Without the need to eliminate host hematopoiesis, the myeloablative conditioning regimen for achieving donor engraftment could be reduced. However, decreasing the intensity of the conditioning regimen would increase the risk of allograft rejection.

In the major histocompatibility complex (MHC) identical setting, host-versus-graft (HVG) and GVH reactions are both mediated by T cells.[46] This fact led to studies that asked if postgrafting immunosuppression designed to control GVHD could simultaneously be given to control the HVG reaction, and thereby enhance allogeneic engraftment. Relying on the postgrafting immune suppression to control the HVG reaction might, in turn, reduce the need for intensive and potentially organ-toxic conditioning. Without ablation of host hematopoiesis before infusion of the donor HSC graft, the use of immunosuppression to control the HVG and GVH reactions would permit establishment of mutual graft–host tolerance as manifested by stable mixed donor–host hematopoietic chimerism (Table 20.3). The state of mixed hematopoietic chimerism could serve as a platform for subsequent adoptive immunotherapy with donor lymphocytes. The following section will define mixed chimerism and review the evidence for the assertion that T cells can mediate the HVG and the GVH reactions.

Definition of mixed chimerism

For the purposes of this discussion, mixed chimerism is defined as the presence of 2.5–97.0% hematopoietic cells of donor origin in a recipient after allogeneic transplantation. Mixed chimerism is assessed by genetic markers that unambiguously distinguish the donor from the recipient cells.[47] Conventional cytogenetics, previously used to assess chimerism after sex-mismatched transplants, have limited sensitivity and permit analysis of small numbers of dividing cells. In sex-mismatched transplants, fluorescent in situ hybridization with X and Y chromosome-specific probes evaluates all nucleated cells regardless of proliferation status and permits the evaluation of large numbers of cells and cell subpopulations after cell sorting. Polymerase chain reaction assays of highly polymorphic mini- or microsatellite markers provide accurate mixed chimerism measurement in both sex-matched and sex-mismatched settings. Percentage donor chimerism is accurately quantified using the storage phosphorimaging technique. Assessment of microchimerism (less than 2.5% donor or host

Table 20.3 Outline for non-myeloablative allografting			
Time course	**Therapy**	**Function**	**Effect**
Pretransplant	Immunosuppression (nonmyeloablative)	Control of HVG reaction	(1) Can be given in outpatient department (2) Less toxic than myeloablative conditioning (3) Can be given to a broad range of patients
Transplant	PBSC Stem cell allograft (T cell replete)	Platform for future adoptive immunotherapy	Induce mixed hematopoietic chimerism
Post-transplant: Day 0 to 35 (or 56)	Immunosuppression: MMF/CSP Increased intensity compared to conventional allografting GVHD prophylaxis (but not T cell ablative)	Control both residual HVG and GVH reactions	(1) Stable mixed chimerism (2) Induction of tolerance
After day 60	(1) DLI *or* (2) Taper pharmacologic immunosuppression	Adoptive anti-tumor therapy	(1) Conversion to complete donor chimerism (2) GVL effect (3) Cure of underlying disease

CSP, Cyclosporine; DLI, Donor lymphocyte infusion; GVH, graft-versus-host; GVHD, graft-versus-host disease; GVL, graft-versus-leukemia; HVG, host-versus-graft; MMF, mycophenolate mofetil; PBSC, peripheral blood stem cells.

cells) can be made with more sensitive assays such as PCR using probes to detect rare Y chromosome sequences of male cells transplanted into a female recipient. The presence of residual host hematopoietic cells of malignant origin can be measured by PCR-based assays such as testing for the *bcr-abl* product in patients who have undergone allotransplant for CML.

EVIDENCE THAT HOST-VERSUS-GRAFT AND GRAFT-VERSUS-HOST REACTIONS ARE MEDIATED BY T CELLS

Host T cells mediate graft rejection

Evidence for implicating T lymphocytes as mediators of the HVG and GVH reactions is derived from experimental animal models as well as results from clinical studies of marrow T cell depletion. Marrow transplantation in MHC-mismatched animal models shows that graft rejection is mediated by natural killer (NK) cells and T cells.[46,48] NK-mediated rejection does not involve immunologic priming and occurs within 1–2 days after transplantation if non-self MHC molecules are encountered.[49] The NK cells are negatively regulated by receptors that recognize the presence of self-MHC molecules on target cells. Conversely, T-cell-mediated rejection involves immunologic priming and does not occur until 7–8 days after transplantation in naïve recipients. Activation of T cells occurs through receptors that recognize the presence of non-self MHC molecules or, in the MHC-matched setting, non-self minor histocompatibility peptide antigens on target cells.

In the HLA-identical setting, T lymphocytes mediate graft rejection.[46] Evidence for this was initially obtained in patients with aplastic anemia, where the risk of allograft rejection was increased by pretransplant transfusion-induced sensitization to alloantigens.[50] Second, there was a high incidence of rejection of T-cell-depleted marrow from HLA-identical donors despite myeloablative conditioning.[51–55] In this setting, the onset of rejection was occasionally delayed until several weeks after transplantation, consistent with a T-cell-mediated process. Retrospective studies have shown lower risks of graft rejection associated with higher doses of TBI exposure in the conditioning regimen.[53,56–58] Finally, host-derived lymphocytes with anti-donor HLA-restricted cytotoxic activity have been identified in the blood of patients with graft rejection after T-cell-depleted HLA-mismatched as well as HLA-identical marrow transplantation.[59–65]

Donor T cells mediate graft-versus-host disease

Graft-versus-host disease is initiated by donor T cells that recognize recipient alloantigens.[46] In the MHC-matched setting the alloantigens are the disparate minor histocompatibility antigens.[66] Minor histocompatibility antigens originate from polymorphic proteins encoded by genes outside the MHC. Polymorphisms that produce a single amino acid substitution in a peptide presented by MHC molecules can be sufficient to generate a T cell alloimmune response.[67] Only a few minor histocompatibility antigens have been defined biochemically.[68,69] Genetic studies in mice have identified more than 40 loci that encode minor histocompatibility antigens, most of which have only two or three known alleles.[66] There are probably many more minor histocompatibility antigens in humans. Since these loci are not genetically linked, there is a high probability of at least some disparity for minor histocompatibility antigens between siblings. Because of the greater diversity of alleles in the general population than within families, the probability of disparity between two unrelated individuals is even higher.[70]

Acute GVHD after myeloablative transplant can be prevented by removal of mature T cells from donor marrow. In HLA-identical recipients given no post-transplant immunosuppression, the incidence of grades II–IV acute GVHD decreased from approximately 80% with unmodified marrow[71] to 20% or less when more than 98% of donor T cells were removed.[53,72–74] The benefit of decreased GVHD risk is offset by an increased risk of graft failure and disease relapse.[15,75,76] To decrease the risk of graft failure, several clinical studies have further intensified the myeloablative preparative regimens. This, in turn, has further increased the risk of regimen-related mortality. Because of the increased risk of graft failure and disease relapse, removal of T cells from the donor marrow to prevent GVHD has not been shown to improve disease-free survival after transplant.

IMMUNE MODULATION: ALLOGRAFTS WITH NON-MYELOABLATIVE PRE- AND POST-TRANSPLANT IMMUNOSUPPRESSION

Given that both HVG and GVH reactions are mediated by T cells, the following section describes a series of experiments designed to test whether improved post-grafting immunosuppression given to control GVHD could concurrently control the HVG reaction and thereby promote allogeneic engraftment. Effective post-grafting immune suppression combined with non-myeloablative pregrafting host immune suppression would allow for the establishment of allogeneic stem cell grafts that would create their own marrow space through subclinical GVH reactions. The net effect would be the establishment of mutual graft–host tolerance that would be manifested by stable donor–host hematopoietic chimerism (Table 20.3). This hypothesis was tested in the preclinical canine model in which post-transplant immune suppression was substituted for intensive pretransplant cytotoxic conditioning therapy in a step-wise manner.

Summary of preclinical studies in dogs

The random-bred preclinical dog model has been critical for the development of clinical HSCT protocols used in Seattle over the past 35 years. These include the development of conditioning regimens that result in consistent allogeneic engraftment. Total body irradiation has been an integral part of most conditioning regimens used in patients as well as in the dog model. One of the features of TBI is the simplicity, accuracy and reproducibility with which it delivers immunosuppression. The marrow toxicity of TBI has been extensively studied in the dog model: doses of 400 cGy or greater were marrow lethal, while 200 cGy was sublethal and non-myeloablative.[77]

Low dose total body irradiation followed by DLA-identical marrow and post-grafting immunosuppression

Table 20.4 summarizes the results of marrow grafts from DLA-identical littermates following conditioning with decreasing doses of TBI: 920 cGy TBI without post-grafting immunosuppression was sufficient for stable engraftment in 95% of transplanted dogs.[78,79] When the TBI dose was decreased to 450 cGy, the rate of sustained engraftment decreased unless cyclosporine (CSP) was given after transplant.[80] When the TBI dose was lowered to 200 cGy, CSP alone given after transplant failed to promote donor engraftment.[81] All dogs quickly rejected their allografts, but survived with autologous hematopoietic recovery. We then enhanced postgrafting immunosuppression by combining a synergistic antimetabolite drug with CSP. Mycophenolate mofetil (MMF) blocks the de novo purine synthesis pathway in T and B cells by binding to inosine monophosphate dehydrogenase (IMPDH), thereby selectively inhibiting lymphocyte replication.[82] MMF has been extensively used in the solid organ transplant setting,[83–90] but until recently there was no clinical experience in the allo-HSCT setting.[91] When combined with CSP, MMF was superior to the combination of methotrexate and CSP in prevention of GVHD in dogs.[92] When MMF plus CSP was given following 200 cGy TBI and DLA-identical marrow, 10 of 11 dogs became long-term stable mixed chimeras without evidence of GVHD.[81]

Role of total body irradiation: immunosuppression

The finding that a non-myeloablative dose of TBI is sufficient to permit establishment of donor engraftment has challenged the previously held notion that TBI is necessary to create marrow space for the graft to home. Instead, what has emerged is the appreciation that the most likely role of TBI is to provide immunosuppression (Table 20.4). To test this question,

Table 20.4 Effect of decreasing total body irradiation (TBI) and increasing postgrafting immunosuppression: marrow grafts from DLA-identical canine littermates after single-dose TBI (7 cGy/min)[78–81,94]

TBI dose (cGy)	Postgrafting immunosuppression	No. of dogs sustained (allografted/studied)
920	–	20/21
450	–	16/39
	Prednisone†	0/5
	CSP‡	7/7
200	CSP	0/4
	MTX§ + CSP	2/5
	MMF¶ + CSP	11/12
100	MMF + CSP	0/6

DLA, dog leukocyte antigen.
† Prednisone: 25 mg/kg per day p.o. days −5 to −3 with tapering to day 32.
‡ Cyclosporine, CSP: 15 mg/kg/b.i.d. p.o. days −1 to 35.
§Methotrexate, MTX: 0.4 mg/kg i.v. days 1, 3, 6 and 11.
¶Mycophenolate mofetil, MMF: 10 mg/kg b.i.d. s.c. days 0 to 27.

dogs were given a non-myeloablative regimen of 450-cGy irradiation to cervical, thoracic and abdominal lymph nodes, while completely shielding most of the marrow-containing bones with lead blocks. Following DLA-identical littermate marrow grafts and post-grafting MMF/CSP, all dogs developed mixed hematopoietic chimerism. Serial marrow samples obtained from unirradiated (shielded) bones showed stable mixed chimerism as early as 4 weeks after transplant.[93] This finding supports the hypothesis that marrow grafts can create their own marrow space, probably through subclinical GVH reactions, and further suggests that pretransplant irradiation can ultimately be replaced by more specific and less toxic means of T cell suppression.

All dogs conditioned with 100-cGy TBI fol-lowed by MMF/CSP rejected their DLA-identi-cal marrow grafts.[94] We asked if stable engraft-ment after 100-cGy TBI could be accomplished by first reducing the HVG reaction with the use of CTLA4Ig. This fusion peptide blocks both T cell costimulation through the B7-CD28 signal pathway and CTLA4-mediated T cell inhibi-tion.[95–101] To induce specific host T cell hypore-sponsiveness, dogs were given CTLA4Ig and donor peripheral blood mononuclear cells before a single dose of 100-cGy TBI. Following transplant of DLA-identical littermate marrow and post-grafting MMF/CSP, all recipients showed initial mixed chimerism and 66% developed long-term stable chimerism.[94] This study suggests that the additional blockade of other costimulatory signals may permit the lowering of the TBI dose further or even the complete elimination of TBI in the current canine model of stem cell transplantation.

Allogeneic transplantation: clinical studies using non-myeloablative total body irradiation and post-grafting immunosuppression

The canine studies were translated to a clinical study of treatment of hematologic malignancies with non-myeloablative allogeneic HSCT for patients who were not eligible for treatment with a conventional allotransplant. The regimen consisted of pretransplant TBI, 200 cGy, given as a single fraction at 7 cGy/min, CSP given at 12.5 mg/kg per day p.o. from day −1 to at least day 35, and MMF at 15 mg/kg per day p.o. b.i.d. from day 0 to day 27. Granulocyte colony stimulating factor (G-CSF) mobilized peripheral blood stem cells from HLA-identical sibling donors were infused on day 0 within 4 h after TBI. From December 1997 to May 1999, 45 patients with a median age of 56 years (range 31–72) were treated using this protocol.[102] Transplants were performed at FHCRC in Seattle and at two collaborating institutions, Stanford University and the University of Leipzig, Germany. Patients were transplanted for AML ($n = 11$), CML ($n = 9$), MM ($n = 8$), CLL ($n = 8$), HD ($n = 4$), Waldenström's macroglobulinemia (WM; $n = 2$), NHL ($n = 1$), ALL ($n = 1$) and advanced MDS ($n = 1$).

The regimen was extremely well tolerated and, in most patients, transplants were performed entirely in the outpatient setting. Patients did not experience mucositis or alopecia, had minimal nausea and vomiting, and had very mild myelosuppression. In those patients who had near normal peripheral blood counts at the time of transplant, there was no need, in most cases, for platelet or red blood cell transfusions. All patients had primary engraftment with mixed or complete donor chimerism present through at least 2 months after transplant.

With a median follow-up of 14 months, some important observations and clinical benefits have become apparent (Table 20.5). Considering the historical results of myeloablative allografting in elderly patients, transplant-related mortality was very low at 6.7%. Death in these three patients occurred at 2, 2 and 12 months and was due to infection following prednisone therapy for GVHD. Relapse mortality was 27%.

Graft rejection occurred in nine of 45 patients between 2 and 4 months after transplant, with recovery of autologous hematopoiesis. Because the preparative regimen was non-myeloablative, all episodes of graft rejection were non-fatal.

Table 20.5 Summary of the first 45 patients with hematologic malignancies treated with 200 cGy total body irradiation (TBI) followed by HLA-identical peripheral blood stem cell transplantation and post-grafting mycophenolate mofetil/cyclosporine

Follow-up	137–586 days
Initial donor engraftment	100%
Graft rejection (non-fatal)	20%
Acute graft-versus-host-disease	47% of patients without rejection
Transplant-related mortality	6.7%
Relapse mortality	27%*

* Includes the two patients with disease relapse who subsequently were treated with myeloablative conventional allogeneic bone marrow transplant.

Rejection occurred in patients who had received no or minimal pretransplant chemotherapy. Among these first 45 patients, the risk of graft rejection was increased for those who had establishment of less than 50% donor T cell chimerism by day 28. It is noteworthy that 28 of 29 (97%) patients with pretransplant exposure to intensive chemotherapy or to multiple cycles of purine analogs had sustained high levels of donor engraftment.[103]

Acute GVHD developed in 47% of patients who did not reject the donor graft. In general, the onset of acute GVHD occurred after the MMF was discontinued on day 27. Of the patients with sustained donor engraftment, 36% and 11% had grade II and III GVHD, respectively. Graft-versus-host disease was readily managed with continuation of cyclosporine and the addition of a course of corticosteroids.

The role of DLI was limited due to the relatively high incidence of clinical or subclinical GVHD. Most patients converted to complete donor chimerism without DLI. In 14 patients, DLI was given for persistent disease or disease progression. Four patients went into complete remission 1–3 months following DLI, five had no disease response and three patients were inevaluable due to concurrent other therapy ($n = 2$) or death from infection ($n = 1$).

Significant disease responses were observed in 16 of 29 patients who had measurable disease pretransplant and who sustained donor engraftment after transplant. These included five CML patients, each of whom achieved a complete molecular response within 6 months after allografting. These patients remain *bcr-abl-*negative by PCR in peripheral blood and bone marrow.

Non-myeloablative allografting has also been achieved in patients with multiple myeloma. Five patients received an autologous PBSC transplant prior to the non-myeloablative allogeneic PBSC transplant. All patients treated in this manner had sustained donor engraftment. Four patients entered into a complete molecular remission following the allograft and one patient died from disease progression.[102]

Summary of clinical non-myeloablative allotransplant results

The results from this study strongly indicate that allografting can be accomplished in the outpatient setting without significant toxicity. It is clear that disease remission can be achieved; however, with limited follow-up, the durability of the complete remissions remains to be determined. None the less, these early responses emphasize the potency of an allogeneic GVL effect independent of cytoreductive therapy. Based on these limited patient data, several observations can be made. The non-myeloablative regimen emphasizes immune modulation, specifically, post-grafting immune suppression, rather than intensive conditioning. The tempo of donor engraftment with the new allogeneic transplantation procedure was more gradual and was completed over a longer time period than the conventional allotransplant method. In most patients there was a gradual progression of increasing donor chimerism combined with the simultaneous progression of a controlled GVH/GVL reaction. Because of the superiority of the synergistic immunosuppression of combined MMF and CSP, there was a delayed onset of occurrence of GVHD which was clinically less severe than would be predicted following myeloablative conditioning. With less organ toxicity from the non-myeloablative TBI, CSP levels were maintained in the high therapeutic range without compromising kidney or hepatic function. For most patients studied, the administration of 200-cGy TBI provided sufficient immunosuppression such that the donor PBSC graft maintained the immunologic advantage during the combined postgrafting MMF/CSP.

Modification of non-myeloablative allotransplant regimen

Based on the successful results of the first 45 patients treated with this well-tolerated non-myeloablative regimen, a modification to the treatment protocol was made, aimed at decreasing the risk of donor graft rejection (Fig. 20.2). Other investigators have reported that fludarabine can be successfully incorporated into a less toxic conditioning regimen for allogeneic HSCT.[104–107] Thus, for patients with CML and those who have not had prior autologous HSCT, we have added a relatively low dose of intravenous fludarabine, 30 mg/m^2 per day given on days −4, −3 and −2, before 200-cGy TBI and donor PBSC. Administration of postgrafting MMF continues as described, with CSP taper beginning on day +56. The addition of fludarabine has not resulted in any apparent increased toxicity.

Preliminary results using matched unrelated donors in establishing mixed chimerism with the non-myeloablative regimen of fludarabine (30 mg/m^2 × 3) and 200-cGy TBI have also shown successful donor engraftment, although the risk of GVHD is likely to be increased.[108] Hence, the postgrafting immunosuppression

with MMF and CSP is extended beyond the 28 and 35+ days, respectively.

FUTURE DIRECTIONS

The development of non-myeloablative conditioning programs will move the stem cell transplants from the current intensive inpatient care setting to the outpatient clinic. Beyond increased safety and patient satisfaction, this approach will significantly reduce the cost of transplants. Establishment of mixed chimerism following non-myelotoxic conditioning could be applied to several settings. These include patients with hematologic malignancies, aplastic anemia, genetic diseases of the hematopoietic system (e.g. sickle cell disease), and severe autoimmune disease (e.g. systemic sclerosis). In

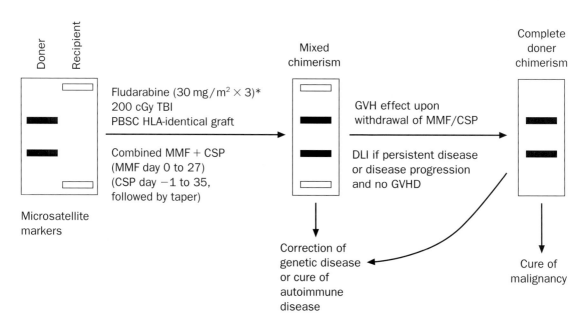

Figure 20.2

Schema for treatment of patients with malignant and non-malignant hematologic diseases with non-myeloablative allogeneic hematopoietic stem cell transplantation.

*The addition of fludarabine is reserved for patients with either no or minimal pretransplant chemotherapy who are at risk for graft rejection.

addition, victims of radiation accidents and candidates for transplants of solid organs may benefit. In patients with hematologic malignancies, achieving mixed chimerism is a temporary goal, with conversion to complete donor chimerism necessary for underlying disease eradication. Some patients will require DLI but many patients achieve complete donor chimerism through a persistent overt or subclinical GVH reaction. In other clinical settings, it is likely that establishing stable mixed chimerism will by itself be sufficient to treat the disease, for example in patients with genetic diseases or aplastic anemia, or in radiation accidents. In these settings, delayed taper of postgrafting immunosuppression to prevent GVHD may be optimal. For patients with T cell immunodeficiency, allogeneic HSCT without pretransplant conditioning and only post-grafting MMF/CSP has achieved mixed chimerism and clinical improvement.[109] In future studies we will assess whether mixed chimerism may serve as a platform for immunotherapy of solid tumors such as melanoma, renal cell carcinoma and gastrointestinal tract malignancies. We will also study whether non-myeloablative allotransplants can improve immune reconstitution in patients with advanced HIV infection. Patients eligible for allotransplant will be those with low CD4+ cells despite good control of viral replication receiving highly active antiretroviral therapy. In addition, we will study whether patients with HIV-related lymphoma may have favorable disease response to an allograft established with the non-myeloablative regimen.

CONCLUSIONS

The concepts presented in this chapter are based on the postulates that the current intensive cytoreductive and toxic conditioning regimens can be replaced by non-myelotoxic immunosuppression and that T-cell-replete allogeneic stem cell grafts can create their own space in the marrow through a GVH reaction. Since HVG and GVH reactions are mediated by T cells,

immunosuppression administered before infusion of donor hematopoietic stem cells is directed exclusively at reducing HVG reactions, while immunosuppression given after transplantation is aimed at both eliminating residual HVG responses and controlling GVH reactions originating in donor cells. Based on results in the dog model with lymph node irradiation, it is clear that pretransplant TBI does not function to create marrow space, but rather to provide immunosuppression. In addition, the results of CTLA4Ig and 100-cGy TBI with postgrafting MMF/CSP suggest that, with improved pretransplant immunosuppression directed at host T cells only, future studies may be able to eliminate TBI altogether. Stable mixed chimerism and mutual graft–host tolerance is achieved because of the successful control of the HVG and GVH reactions. Results from the clinical study suggest that in many cases some GVH reactions persist after withdrawal of MMF – either overtly as readily controlled GVHD, or subclinically as gradual conversion to complete donor chimerism. In addition, conversion to complete donor chimerism and eradication of residual diseases can be induced by subsequent adoptive immunotherapy with infusion of donor lymphocytes.

REFERENCES

1. Jacobson LO, Marks EK, Robson MJ et al. Effect of spleen protection on mortality following X-irradiation. J Lab Clin Med 1949;34:1538–43.
2. Nowell PC, Cole LJ, Habermeyer JG, Roan PL. Growth and continued function of rat marrow cells in x-radiated mice. Cancer Res 1956;16:258–61.
3. Ford CE, Hamerton JL, Barnes DWH, Loutit JF. Cytological identification of radiation-chimaeras. Nature 1956;177:452–4.
4. Main JM, Prehn RT. Successful skin homografts after the administration of high dosage X radiation and homologous bone marrow. J Natl Cancer Inst 1955;15:1023–9.
5. Thomas ED, Storb R, Clift RA et al. Bone-marrow transplantation. N Engl J Med 1975; 292:832–43, 895–902.

6. Ringdén O, Horowitz MM, Gale RP et al. Outcome after allogeneic bone marrow transplant for leukemia in older adults. JAMA 1993;270:57–60.

7. Hansen JA, Gooley TA, Martin PJ et al. Bone marrow transplants from unrelated donors for patients with chronic myeloid leukemia. N Engl J Med 1998;338:962–8.

8. Clift RA, Buckner CD, Storb R et al. The influence of patient age on the outcome of transplantation during chronic phase (CP) of chronic myeloid leukemia (CML). Blood 1995;86:617 (abstract).

9. SEER Cancer Statistics Review, 1973–1992. Tables and Graphs. Bethesda: NCI, 1995.

10. Burchenal JH, Oettgen HF, Holmberg EAD et al. Effect of total body irradiation on the transplantability of mouse leukemias. Cancer Res 1960;20:425.

11. Barnes DWH, Corp MJ, Loutit JF, Neal FE. Treatment of murine leukaemia with X-rays and homologous bone marrow. Preliminary communication. BMJ 1956;2:626–7.

12. Mathe G, Amiel JL, Schwarzenberg L et al. Adoptive immunotherapy of acute leukemia: Experimental and clinical results. Cancer Res 1965;25:1525–31.

13. Weiden PL, Flournoy N, Thomas ED et al. Antileukemic effect of graft-versus-host disease in human recipients of allogeneic-marrow grafts. N Engl J Med 1979;300:1068–73.

14. Weiden PL, Sullivan KM, Flournoy N et al. Antileukemic effect of chronic graft-versus-host disease. Contribution to improved survival after allogeneic marrow transplantation. N Engl J Med 1981;304:1529–33.

15. Horowitz MM, Gale RP, Sondel PM et al. Graft-versus-leukemia reactions after bone marrow transplantation. Blood 1990;75:555–62.

16. Butturini A, Bortin MM, Gale RP. Graft-versus-leukemia following bone marrow transplantation. Bone Marrow Transplant 1987;2:233–42.

17. Kersey JH, Weisdorf D, Nesbit ME et al. Comparison of autologous and allogeneic bone marrow transplantation for treatment of high-risk refractory acute lymphoblastic leukemia. N Engl J Med 1987;317:461–7.

18. Weisdorf DJ, Nesbit ME, Ramsay NKC et al. Allogeneic bone marrow transplantation for acute lymphoblastic leukemia in remission: prolonged survival associated with acute graft-versus-host disease. J Clin Oncol 1987;5:1348–55.

19. Sullivan KM, Weiden PL, Storb R et al. Influence of acute and chronic graft-versus-host disease on relapse and survival after bone marrow transplantation from HLA-identical siblings as treatment of acute and chronic leukemia. Blood 1989;73:1720–8.

20. Storb R, Doney KC, Thomas ED et al. Marrow transplantation with or without donor buffy coat cells for 65 transfused aplastic anemia patients. Blood 1982;59:236–46.

21. Sullivan KM, Storb R, Buckner CD et al. Graft-versus-host disease as adoptive immunotherapy in patients with advanced hematologic neoplasms. N Engl J Med 1989;320:828–34.

22. Kolb HJ, Mittermüller J, Clemm Ch et al. Donor leukocyte transfusions for treatment of recurrent chronic myelogenous leukemia in marrow transplant patients. Blood 1990;76:2462–5.

23. Porter DL, Roth MS, McGarigle C et al. Induction of graft-versus-host disease as immunotherapy for relapsed chronic myeloid leukemia. N Engl J Med 1994;330:100–6.

24. Kolb HJ, Schattenberg A, Goldman JM et al. Graft-versus-leukemia effect of donor lymphocyte transfusions in marrow grafted patients. European Group for Blood and Marrow Transplantation Working Party Chronic Leukemia. Blood 1995;86:2041–50.

25. Giralt S, Hester J, Huh Y et al. CD8-Depleted donor lymphocyte infusion as treatment for relapsed chronic myelogenous leukemia after allogeneic bone marrow transplantation. Blood 1995;86:4337–43.

26. Collins RH, Jr., Shpilberg O, Drobyski WR et al. Donor leukocyte infusions in 140 patients with relapsed malignancy after allogeneic bone marrow transplantation. J Clin Oncol 1997;15:433–44.

27. MacKinnon S, Papadopoulos EB, Carabasi MH et al. Adoptive immunotherapy evaluating escalating doses of donor leukocytes for relapse of chronic myeloid leukemia after bone marrow transplantation: separation of graft-versus-leukemia responses from graft-versus-host disease. Blood 1995;86:1261–8.

28. Wright SE, Thomas ED, Buckner CD et al. Experience with second marrow transplants. Exp Hematol 1976;4:221–6.

29. Atkinson K, Biggs J, Concannon A et al. Second marrow transplants for recurrence of haematological malignancy. Bone Marrow Transplant 1986;1:159–66.

30. Blume KG, Forman SJ. High dose busulfan/ etoposide as a preparatory regimen for second bone marrow transplants in hematologic malignancies. Blut 1987;55:49–53.

31. Champlin RE, Ho WG, Lenarsky C et al. Successful second bone marrow transplants for treatment of acute myelogenous leukemia or acute lymphoblastic leukemia. Transplant Proc 1985;17:496–9.

32. Radich JP, Sanders JE, Buckner CD et al. Second allogeneic marrow transplantation for patients with recurrent leukemia after initial transplant with total-body irradiation-containing regimens. J Clin Oncol 1993;11:304–13.

33. Mrsic M, Horowitz MM, Atkinson K et al. Second HLA-identical sibling transplants for leukemia recurrence. Bone Marrow Transplant 1992;9:269–75.

34. Kolb H-J. Management of relapse after hematopoietic cell transplantation. In: Thomas ED, Blume KG, Forman SJ, editors. Hematopoietic cell transplantation, 2nd edn. Boston: Blackwell Science, 1999:929–36.

35. Rondon G, Giralt S, Huh Y et al. Graft-versus-leukemia effect after allogeneic bone marrow transplantation for chronic lymphocytic leukemia. Bone Marrow Transplant 1996;18: 669–72.

36. Bertz H, Burger JA, Kunzmann R et al. Adoptive immunotherapy for relapsed multiple myeloma after allogeneic bone marrow transplantation (BMT): evidence for a graft-versus-myeloma effect. Leukemia 1997;11:281–3.

37. Tricot G, Vesole DH, Jagannath S et al. Graft-versus-myeloma effect: proof of principle. Blood 1996;87:1196–8.

38. Lokhorst HM, Schattenberg A, Cornelissen JJ et al. Donor leukocyte infusions are effective in relapsed multiple myeloma after allogeneic bone marrow transplantation. Blood 1997;90: 4206–11.

39. Aschan J, Lonnqvist B, Ringden O et al. Graft-versus-myeloma effect [Letter]. Lancet 1996;348: 346.

40. Alyea EP, Soiffer RJ, Canning C et al. Toxicity and efficacy of defined doses of CD+ donor lymphocytes for treatment of relapse after allogeneic bone marrow transplant. Blood 1998;91: 3671–80.

41. van Rhee F, Lin F, Cullis JO et al. Relapse of chronic myeloid leukemia after allogeneic bone marrow transplant: the case for giving donor leukocyte transfusions before the onset of hematologic relapse. Blood 1994;83:3377–83.

42. Keil F, Haas OA, Fritsch G et al. Donor leukocyte infusion for leukemic relapse after allogeneic marrow transplantation: lack of residual donor hematopoiesis predicts aplasia. Blood 1997;89:3113–17.

43. Bonini C, Ferrari G, Verzeletti S et al. HSV-TK gene transfer into donor lymphocytes for control of allogeneic graft-versus leukemia. Science 1997;276:1719–24.

44. Andreani M, Manna M, Lucarelli G et al. Persistence of mixed chimerism in patients transplanted for the treatment of thalassemia. Blood 1996;87:3494–9.

45. Walters MC, Patience M, Leisenring W et al. Bone marrow transplantation for sickle cell disease. N Engl J Med 1996;335:369–76.

46. Martin PJ. Overview of marrow transplantation immunology. In: Thomas ED, Blume KG, Forman SJ, editors. Hematopoietic cell transplantation, 2nd edn. Boston: Blackwell Science, 1999:19–27.

47. Bryant E, Martin PJ. Documentation of engraftment and characterization of chimerism following hematopoietic cell transplantation. In: Thomas ED, Blume KG, Forman SJ, editors. Hematopoietic cell transplantation, 2nd edn. Boston: Blackwell Science, 1999:197–206.

48. Murphy WJ, Kumar V, Bennett M. Acute rejection of murine bone marrow allografts by natural killer cells and T cells. Differences in kinetics and target antigens recognized. J Exp Med 1987;166:1499–509.

49. Murphy WJ, Kumar V, Cope JC, Bennett M. An absence of T cells in murine bone marrow allografts leads to an increased susceptibility to rejection by natural killer cells and T cells. J Immunol 1990;144:3305–11.

50. Doney K, Leisenring W, Storb R et al. Primary treatment of acquired aplastic anemia: outcomes with bone marrow transplantation and immunosuppressive therapy. Ann Intern Med 1997;126:107–15.

51. O'Reilly RJ, Collins NH, Kernan N et al. Transplantation of marrow-depleted T cells by soybean lectin agglutination and E-rosette depletion: major histocompatibility complex-related graft resistance in leukemic transplant recipients. Transplant Proc 1985;17:455–9.

52. Martin PJ, Hansen JA, Buckner CD et al. Effects of in vitro depletion of T cells in HLA-identical allogeneic marrow grafts. Blood 1985;66:664–72.

53. Marmont AM, Horowitz MM, Gale RP et al. T-Cell depletion of HLA-identical transplants in leukemia. Blood 1991;78:2120–30.

54. Wagner JE, Donnenberg AD, Noga SJ et al. Lymphocyte depletion of donor bone marrow by counterflow centrifugal elutriation: results of a phase I clinical trial. Blood 1988;72:1168–76.

55. Kernan NA, Bordignon C, Heller G et al. Graft failure after T-cell-depleted human leukocyte antigen identical marrow transplants for leukemia: I. Analysis of risk factors and results of secondary transplants. Blood 1989;74:2227–36.

56. Burnett AK, Robertson AG, Hann IM et al. In vitro T-depletion of allogeneic bone marrow prevention of rejection in HLA-matched transplants by increased TBI. Bone Marrow Transplant 1986;1(suppl 1):121.

57. Martin PJ, Hansen JA, Torok-Storb B et al. Graft failure in patients receiving T cell-depleted HLA-identical allogeneic marrow transplants. Bone Marrow Transplant 1988;3:445–56.

58. Patterson J, Prentice HG, Brenner MK et al. Graft rejection following HLA-matched T-lymphocyte depleted bone marrow transplantation. Br J Haematol 1986;63:221–30.

59. Kernan NA, Flomenberg N, Dupont B, O'Reilly RJ. Graft rejection in recipients of T-cell-depleted HLA-nonidentical marrow transplants for leukemia. Transplantation 1987;43:842–7.

60. Donohue J, Homge M, Kernan NA. Characterization of cells emerging at the time of graft failure after bone marrow transplantation from an unrelated marrow donor. Blood 1993;82:1023–9.

61. Bosserman LD, Murray C, Takvorian T et al. Mechanism of graft failure in HLA-matched and HLA-mismatched bone marrow transplant recipients. Bone Marrow Transplant 1989;4:239–45.

62. Bordignon C, Keever CA, Small TN et al. Graft failure after T-cell-depleted human leukocyte antigen identical marrow transplants for leukemia: II. In vitro analyses of host effector mechanisms. Blood 1989;74:2237–43.

63. Voogt PJ, Fibbe WE, Marijt WAF et al. Rejection of bone-marrow graft by recipient-derived cytotoxic T lymphocytes against minor histocompatibility antigens. Lancet 1990;i:131–4.

64. Marijt WA, Kernan NA, Diaz-Barrientos T et al. Multiple minor histocompatibility antigen-specific cytotoxic T lymphocyte clones can be generated during graft rejection after HLA-identical bone marrow transplantation. Bone Marrow Transplant 1995;16:125–32.

65. Bunjes D, Heit W, Arnold R et al. Evidence for the involvement of host-derived OKT8-positive T cells in the rejection of T-depleted, HLA-identical bone marrow grafts. Transplantation 1987;43:501–5.

66. Simpson E. Minor transplantation antigens: animal models for human host-versus-graft, graft-versus-host, and graft-versus-leukemia reactions [Review]. Transplantation 1998;65:611–16.

67. den Haan JM, Meadows LM, Wang W et al. The minor histocompatibility antigen HA-1: a diallelic gene with a single amino acid polymorphism. Science 1998;269:1054–7.

68. Goulmy E, Schipper J, Pool J et al. Mismatches of minor histocompatibility antigens between HLA-identical donors and recipients and the development of graft-versus-host disease after bone marrow transplantation. N Engl J Med 1996;334:281–5.

69. den Haan JM, Sherman NE, Blokland E et al. Identification of a graft versus host disease-associated human minor histocompatibility antigen. Science 1995;268:1476–80.

70. Martin PJ. Increased disparity for minor histocompatibility antigens as a potential cause of increased GVHD risk in marrow transplantation from unrelated donors compared with related donors. Bone Marrow Transplant 1991; 8:217–23.

71. Sullivan KM, Deeg HJ, Sanders J et al. Hyperacute graft-v-host disease in patients not given immunosuppression after allogeneic marrow transplantation [Concise report]. Blood 1986;67:1172–5.

72. Antin JH, Bierer BE, Smith BR et al. Selective depletion of bone marrow T lymphocytes with anti-CD5 monoclonal antibodies: effective prophylaxis for graft-versus-host disease in patients with hematologic malignancies. Blood 1991;78:2139–49.

73. Soiffer RJ, Murray C, Mauch P et al. Prevention of graft-versus-host disease by selective depletion of CD6-positive T lymphocytes from donor bone marrow. J Clin Oncol 1992;10:1191–200.

74. Young JW, Papadopoulos EB, Cunningham I et al. T-cell-depleted allogeneic bone marrow transplantation in adults with acute nonlymphocytic leukemia in first remission. Blood 1992;79:3380–7.

75. Goldman JM, Gale RP, Horowitz MM et al. Bone marrow transplantation for chronic myelogenous leukemia in chronic phase: increased risk of relapse associated with T-cell depletion. Ann Intern Med 1988;108:806–14.

76. Martin PJ, Clift RA, Fisher LD et al. HLA-Identical marrow transplantation during accelerated phase chronic myelogenous leukemia: analysis of survival and remission duration. Blood 1988;72:1978–84.

77. Storb R, Raff RF, Graham T et al. Marrow toxicity of fractionated versus single dose total body irradiation is identical in a canine model. Int J Radiat Oncol Biol Phys 1993;26:275–83.

78. Storb R, Raff RF, Appelbaum FR et al. What radiation dose for DLA-identical canine marrow grafts? Blood 1988;72:1300–4.

79. Storb R, Raff RF, Appelbaum FR et al. DLA-Identical bone marrow grafts after low-dose total body irradiation: the effect of canine recombinant hematopoietic growth factors. Blood 1994;84:3558–66.

80. Yu C, Storb R, Mathey B et al. DLA-Identical bone marrow grafts after low-dose total body irradiation: effects of high-dose corticosteroids and cyclosporine on engraftment. Blood 1995;86:4376–81.

81. Storb R, Yu C, Wagner JL et al. Stable mixed hematopoietic chimerism in DLA-identical littermate dogs given sublethal total body irradiation before and pharmacological immunosuppression after marrow transplantation. Blood 1997;89:3048–54.

82. Allison AC, Eugui EM. Purine metabolism and immunosuppressive effects of mycophenolate mofetil (MMF) [Review]. Clin Transplant 1996;10:77–84.

83. Sollinger HW, for the US Renal Transplant Mycophenolate Mofetil Study Group. Mycophenolate mofetil for the prevention of acute rejection in primary cadaveric renal allograft recipients. Transplantation 1995;60:225–32.

84. Sollinger HW. Update on preclinical and clinical experience with mycophenolate mofetil [Review]. Transplant Proc 1996;28:24–9.

85. Shapiro R, Jordan ML, Scantlebury VP et al. A prospective, randomized trial to compare tacrolimus and prednisone with and without mycophenolate mofetil in patients undergoing renal transplantation: first report. J Urol 1998;160:1982–5.

86. Mathew TH. A blinded, long-term, randomized multicenter study of mycophenolate mofetil in cadaveric renal transplantation: results at three years. Transplantation 1998;65:1450–4.

87. US Renal Transplant Mycophenolate Mofetil Study Group. Mycophenolate mofetil in cadaveric renal transplantation. Am J Kidney Dis 1999;34:296–303.

88. European Mycophenolate Mofetil Cooperative Study Group. Mycophenolate mofetil in renal transplantation: 3-year results from the placebo-controlled trial. Transplantation 1999;68:391–6.

89. Jain AB, Hamad I, Rakela J et al. A prospective randomized trial of tacrolimus and prednisone versus tacrolimus, prednisone, and mycophenolate mofetil in primary adult liver transplant recipients: an interim report. Transplantation 1998;66:1395–8.

90. Fisher RA, Ham JM, Marcos A et al. A prospective randomized trial of mycophenolate mofetil with neoral or tacrolimus after orthotopic liver transplantation. Transplantation 1998;66:1616–21.

91. Mookerjee B, Altomonte V, Vogelsang G. Salvage therapy for refractory chronic graft-versus-host disease with mycophenolate mofetil and tacrolimus. Bone Marrow Transplant 1999;24:517–20.

92. Yu C, Seidel K, Nash RA et al. Synergism between mycophenolate mofetil and cyclosporine in preventing graft-versus-host disease among lethally irradiated dogs given DLA-nonidentical unrelated marrow grafts. Blood 1998;91:2581–7.

93. Storb R, Yu C, Barnett T et al. Stable mixed hematopoietic chimerism in dog leukocyte antigen-identical littermate dogs given lymph node irradiation before and pharmacologic immunosuppression after marrow transplantation. Blood 1999;94:1131–6.

94. Storb R, Yu C, Zaucha JM et al. Stable mixed hematopoietic chimerism in dogs given donor antigen, CTLA4Ig, and 100 cGy total body irradiation before and pharmacologic immunosuppression after marrow transplant. Blood 1999;94:2523–9.

95. Allison JP, Krummel MF. The Yin and Yang of T cell costimulation [Review]. Science 1995;270:932–3.

96. Lee KM, Chuang E, Griffin M et al. Molecular basis of T cell inactivation by CTLA-4. Science 1998;282:2263–6.

97. Shahinian A, Pfeffer K, Lee KP et al. Differential

T cell costimulatory requirements in CD28-deficient mice. Science 1993;261:609–12.

98. Kundig TM, Shahinian A, Kawai K et al. Duration of TCR stimulation determines costimulatory requirement of T cells. Immunity 1996;5:41–52.

99. Judge TA, Tang A, Spain LM et al. The in vivo mechanism of action of CTLA4Ig. J Immunol 1996;156:2294–9.

100. Gribben JG, Guinan EC, Boussiotis VA et al. Complete blockade of B7 family-mediated costimulation is necessary to induce human alloantigen-specific anergy: a method to ameliorate graft-versus-host disease and extend the donor pool. Blood 1996;87:4887–93.

101. Gribben JG, Freeman GJ, Boussiotis VA et al. CTLA4 mediates antigen-specific apoptosis of human T cells. Proc Natl Acad Sci USA 1995; 92:811–15.

102. McSweeney P, Niederwiser D, Shizuru JA et al. Hematopoietic cell transplantation in older patients with hematogic malignancies: replacing high-dose cytotoxic therapy with graft-versus-tumor effects. Blood 2001;97:3390–400.

103. Molina A, McSweeney P, Maloney DG et al. Degree of early donor T-cell chimerism predicts GVHD and graft rejection in patients with non-myeloablative hematopoietic stem cell allografts. Blood 1999;94 (suppl 1):394 (abstract 1745).

104. Giralt S, Estey E, Albitar M et al. Engraftment of allogeneic hematopoietic progenitor cells with purine analog-containing chemotherapy: harnessing graft-versus-leukemia without myeloablative therapy. Blood 1997;89:4531–6.

105 Khouri IF, Keating M, Körbling M et al. Transplant-lite: induction of graft-versus-malignancy using fludarabine-based nonablative chemotherapy and allogeneic blood progenitor-cell transplantation as treatment for lymphoid malignancies. J Clin Oncol 1998;16:2817–24.

106. Slavin S, Nagler A, Naparstek E et al. Nonmyeloablative stem cell transplantation and cell therapy as an alternative to conventional bone marrow transplantation with lethal cytoreduction for the treatment of malignant and nonmalignant hematologic diseases. Blood 1998;91:756–63.

107. Childs R, Clave E, Contentin N et al. Engraftment kinetics after nonmyeloablative allogeneic peripheral blood stem cell transplantation: full donor T-cell chimerism precedes alloimmune responses. Blood 1999;94:3234–41.

108. Niederwieser D, Wolff D, Hegenbart U et al. Hematopoietic stem cell transplants (HSCT) from HLA-matched and one-allele mismatched unrelated donors using a nonmyeloablative regimen. Blood 1999;94(suppl 1):561 (abstract 2506).

109. Woolfrey AE, Nash RA, Frangoul HA et al. Non-myeloablative transplant regimen used for induction of multi-lineage allogeneic hematopoietic mixed donor-host chimerism in patients with T-cell immunodeficiency. Blood 1998;92 (suppl 1):520 (abstract).

Part 4

Current and future developments

21

Gene therapy of cancer

Stephen Devereux

CONTENTS Introduction • Vector technology • Strategies for gene therapy of cancer • Ethical, regulatory and safety issues • Future prospects

INTRODUCTION

Malignant tumours develop through the accumulation of mutations in critical genes controlling cell growth, differentiation or apoptosis, and the ideal cancer therapy should therefore target these abnormalities. This might be achieved by chemically inhibiting or bypassing abnormal gene products or by correcting the underlying genetic lesions in each tumour cell. The former lies within the remit of conventional pharmacology, and exciting new drugs such as the tyrosine kinase inhibitor STI-571 in chronic myeloid leukaemia look extremely promising in this regard.[1] The latter is more challenging since it will require the development of a new technology, that of gene therapy, with the ability to target, repair or replace damaged genes. Gene therapy may also be used to modify cellular function in ways that assist cancer treatment, for example by promoting the anti-tumour effects of the immune system or of other more conventional modalities such as chemotherapy. Although there is much to learn, the first steps towards the gene therapy of cancer have been taken and important lessons learnt. This chapter will summarize progress to date, focus on some of the areas that are currently limiting progress and illustrate some of the gene therapy strategies that may be useful

in future. Anti-sense therapy with synthetic oligonucleotides is not discussed as it depends on different technology and is subject to different regulatory rules.

VECTOR TECHNOLOGY

The primary requirement for gene therapy is for a safe and efficient method of delivering the therapeutic gene to the target cell. Whilst physical or chemical gene transfer methods such as electroporation or calcium phosphate-mediated transfection are usually adequate for in vitro experiments, primary cells generally require the use of viral vectors. Although it may eventually be possible to design completely synthetic agents, current vectors are based on well-studied human or animal viruses. Vectors based on murine retroviruses were first developed in the 1980s by replacing viral structural genes with the gene of interest and using a packaging or helper cell line transfected with the deleted genes to provide the molecules required for virus production.[2] Provided that recombination between packager and viral genomes does not occur, the resulting viruses do not carry structural genes and should be incapable of replication. Similar systems have been devised for other viruses; however, none of the current

Table 21.1 Current gene therapy vectors

Vector	Advantage	Disadvantage	Application
Murine leukaemia virus based retroviruses	Well characterized. Integrates into genome. Pseudotypes available	Low titre. Ineffective in non-dividing cells. Low receptor expression in some cells. Small insert size. Poor expression of protein	Marker and suicide gene studies. Vaccines
Lentiviruses	Infects non-dividing cells	More complex genome. Low titre	Stem cells. Post-mitotic cells
Adenovirus	High titre. Efficient infection of most cells	Replication-competent virus always present. Immunogenic	Vaccines and other localized applications requiring transient expression
Adenoassociated virus	Integrates into specific site	Small insert size. No packaging cells and requires adenovirus for production. No site-specific integration unless viral genes present	Expression in some post-mitotic cells, e.g. retina. Vaccines and other local applications
Herpes virus	Efficient entry into neurons	Complex genome and vector construction. Non-integrating	CNS-directed therapy
Plasmid vectors	Simple to construct and prepare. Well characterized	Low efficiency. Transient expression	Topical or local application. Vaccines

vectors is ideal and the development of better agents is a major priority in commercial and academic gene therapy laboratories across the world. The properties of the most commonly used vectors are described below and summarized in Table 21.1.

DNA-based vectors

Introduction

The simplest method of transferring genetic material is to use isolated DNA. In order for this to be effective, the DNA must carry the regulatory sequences necessary for gene transcrip-

tion and translation, and an efficient method of introducing the vector into target cells is required. Clearly, unless the DNA is capable of replication or becomes integrated into the genome of the target cell, this method of gene transfer is always transient, especially in dividing cells in which copy number halves with each generation. In addition, unlike bacteria, mammalian cells do not have a mechanism for passing DNA from cell to cell, so gene expression is restricted to those cells initially transfected. Despite these drawbacks, 'naked DNA' vectors are suitable for applications requiring localized gene expression, such as vaccination, and have already been used in clinical trials.

Methods of introducing DNA into target cells

There are a number of methods for facilitating DNA uptake by cells. In general these work best in immortalized cell lines, but less well in the primary cells of interest in gene therapy, and all involve some degree of cellular toxicity. Direct micro-injection is the best technique for introducing very large genetic elements such as artificial chromosomes; however, its exploitation in gene therapy is limited by the small cell numbers involved. Ballistic transfection involves coating DNA onto gold or tungsten microbeads which are accelerated through the cell membrane using a 'gene gun' driven by compressed gas.[3] This method achieves effective local gene transfer and has been studied as a method for introducing genes through the skin for vaccination. The standard methods of achieving in vitro gene transfer in laboratory studies, such as calcium phosphate-mediated gene transfer and electroporation, have not been useful in gene therapy, mainly because of poor efficiency and toxicity to target cells. Lipofection,[4] in which DNA complexed to cationic lipid enters the cell through an ill-defined route, is less toxic and may be useful in gene therapy

Plasmid vectors

These are double-stranded circular DNA molecules originally identified as mediators of gene transfer between bacteria. They replicate within bacteria, often to very high copy number, and are crucial to recombinant DNA technology since they provide a simple means of cutting, pasting and amplifying DNA fragments. Although bacterial in origin, they may be modified to include appropriate transcription and translation signals so that when introduced into mammalian cells they express exogenous genes. Plasmid vectors integrate into mammalian genomes with very low efficiency and are normally maintained as non-replicating episomes. Inclusion of certain viral sequences allows plasmid replication; for example, the Epstein–Barr virus origin of replication causes plasmids to amplify and maintain transgene expression in cells expressing Epstein–Barr nuclear antigen.[5]

The practical size limit for plasmid vectors is 10–12 kb; taking into account sequences necessary for bacterial replication and selection, transgene(s) up to 8 kb may be inserted. This effectively restricts the regulatory sequences to simple constitutive promoters and enhancers that are not subject to normal regulation in the target cell.

Artificial chromosomes

A potential means of overcoming the above shortcomings would be to construct artificial chromosomes that could contain all of the normal regulatory sequences of the gene, ensuring the correct pattern of tissue expression. It is possible to construct both yeast and murine artificial chromosomes and these might ultimately prove to be useful in situations requiring gene transfer into a small population of cells with a high replicative potential, such as haemopoietic stem cells.

Retroviral vectors

The life cycle of retroviruses[6] makes them particularly useful as gene transfer vehicles. They have evolved efficient mechanisms for cellular entry and integrate into the genome of the host cell so that both the initial target cell and its progeny will carry virus-derived sequence. They also have important limitations, however, and their ability to integrate and recombine raises important safety issues.

Murine leukaemia virus
Retroviral life cycle
The simplest, best characterized and most frequently used retroviral vectors are based on murine leukaemia virus (MLV), a group C oncogenic retrovirus. The MLV virion comprises a double-stranded RNA genome associated with structural proteins and enzymes. The viral envelope protein (env) has two components, a surface receptor binding (SU) portion and a transmembrane (TM) domain that are linked by a disulphide bridge and inserted as trimers in the packaging-cell-derived viral

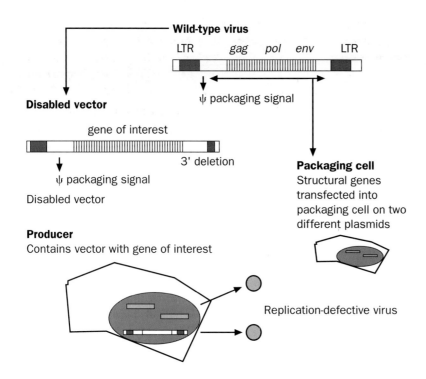

Figure 21.1
A typical retroviral packaging system. The viral structural genes *gag*, *pol* and *env* are deleted from the viral vector and provided 'in-trans' in a helper packaging cell. The possibility of generating replication-competent retrovirus is reduced by separating *gag/pol* and *env* on separate plasmids, by deleting the 3' LTR from the vector and by minimizing any homology between the sequences in the vector and the structural gene constructs.

membrane. Env molecules from a variety of viruses may be incorporated into MLV, resulting in 'pseudotypes' with altered species and tissue tropism. The viral core comprises double-stranded RNA, capsid, nucleocapsid and matrix proteins. The genome is relatively simple and comprises regulatory sequences necessary for transcription, translation, packaging, reverse transcription and integration, as well as the three structural genes *gag*, *pol* and *env*. In viral gene transfer vectors, a helpful packaging cell line transfected with the appropriate genes provides structural proteins allowing the viral backbone to accommodate the gene of interest (Fig. 21.1).

The viral env protein is required for entry into the target cell and determines the cellular tropism. Although initial attachment appears to be env-independent,[7] membrane fusion and virus entry depend on an interaction between env and a specific cell surface receptor.[8] Several retroviral receptors have now been character-

ized and specific envelope–receptor interactions are responsible for species restriction. In addition, the density of retroviral receptor is an important determinant of the efficiency of transduction.[9,10] Since this may vary between cell types, selection of the most appropriate env molecule is an important consideration in the design of vectors for gene therapy. Receptor deficiency may be bypassed to some extent by using the fibronectin fragment CH296 which co-localizes vector and cell through its heparin and integrin binding domains.[11]

Once the viral core is released into the cytoplasm, viral RNA undergoes reverse transcription, primed by a tRNA molecule. During this process the 3' LTR is transposed to the 5' position of the proviral cDNA. This fact has been exploited in the construction of self-inactivating vectors in which the 3' LTR is replaced by a heterologous promoter molecule. Once transposed to the 5' region, the heterologous promoter functions for gene transcription but renders the viral genome incapable of further propagation.[12] Following reverse transcription, the proviral cDNA must gain access to the cell genome in order for integration to occur. The MLV provirus does not possess a nuclear localization signal and so depends upon breakdown of the nuclear pore membrane during cell division.[13] This is an important limitation because it renders MLV-based vectors highly inefficient in targets that divide only infrequently, such as haemopoietic stem cells.[14] Lentiviral vectors based on HIV or similar animal viruses do not have this limitation and considerable progress has been made in developing systems, based on these agents, suitable for use in gene therapy.[15,16]

Safety considerations

The properties of retroviruses make them suitable for gene therapy but also raise important safety concerns. Random integration into the genome might modify genes critical for cell growth and lead to malignant transformation; however, in practice, the chances of this appear to be very low.[17] A more serious concern is the potential for generating replication-competent retrovirus (RCR). Disabled retroviruses may regain their structural genes by recombining with transfected *gag/pol/env* or with homologous endogenous genes. When RCR is present, the risk of insertional mutagenesis is real, as was demonstrated in a study in monkeys in which T cell lymphoma developed in three monkeys after gene transfer using a helper virus-contaminated retroviral producer cell line.[18] More recently a spongiform encephalopathy was described in mice infected with RCR.[19]

Numerous strategies for reducing the risk of RCR have been described, including separation of viral structural genes on different plasmids[20] and minimizing any overlap between cellular and vector sequence by deletion (see Fig. 21.1) or by using human packaging cells that carry fewer endogenous retroviral sequences.[21,22] Needless to say, rigorous testing for RCR by at least two methods is mandatory for all preparations of retroviral vector destined for clinical use.

Adenovirus and adenoassociated virus

Adenoviruses are a common cause of upper respiratory illness in humans and have been used as vaccines for a number of years. They are enveloped double-stranded DNA viruses with a 36 kb genome that can be readily manipulated using standard molecular biological techniques.[23] Replication-defective vectors have been produced for use in gene therapy by deletion of the *E1A* and *E1B* genes which are provided by the human embryonic kidney HEK 293 packaging cell line. Adenoviral vectors have several advantages over retroviruses. They can be produced to very high titres, in excess of 10^6 infectious particles per millilitre, and can infect a wide variety of cell types, including non-dividing cells. Disadvantages include immune responses to viral proteins[24] and, as the vector does not integrate into the host genome, transient expression of the transgene. Current vectors all result in generation of some replication-competent adenovirus (RCA) although, because adenoviruses are so ubiquitous, this has not precluded their use in gene therapy. The first gene therapy death was recently recorded in a patient with ornithine transcarbamylase deficiency who received high dose recombinant adenovirus in an attempt to correct the enzyme defect.[25] Although the cause of death is not fully clear, it seems likely to relate to the dose of virus, and reconsideration of the use of adenoviruses in gene therapy is certain to result. A new generation of 'gutless' vectors are under development which have no RCA, have high-level gene expression and have minimal inflammatory response, and these will likely supersede current systems.

Adenoassociated virus (AAV) is a non-pathogenic single-stranded DNA parvovirus that has many attractive properties as a gene therapy vector.[26] Wild-type AAV is defective, relying on the presence of adenovirus for replication, and recombinant AAV vectors are further disabled by removal of most of the genome. AAV can integrate into non-dividing cells at a specific site on human chromosome 19; however, it can also exist for prolonged periods as an episome and it is important to distinguish the two.[27] At present the most significant limitation of these agents centres around the development of methods for generating viral stocks free of adenovirus and wild-type AAV, since the former raises safety issues and the latter might reduce the efficiency of gene transfer.

Other viruses

A variety of other viruses are under study as possible vectors for gene therapy. These include herpes simplex virus, which is of interest because of its tropism for the central nervous system (CNS) and ability to infect non-dividing cells,[6,28] and vaccinia, which has a well-established safety record and potential use in immune gene therapy.

Vector targeting

Because failure to restrict gene transfer to the desired target cells is both wasteful and potentially hazardous, considerable efforts have been made to develop targeted vectors. The simplest method of directing a vector is to harvest and purify the target cells and perform gene transfer ex vivo, removing remaining vector prior to administration of the gene-modified cells. This method has been widely used in the haemopoietic system because the cells are readily accessible, clinically applicable cell purification systems are available[29] and transplantation technology is well established. Direct injection of vectors or producer cell lines into tumour masses has also been proposed and several pilot clinical studies have been performed in this way. Vectors suitable for in vivo administration with more sophisticated cell targeting capabilities will, however, be required for many applications, including cancer gene therapy. Retroviral and adenoviral vectors can be targeted by modifying their envelope or spike proteins, although in the case of retrovirus this has proved problematic since even minor modifications to env can interfere with membrane fusion. Targeting may also be achieved using tissue-specific promoters in either plasmid or retroviral vectors.[30,31] In addition, recently, it has been shown that an attenuated vaccine strain of measles virus selectively replicates in human myeloma cell lines and can inhibit the growth of myeloma xenografts in mice.[32]

Choice of vector

The choice of gene therapy vector depends on safety considerations, on the desired duration of gene expression and on the target tissue. Vector technology is in its infancy and none of the available vectors are ideal. At present, safety considerations preclude the use of replicating vectors; thus retroviruses and AAV are the only candidates for long-term expression. A variety of MLV pseudotypes are now available with different cell tropism; for example, GALV-1 and RD114 appear superior to amphotropic env in the haemopoietic system.[33,34] For transient gene expression, adenovirus is currently the best option; however, safety concerns have recently been raised after the recent death of a patient[25] and there is concern about immune responses following repeated administration.[24,35] For localized transient gene expression, the naked DNA vectors or adenovirus may be suitable. Although inefficient, plasmid DNA is probably safer than adenovirus and it is far simpler to produce purified plasmid than viral stocks.

STRATEGIES FOR GENE THERAPY OF CANCER

Gene marking studies

Probably the most useful contribution of gene transfer technology to the treatment of human disease to date have been experiments in which the transgene functions as a cell marker.

Autologous bone marrow transplantation

The first bone marrow gene marking study[36] demonstrated that following autologous transplantation for acute myeloblastic leukaemia or neuroblastoma, infused tumour cells contribute to relapse. The marker gene persisted in bone marrow as well as peripheral blood mononuclear cells and neutrophils for at least 18 months, thus demonstrating that autologous bone marrow is able to restore long-term haemopoiesis.[37] A similar study performed in adults undergoing high dose therapy for breast cancer or myeloma involved marking purified CD34 cells from blood or bone marrow with different vectors.[38] Although 10/10 patients had detectable marker genes at the time of engraftment, by 18 months only 3/9 were PCR-positive at a level of 1:1000 to 1:10 000 bone marrow cells.

Adoptive immunotherapy

Cell marking has been particularly helpful in the study of immunotherapy for Epstein–Barr virus (EBV) associated post-transplant lymphoproliferative disorder. The incidence of this condition after allogeneic bone marrow transplantation relates to the degree of immunosuppression and can be as high as 30% in the unrelated or mismatched donor setting. Infusions of donor leukocytes are effective in this situation[39] but carry the risk of graft-versus-host disease. Specific cytotoxic T cell lines raised from the donor against EBV-infected lymphoblastoid cells are also effective and can be marked with a retroviral vector to determine their persistence and behaviour in vivo.[40] Cytotoxic T cells specific for EBV (EBV-CTLs) are also effective at preventing EBV lymphoproliferation.[41] Reinfused EBV-CTLs marked with the neomycin resistance gene (*Neo*[r]) were shown to expand in vivo by a factor of 100- to 1000-fold and to persist for up to 5 months. In one of the 14 patients treated in this study, *Neo*[r]-marked T cells were detectable for 14 weeks after transplant but could not be detected for the next 18 months, during which time the levels of EBV DNA in the blood were low. Reactivation of latent EBV at 18 months, indicated by a rise in EBV DNA level, was associated with the reappearance of marked T cells, indicating that there had been expansion from a long-lived population of infused cells.

Correction of genetic defect

As discussed above, the ideal cancer treatment would correct the underlying genetic defect(s) within the cell. In vivo administration of a replication-competent vector would be the most effective way of achieving gene transfer into the highest number of tumour cells. Whilst this is not yet possible, a number of clinical trials are underway which show the way forward.

p53

The most common genetic defect in human cancer involves the p53 tumour suppressor gene, which is mutated in about 50% of tumours. The p53 protein is involved in the detection of DNA damage, cell cycle checkpoint control and apoptosis, and cells with p53 abnormalities are resistant to the effects of chemotherapy and radiotherapy. Numerous in vitro and animal studies have demonstrated that restoration of wild-type p53 protein reduces tumourgenicity and increases the sensitivity of malignant cells to chemotherapy and radiotherapy. In addition, there is evidence for a bystander effect, possibly due to effects on angiogenesis,[42] in which there is death of non-p53-corrected cells in p53-deficient tumours treated with wild-type p53 bearing adenoviral vectors. Clinical trials of two approaches to p53-directed cancer therapy are currently underway.

E1B, 55-kDa gene-attenuated adenovirus

During infection with wild-type adenovirus, the *E1B* gene product binds to and inactivates p53, resulting in virus replication and cell death. Adenovirus with a deletion of *E1B* replicates and induces cytotoxicity in p53-deficient cells but cannot replicate in cells with wild-type p53.[43] An adenovirus of this type has been developed for clinical use (ONYX-015); encouraging results have been obtained in animals bearing human tumours[44] and clinical trials are currently underway. Although not strictly gene therapy, this approach illustrates how suitably targeted replicating vectors might be used in future.

p53 adenovirus

A second p53-based strategy employs adenoviral vector engineered to express normal p53 (Ad-p53). Since they employ nominally replication defective adenovirus (albeit usually contaminated by RCA) and are not targeted, these studies have relied on direct injection into the tumour.

Non-small cell lung cancer

A dose escalation study of direct Ad-p53 injection into incurable non-small cell lung cancer lesions demonstrated gene transfer at the highest virus dose. Tumour responses were seen in four out of six patients in whom gene transfer was successful and not at any untreated sites.[45] No significant toxicity was observed. A similar study in 28 patients with similar tumours showed vector DNA in 18/21 evaluable biopsies and vector mRNA in 12/26. Responses were seen in two cases, disease stabilization in 16 and progression in seven, and toxicity was described as minimal.[46]

Head and neck cancer

A similar approach has been taken to the therapy of head and neck cancer, either as an adjuvant to surgery[47] or in recurrent disease.[48] In the adjuvant setting, four of 15 patients were disease-free at a mean of 18 months, whilst in recurrent disease, two of 17 showed regression, six of 17 had stable disease for up to 3.5 months and the remainder had disease progression. Somewhat alarmingly, infectious Ad-p53 was present in blood and urine in proportion to the dose of virus injected. No adverse effects due to this were reported; however, the possibility of infecting the wider population with a virus encoding an oncogene must be a cause for concern.

Modulation of drug resistance

Current cancer therapy involves the use of relatively non-specific drugs or radiation to destroy malignant cells. A number of gene therapy strategies have therefore been devised to increase the narrow therapeutic window of such treatment, either by increasing the resistance of normal tissues or by increasing the sensitivity of the tumour to the effects of chemotherapy.

Chemoprotection

The haemopoietic system is the tissue most sensitive to chemotherapy, and myelosuppression is thus its most important dose-limiting toxicity. A number of groups have sought to protect the haemopoietic system from drug toxicity by transferring drug resistance genes into haemopoietic stem cells.

Multi-drug resistance gene

The multi-drug resistance gene (MDR1) encodes the ATP-dependent membrane efflux transporter P-glycoprotein (PGP). Overexpression of MDR1 is a common cause of tumour resistance to a variety of chemotherapeutic drugs, including the anthracyclines, vinca alkaloids, taxanes and epidophylotoxins. Normal haemopoietic stem cells, but not the progenitor pool, express high levels of MDR1, so that MDR1 substrate drugs cause myelosuppression but not ablation. Constitutive expression of MDR1 in murine haemopoietic cells protects against the toxic effects of MDR1 substrate drugs and selects for transduced cells.[49,50] Transfer of the MDR1 gene into human haemopoietic cells should both protect the bone marrow against the toxicity of MDR1 substrate drugs and enable selection for transduced cells. Several groups have performed pilot clinical trials of MDR1 gene transfer in patients undergoing high dose chemotherapy and autologous stem cell transplantation.[51–53] Despite relatively efficient gene transfer in the latter study, there has been no convincing evidence for chemoprotection or selection of transduced cells. A selective expansion of MDR1-transduced stem cells and the development of a myeloproliferative disorder was recently reported in a murine bone marrow transplant model.[54] Whilst the significance of this remains uncertain it raises questions over the wisdom of attempts to constitutively overexpress MDR1 in human stem cells.

Other potential chemoprotectant drugs

Several other molecules have the potential for protecting against drug-induced myelotoxicity. These include: multi-drug resistance-associated protein (MRP),[55] aldehyde dehydrogenase (ALDH),[56] dihydrofolate reductase (DHFR),[57] methyl guanine methyltransferase (MGMT)[58] and glutathione S-transferase (GST).[58] MRP enhances resistance to the same drugs as MDR1, ALDH inactivates the active cyclophosphamide metabolites, DHFR prevents methotrexate toxicity, MGMT removes the DNA alkyl adducts produced by the nitrosoureas, and GST detoxifies a range of alkylating agents. Of all the potential chemoprotection genes, MGMT is the most attractive because the nitrosoureas are true stem cell toxins and it should be possible to achieve stem cell protection by successful gene transfer.[60] The cellular toxicity of nitrosoureas is increased by pretreatment with O6-benzylguanine, which further enhances the differential sensitivity between MGMT-transduced and untransduced cells.[61]

Pro-drug activation

There are several enzymes that convert inactive pro-drugs to toxic metabolites, and transfer of these genes into tumour cells is a strategy for achieving selective tumour killing. This strategy, known as gene-directed enzyme pro-drug therapy (G-DEPT), has been widely studied in vitro and in a number of clinical trials. The most commonly used system is the herpes simplex thymidine kinase gene (HSV-TK) which converts ganciclovir and aciclovir to toxic phosphorylated metabolites.[62] Other less widely used enzymes include cytosine deaminase,[63] which converts 5-fluorocytosine to 5-fluorouracil, and xanthine phosphoribosyl transferase, which converts 6-thioxanthine to 6-thioxanthine triphosphate. Although in theory G-DEPT requires that the enzyme is transferred into every tumour cell, in practice there is a 'bystander effect', characterized by apoptosis of the affected cells.

HSV-TK therapy of malignant brain tumours

Several groups have conducted clinical trials of HSV-TK/ganciclovir therapy for poor-prognosis brain tumours. These have involved implantation of HSV-TK retroviral producer cells[64-67] or, in a proposed study, an adenoviral vector.[68] In the retroviral studies, a total of 70 patients have been reported in whom vector producers were instilled following either resection or recurrence. Follow-up information is limited; however, the beneficial effects seem to have been marginal and restricted to those patients with the smallest tumours. A recent report in mice with syngeneic gliomas treated with a single injection of an adenoviral HSV-TK vector followed by ganciclovir showed chronic brain inflammation and demyelination at the original tumour site. The reason for this finding is unclear but it may be due to a bystander immune response to tumour or adenoviral antigens, and it signals caution in human studies of this type.[69]

HSV-TK transduction of T lymphocytes for adoptive immunotherapy

A further application of the 'suicide gene' strategy is as an adjunct to adoptive immunotherapy following allogeneic haemopoietic cell transplantation. Infusion of donor lymphocytes (DLI) is an effective means of augmenting the graft-versus-tumour effect of allogeneic transplantation, even following relapse of the original disease.[70] Unfortunately, DLI also frequently results in graft-versus-host disease (GVHD), particularly when given within 6 months of the original transplant. Transduction of T cells with the HSV-TK gene prior to reinfusion provides a potential method for rescuing the patient from GVHD by eliminating donor T cells using ganciclovir.[71] Since only a small number of T cells can cause significant GVHD, the success of this approach depends on achieving transduction efficiencies close to 100%. Although described in principle some time ago, the effectiveness of this approach has yet to be proved in larger studies.

Immune gene therapy

In recent years tumour immunotherapy has received a great deal of attention. Two developments have contributed to this. The first is the identification of target antigens expressed by tumours that can be recognized by cytotoxic T cells. Tumour antigens may arise through point mutation, the formation of fusion genes by chromosomal translocation, by over- or aberrant expression of differentiation gene products, by virally encoded proteins, or by aberrant post-translational modification. So far, over- or aberrantly expressed normal antigens have proved the most promising therapeutic targets, because, in contrast to point mutations, they usually provide a relatively large number of potential T cell epitopes. The second area of progress has been the increased understanding of factors regulating the immune response. Over the last decade there have been great strides in elucidating the nature of thymic selection and the heterogeneity of peripheral lymphocytes, including the recognition of effector cells with distinct Th1 and Th2 cytokine production profiles. Of particular importance to tumour immunology have been advances in the understanding of antigen presentation. The realization that T cells can 'see' intracellular antigens means that tumour proteins are now potential targets for immunotherapy. A considerable body of work has shown that the immune repertoire of individuals who have tumours contains both T and B cells capable of responding to antigens present within malignant cells.[72–74] Immunotherapeutic approaches to cancer therapy are thus aimed at improving tumour antigen presentation, enhancing effector cell responses or both. A number of these strategies have employed gene transfer techniques, and an outline of these along with data on some of the clinical trials is given below.

Antigen presentation

Antigen is presented to cytotoxic or helper T lymphocytes as peptides associated with MHC class 1 or 2 molecules and the CD3 antigen receptor. Professional antigen-presenting cells such as dendritic cells (DCs) possess an array of co-stimulatory molecules capable of activating naïve T cells.[75] Tumour antigenicity might therefore be enhanced either by expressing the tumour antigen in DCs that already possess the requisite signals or by transducing the tumour itself with co-stimulatory molecules such as CD80 and CD86. The mechanism of CD80-induced T cell activation has been well studied in vitro; however, the situation may be more complex in tumours. In vitro incubation of T cells and leukaemic blasts engineered to express CD80 results in T cell activation and survival, but soluble factors secreted by the leukaemic cells inhibit generation of the Th1 cytokines necessary for cytotoxic responses.[76] Finally, certain cytokines such as granulocyte–macrophage colony stimulating factor (GM-CSF) modulate dendritic cell function, and transduction of tumour cells with GM-CSF is a further method of augmenting antigen presentation.[77] Tumour cells or DCs modified in the ways described may be used either as cellular vaccines or as a means of generating T cell lines ex vivo for use in adoptive immunotherapy.

Effector function

An alternative strategy is to enhance antitumour responses by increasing the level of T cell activation more directly. The earliest attempts at this involved transduction of tumour cells with cytokines such as interleukin-2 (IL-2) or IL-7. More sophisticated approaches include the construction of T cell lines with hybrid T cell receptors in which the signal-transducing zeta chain, for example, is fused to a ligand-binding extracellular domain that dimerizes and activates the T cell when it binds to the tumour antigen.[78]

Clinical trials

Tumour vaccination in melanoma

Malignant melanoma has historically been one of the tumours most responsive to immunotherapy and this, coupled with the poor prognosis of patients with metastatic disease, has encouraged the clinical trials of immune gene therapy. Protocols have involved either ex vivo transduction of autologous tumour cells with the cDNAs for IL-2,[79] IL-7[80] or interferon-γ (IFN-γ),[81] or direct intratumour injection of IL-2 adenovirus.[82] Others have used HLA-A2-compatible allogeneic melanoma cells[83] or fibroblasts engineered to secrete IL-2.[84] In general the vaccinations were well tolerated but the responses minor and confined to local erythema and infiltration by T cells at the injection site or detectable in vitro responses, such as anti-tumour cytotoxic T cells or antibodies. The best responses were seen in the Ad-IL-2 study, in which 24% of patients had local regression at the site of injection.

Idiotypic vaccination in non-Hodgkin's lymphoma

Vaccination with idiotypic protein is known to induce anti-tumour immune responses in B cell lymphomas;[85] however, purification of idiotype protein is cumbersome and not feasible on a large scale. An alternative approach is to use the polymerase chain reaction to amplify the V_H and V_L portions of the tumour immunoglobulin cloned into a plasmid construct capable of expressing single chain antibody (sFv). Fusion of the tetanus toxin fragment C chain to the sFv construct results in greatly enhanced immunogenicity when then used as a DNA vaccine and protects against experimental lymphoma and myeloma in an animal model.[86] Phase I clinical trials of this approach are underway in patients with B cell lymphoma.

Adenovirus CD40L gene therapy for B cell chronic lymphocytic leukaemia

The malignant B cells in chronic lymphocytic leukaemia (B-CLL) express a unique immunoglobulin idiotype, which is a potential tumour antigen, as well as high levels of class 1 and 2 MHC proteins. However, B-CLL cells are poor antigen-presenting cells, in part because of a lack of co-stimulatory molecules. Activated CD4 T cells normally express CD40L, which activates CD40+ B cells, monocytes and dendritic cells, upregulating co-stimulatory molecules such as CD54, 80 and 86. In B-CLL, CD4 cells fail to express CD40L, leading to deficient antigen presentation and an immunodeficiency state.[87] Transfer of CD40L into B-CLL cells using an adenoviral vector has been shown to correct this defect through its effects on bystander leukaemic cells.[88] A clinical trial based on this observation has been initiated; initial reports show evidence of anamnestic T cell responses and the generation of autologous anti-tumour CTLs.[89]

ETHICAL, REGULATORY AND SAFETY ISSUES

Since gene therapy became a practical possibility over a decade ago there has been widespread concern over its ethics and safety. Provided safety can be assured, somatic gene therapy, in which only the somatic cells of the individual subject are modified, is now viewed as no more ethically challenging than blood transfusion. Gene therapy studies of this type have therefore been allowed to proceed in most countries subject to formal review of the protocol and safety issues. An embargo has been placed on attempts at germ line gene therapy where the objective is to modify genes in an individual subject and his or her progeny. Apart from the fact that the technology to do this does not yet exist, such interventions raise more fundamental questions about the effects on the human gene pool and the impossibility of obtaining consent from the subjects affected.

Most countries have followed the lead of the USA by establishing formalized procedures for protocol review and by subjecting any vectors and modified cells to the same rigour of manufacturing regulation as more conventional pharmaceuticals. In the UK, gene therapy studies must be approved by the Gene Therapy Advisory Committee, a body which has scientific members as well as representatives from industry, the law, the media and religious bodies. Vector manufacture and cell processing are regulated by the Medicines Control Agency, and the prospective gene therapist must also gain approval from local research and ethics and genetic modification safety committees. Regulation of this type, combined with an open debate and transparency, is essential if the field of gene therapy is to keep public confidence. It is usual for protocols to be published in gene therapy journals prior to commencement and for the deliberations of the regulatory authorities to be made public.

FUTURE PROSPECTS

Considering the huge investment of time and money, the initial results of clinical gene therapy studies have been most disappointing. Prompted by this, a detailed review of the field, conducted by the US National Institutes of Health (NIH), made a number of key recommendations for the future direction of research.[90] These included a greater attention to the basic biology of vector design and the cellular targets and the molecular pathology of the diseases under study. Although the need for animal experimentation was emphasized, it was also recognized that in some disorders, such as HIV, cystic fibrosis and cancer, progress would require carefully conducted clinical trials.

In the short and medium term, the future of cancer gene therapy is likely to follow the direction outlined in the NIH review. In the longer term, the results of human genome sequencing efforts seem likely to expand the molecular targets of cancer therapy, and the ability to rapidly screen tumours for these defects using microarray technology should make it possible to design rational and specific treatments for individual patients. Whether these are drug or vector based will depend on the rate of progress in pharmacology and gene therapy. In the meantime the development of chemoprotection, G-DEPT and immune gene therapy strategies will continue and, although none of these approaches are likely to be curative, they may prove useful adjuncts to conventional therapy.

REFERENCES

1. Druker B, Talpaz M, Resta D et al. Efficacy and safety of a specific inhibitor of BCR-ABL tyrosine kinase in chronic myeloid leukemia. N Engl J Med 2001;344:1031–7.
2. Mann R, Mulligan RC, Baltimore D. Construction of a retrovirus packaging mutant and its use to produce helper-free defective retrovirus. Cell 1983;33:153–9.
3. Yang NS, Burkholder J, Roberts B, Martinell B, McCabe D. In vivo and in vitro gene transfer to mammalian somatic cells by particle bombardment. Proc Natl Acad Sci USA 1990;87:9568–72.
4. Felgner P, Gadek T, Holm M et al. A highly efficient lipid mediated DNA transfection procedure. Proc Nat Acad Sci USA 1987;84:7413–17.
5. Sugden B, Marsh K, Yates J. A vector that replicates as a plasmid and can be efficiently selected in B-lymphoblasts transformed by Epstein–Barr virus. Mol Cell Biol 1985;5:410–3.
6. Coffin J. Retroviridae and their replication. In: Fields B, Knipe D, editors. Virology (2nd edn). New York: Raven Press Ltd, 1990: 1437–500.
7. Pizzato M, Marlow SA, Blair ED, Takeuchi Y. Initial binding of murine leukemia virus particles to cells does not require specific Env-receptor interaction. J Virol 1999;73:8599–611.
8. Weiss R, Tailor C. Retrovirus receptors. Cell 1995;82:531–3.
9. Kurre P, Kiem H, Morris J, Heyward S, Battini J, Miller A. Efficient transduction by an amphotropic retrovirus vector is dependent on high level expression of the cell surface virus receptor. J Virol 1999;73:495–500.
10. Macdonald C, Walker S, Watts M, Ings S, Linch D, Devereux S. Effect of changes in expression of the amphotropic retroviral receptor Pit-2 on transduction efficiency and viral titre; implications for gene therapy. Hum Gene Ther, 2002, in press.
11. Hanenberg H, Xiao XL, Dilloo D et al. Colocalization of retrovirus and target cells on specific fibronectin fragments increases genetic transduction of mammalian cells. Nature Med 1996;2:876–82.
12. Yu SF, von Ruden T, Kantoff PW et al. Self-inactivating retroviral vectors designed for transfer of whole genes into mammalian cells. Proc Natl Acad Sci USA 1986;83:3194–8.
13. Roe T, Reynolds TC, Yu G, Brown PO. Integration of murine leukemia virus DNA depends on mitosis. EMBO J 1993;12:2099–108.

14. Abkowitz JL, Catlin SN, Guttorp P. Evidence that hematopoiesis may be a stochastic-process in-vivo. Nature Med 1996;2:190–7.

15. Naldini L, Blomer U, Gallay P et al. In vivo gene delivery and stable transduction of nondividing cells by a lentiviral vector (see comments). Science 1996;272:263–7.

16. Kim VN, Mitrophanous K, Kingsman SM, Kingsman AJ. Minimal requirement for a lentivirus vector based on human immunodeficiency virus type 1. J Virol 1998;72:811–6.

17. Temin H. Safety considerations in somatic gene therapy of human disease with retroviral vectors. Hum Gene Ther 1990;1:123.

18. Donahue RE, Kessler SW, Bodine D et al. Helper virus induced T cell lymphoma in nonhuman primates after retroviral mediated gene transfer. J Exp Med 1992;176:1125–35.

19. Munk C, Lohler J, Prassolov V, Just U, Stockschlader M, Stocking C. Amphotropic murine leukemia viruses induce spongiform encephalomyelopathy. Proc Natl Acad Sci USA 1997;94:5837–42.

20. Markowitz D, Goff S, Bank A. A safe packaging line for gene-transfer – separating viral genes on 2 different plasmids. J Virol 1988;62:1120–4.

21. Cosset FL, Takeuchi Y, Battini JL, Weiss RA, Collins MKL. High titer packaging cells producing recombinant retroviruses resistant to human serum. J Virol 1995;69:7430–6.

22. Patience C, Takeuchi Y, Cosset FL, Weiss RA. Packaging of endogenous retroviral sequences in retroviral vectors produced by murine and human packaging cells. J Virology 1998;72:-2671–6.

23. Kovesdi I, Brough D, Bruder J, Wickham T. Adenoviral vectors for gene transfer. Curr Opin Biotechnol 1997;8:583–9.

24. Tripathy SK, Black HB, Goldwasser E, Leiden JM. Immune responses to transgene-encoded proteins limit the stability of gene expression after injection of replication-defective adenovirus vectors. Nature Med 1996;2:545–50.

25. Hollon T. Researchers and regulators reflect on the first gene therapy death. Nature Med 2000;6:6.

26. Rabinowitz J, Samulski J. Adenoassociated virus expression systems for gene transfer. Curr Opin Biotechnol 1998;9:470–5.

27. Malik P, McQuiston SA, Yu XJ et al. Recombinant adeno-associated virus mediates a high level of gene transfer but less efficient integration in the K562 human hematopoietic cell line. J Virol 1997;71:1776–83.

28. Dilloo D, Rill D, Entwistle C et al. A novel herpes vector for the high-efficiency transduction of normal and malignant human hematopoietic cells. Blood 1997;89:119–27.

29. Watts M, Sullivan A, Ings S et al. Evaluation of clinical scale CD34+ cell purification: experience of 71 immunoaffinity column procedures. Bone Marrow Transplant 1997;20:157–62.

30. Vile RG, Hart IR. Use of tissue-specific expression of the herpes-simplex virus thymidine kinase gene to inhibit growth of established murine melanomas following direct intratumoral injection of DNA. Cancer Res 1993;53:3860–4.

31. Huber BE, Richards CA, Krenitsky TA. Retroviral-mediated gene-therapy for the treatment of hepatocellular carcinoma – an innovative approach for cancer therapy. Proc Natl Acad Sci USA 1991;88:8039–43.

32. Peng KW, Ahmann GJ, Pham L et al. Systemic therapy of myeloma xenografts by an attenuated measles virus. Blood 2001;98:2002–7.

33. Kiem HP, Heyward S, Winkler A et al. Gene transfer into marrow repopulating cells: comparison between amphotropic and gibbon ape leukemia virus pseudotyped retroviral vectors in a competitive repopulation assay in baboons. Blood 1997;90:4638–45.

34. Kelly P, Vandergriff J, Vanin E, Nienhuis A. Efficient transduction of CD34+ and CD34+ CD38− human hematopoietic cells with a SCID repopulating cell (SRC) potential with an oncoretroviral vector pseudotyped with a feline endogenous virus (RD114) evelope protein. Blood 1999;94:2718 (abstract).

35. Knowles MR, Hohneker KW, Zhou Z et al. A controlled study of adenoviral-vector-mediated gene transfer in the nasal epithelium of patients with cystic fibrosis (see comments). N Engl J Med 1995;333:823–31.

36. Brenner M, Rill D, Moen R. Gene marking to trace origin of relapse after autologous bone marrow transplantation. Lancet 1993;341:85–6.

37. Brenner MK, Rill DR, Holladay MS et al. Gene marking to determine whether autologous marrow infusion restores long-term hematopoiesis in cancer patients. Lancet 1993;342:1134–7.

38. Dunbar CE, Cottler-Fox M, O'Shaughnessy JA et al. Retrovirally marked CD34-enriched peripheral blood and bone marrow cells contribute to long-term engraftment after autologous trans-

plantation. Blood 1995;85:3048–57.

39. Papadopoulos EB, Ladanyi M, Emanuel D et al. Infusions of donor leukocytes to treat Epstein–Barr virus-associated lymphoproliferative disorders after allogeneic bone-marrow transplantation. N Engl J Med 1994;330:1185–91.

40. Rooney CM, Smith CA, Ng CYC et al. Use of gene-modified virus-specific T-lymphocytes to control Epstein–Barr-virus-related lymphoproliferation. Lancet 1995;345:9–13.

41. Heslop HE, Ng CYC, Li CF et al. Long-term restoration of immunity against Epstein–Barr-virus infection by adoptive transfer of gene-modified virus-specific T-lymphocytes. Nature Med 1996;2:551–5.

42. Bouvet M, Ellis LM, Nishizaki M et al. Adenovirus-mediated wild-type p53 gene transfer down-regulates vascular endothelial growth factor expression and inhibits angiogenesis in human colon cancer. Cancer Res 1998;58:2288–92.

43. Bischoff JR, Kirn DH, Williams A et al. An adenovirus mutant that replicates selectively in p53-deficient human tumor cells. Science 1996;274:373–6.

44. Heise C, Sampson-Johannes A, Williams A, McCormick F, Von Hoff DD, Kirn DH. ONYX-015, an E1B gene-attenuated adenovirus, causes tumor-specific cytolysis and antitumoral efficacy that can be augmented by standard chemotherapeutic agents (see comments). Nature Med 1997;3:639–45.

45. Schuler M, Rochlitz C, Horowitz JA et al. A phase I study of adenovirus-mediated wild-type p53 gene transfer in patients with advanced non-small cell lung cancer. Hum Gene Ther 1998;9:2075–82.

46. Swisher SG, Roth JA, Nemunaitis J et al. Adenovirus-mediated p53 gene transfer in advanced non-small-cell lung cancer. J Natl Cancer Inst 1999;91:763–71.

47. Clayman GL, Frank DK, Bruso PA, Goepfert H. Adenovirus-mediated wild-type p53 gene transfer as a surgical adjuvant in advanced head and neck cancers. Clin Cancer Res 1999;5:1715–22.

48. Clayman GL, el-Naggar AK, Lippman SM et al. Adenovirus-mediated p53 gene transfer in patients with advanced recurrent head and neck squamous cell carcinoma. J Clin Oncol 1998;16:2221–32.

49. Podda S, Ward M, Himelstein A et al. Transfer and expression of the human multiple drug resistance gene into live mice. Proc Natl Acad Sci USA 1992;89:9676–80.

50. Sorrentino B, Brandt S, Bodine D et al. Selection of drug resistant bone marrow cells in-vivo after retroviral transfer of human MDR1. Science 1992;257:99–103.

51. Hesdorffer C, Ayello J, Ward M et al. Phase I trial of retroviral-mediated transfer of the human MDR1 gene as marrow chemoprotection in patients undergoing high-dose chemotherapy and autologous stem-cell transplantation. J Clin Oncol 1998;16:165–72.

52. Devereux S, Corney C, Macdonald C et al. Feasibility and preliminary results of multi-drug resistance (MDR-1) gene transfer in patients undergoing high dose therapy and peripheral blood stem cell transplantation for lymphoma. Gene Ther 1998;5:403–8.

53. Moscow JA, Huang H, Carter C et al. Engraftment of MDR1 and NeoR gene-transduced hematopoietic cells after breast cancer chemotherapy. Blood 1999;94:52–61.

54. Bunting KD, Galipeau J, Topham D, Benaim E, Sorrentino BP. Transduction of murine bone marrow cells with an MDR1 vector enables ex vivo stem cell expansion, but these expanded grafts cause a myeloproliferative syndrome in transplanted mice. Blood 1998;92:2269–79.

55. Dhondt V, Caruso M, Ward M, Cole S, Deeley R, Bank A. Expression of the Multidrug-Resistance Protein (MRP) gene using retroviral vectors. Blood 1995;86:1849.

56. Magni M, Shammah S, Schiro R, Mellado W, Dallafavera R, Gianni AM. Induction of cyclophosphamide-resistance by aldehyde-dehydrogenase gene-transfer. Blood 1996;87:1097–103.

57. Lo KM, Lynch CA, Gillies SD. The use of a wild-type dihydrofolate reductase-encoding cdna as a dominant selectable marker and induction of expression by methotrexate. Gene 1992;121:365–9.

58. Dumenco LL, Warman B, Hatzoglou M, Lim IK, Abboud SL, Gerson SL. Increase in nitrosourea resistance in mammalian cells by retrovirally mediated gene transfer of bacterial O6-alkylguanine-DNA alkyltransferase. Cancer Res 1989;49:6044–51.

59. Puchalski RB, Fahl WE. Expression of recombinant glutathione S-transferase-Pi, Ya, or Yb-1 confers resistance to alkylating agents. Proc Natl Acad Sci USA 1990;87:2443–7.

60. Chinnasamy N, Rafferty JA, Hickson I et al.

Chemoprotective gene transfer II: multilineage in vivo protection of haemopoiesis against the effects of an antitumour agent by expression of a mutant human O6-alkylguanine-DNA alkyl-transferase. Gene Ther 1998;5:842–7.

61. Chinnasamy N, Rafferty JA, Hickson I et al. O6-Benzylguanine potentiates the in vivo toxicity and clastogenicity of temozolomide and BCNU in mouse bone marrow. Blood 1997;89:1566–73.

62. Moolten FL. Tumor chemosensitivity conferred by inserted herpes thymidine kinase genes – paradigm for a prospective cancer control strategy. Cancer Res 1986;46:5276–81.

63. Mullen CA, Kilstrup M, Blaese RM. Transfer of the bacterial gene for cytosine deaminase to mammalian cells confers lethal sensitivity to 5-fluorocytosine – a negative selection system. Proc Natl Acad Sci USA 1992;89:33–7.

64. Izquierdo M, Martin V, de Felipe P et al. Human malignant brain tumor response to herpes simplex thymidine kinase (HSVtk)/ganciclovir gene therapy. Gene Ther 1996;3:491–5.

65. Klatzmann D, Valery CA, Bensimon G et al. A phase I/II study of herpes simplex virus type 1 thymidine kinase 'suicide' gene therapy for recurrent glioblastoma. Study Group on Gene Therapy for Glioblastoma. Hum Gene Ther 1998;9:2595–604.

66. Ram Z, Culver KW, Oshiro EM et al. Therapy of malignant brain tumors by intratumoral implantation of retroviral vector-producing cells. Nature Med 1997;3:1354–61.

67. Shand N, Weber F, Mariani L et al. A phase 1–2 clinical trial of gene therapy for recurrent glioblastoma multiforme by tumor transduction with the herpes simplex thymidine kinase gene followed by ganciclovir. GLI328 European–Canadian Study Group. Hum Gene Ther 1999; 10:2325–35.

68. Eck SL, Alavi JB, Alavi A et al. Treatment of advanced CNS malignancies with the recombinant adenovirus H5.010RSVTK: a phase I trial. Hum Gene Ther 1996;7:1465–82.

69. Dewey RA, Morrissey G, Cowsill CM et al. Chronic brain inflammation and persistent herpes simplex virus 1 thymidine kinase expression in survivors of syngeneic glioma treated by adenovirus-mediated gene therapy: implications for clinical trials. Nature Med 1999;5:1256–63.

70. Kolb HJ, Mittermuller J, Clemm C et al. Donor leukocyte transfusions for treatment of recurrent chronic myelogenous leukemia in marrow transplant patients. Blood 1990;76:2462–5.

71. Bonini C, Ferrari G, Verzeletti S et al. HSV-TK gene transfer into donor lymphocytes for control of allogeneic graft-versus-leukemia (see comments). Science 1997;276:1719–24.

72. Vanderbruggen P, Traversari C, Chomez P et al. A gene encoding an antigen recognized by cytolytic lymphocytes-T on a human melanoma. Science 1991;254:1643–7.

73. Coulie PG, Brichard V, Vanpel A et al. A new gene coding for a differentiation antigen recognized by autologous cytolytic T-lymphocytes on HLA-A2 melanomas. J Exp Med 1994;180:35–42.

74. Kawakami Y, Eliyahu S, Sakaguchi K et al. Identification of the immunodominant peptides of the MART-1 human melanoma antigen recognized by the majority of HLA-A2-restricted tumor-infiltrating lymphocytes. J Exp Med 1994; 180:347–52.

75. Steinman R. The dendritic cell system and its role in immunogenicity. Annu Rev Immunol 1991;9:271–96.

76. Buggins AG, Lea N, Gaken J et al. Effect of co-stimulation and the microenvironment on antigen presentation by leukemic cells. Blood 1999;94: 3479–90.

77. Dranoff G, Jaffee E, Lazenby A et al. Vaccination with irradiated tumor-cells engineered to secrete murine granulocyte–macrophage colony-stimulating factor stimulates potent, specific, and long-lasting antitumor immunity. Proc Natl Acad Sci USA 1993;90:3539–43.

78. Eshhar Z, Waks T, Gross G, Schindler DG. Specific activation and targeting of cytotoxic lymphocytes through chimeric single chains consisting of antibody-binding domains and the gamma or zeta subunits of the immunoglobulin and T-cell receptors. Proc Natl Acad Sci USA 1993;90:720–4.

79. Palmer K, Moore J, Everard M et al. Gene therapy with autologous, interleukin 2-secreting tumor cells in patients with malignant melanoma. Hum Gene Ther 1999;10:1261–8.

80. Moller P, Sun Y, Dorbic T et al. Vaccination with IL-7 gene-modified autologous melanoma cells can enhance the anti-melanoma lytic activity in peripheral blood of patients with a good clinical performance status: a clinical phase I study. Br J Cancer 1998;77:1907–16.

81. Abdel-Wahab Z, Weltz C, Hester D et al. A phase I clinical trial of immunotherapy with interferon-gamma gene-modified autologous

melanoma cells: monitoring the humoral immune response. Cancer 1997;80:401–12.

82. Stewart AK, Lassam NJ, Quirt IC et al. Adenovector-mediated gene delivery of inter-leukin-2 in metastatic breast cancer and melanoma: results of a phase 1 clinical trial. Gene Ther 1999;6:350–63.

83. Belli F, Arienti F, Sule-Suso J et al. Active immunization of metastatic melanoma patients with interleukin-2-transduced allogeneic melanoma cells: evaluation of efficacy and tolerability [published erratum appears in Cancer Immunol Immunother 1997 Oct;45(2):119]. Cancer Immunol Immunother 1997;44:197–203.

84. Veelken H, Mackensen A, Lahn M et al. A phase-I clinical study of autologous tumor cells plus interleukin-2-gene-transfected allogeneic fibroblasts as a vaccine in patients with cancer. Int J Cancer 1997;70:269–77.

85. Hsu FJ, Caspar CB, Czerwinski D et al. Tumor-specific idiotype vaccines in the treatment of patients with B-cell lymphoma – Long-term results of a clinical trial. Blood 1997;89:3129–35.

86. King CA, Spellerberg MB, Zhu D et al. DNA vaccines with single-chain Fv fused to fragment C of tetanus toxin induce protective immunity against lymphoma and myeloma. Nature Med 1998;4:1281–6.

87. Cantwell M, Hua T, Pappas J, Kipps TJ. Acquired CD40-ligand deficiency in chronic lymphocytic leukemia. Nature Med 1997;3: 984–9.

88. Kato K, Cantwell MJ, Sharma S, Kipps TJ. Gene transfer of CD40-ligand induces autologous immune recognition of chronic lymphocytic leukemia B cells. J Clin Invest 1998;101:1133–41.

89. Rassenti L, Cielinska S, Kipps T. CD154 gene therapy of chronic lymphocytic leukemia patients leads to anamnestic T cell responses. Blood 1999;94:2675 (abstract).

90. Orkin S, Motulsky A. Report and recommendations of the panel to assess the NIH investment in research on gene therapy, 1995. http://www.nih.gov/news/panelrep.html

22

Cost-effectiveness of high dose chemotherapy in non-Hodgkin's lymphoma, Hodgkin's disease and multiple myeloma

Fiona Sampson, Stephen Beard and Paul Lorigan

CONTENTS Introduction • Appropriate form of evaluation • Identifying and interpreting evidence of clinical effectiveness • Measurement of health benefit • Estimating marginal cost of HDC • Results • Discussion

INTRODUCTION

Role of economic evaluation

Increasing concern over the financial limitations of healthcare resources, together with progressive moves towards more evidence-based clinical practice, have elevated the importance of health economic considerations in the evaluation of new healthcare technologies. The need to consider both the costs and benefits of these novel and frequently expensive interventions is now widely recognized and advocated, alongside the evaluation of clinical efficacy and the development of clear clinical guidelines.[1-3]

The vast majority of such health economic evaluations are necessarily performed as secondary analyses. These studies use a variety of analytical approaches and draw from a wide spectrum of available data, including outcomes of primary research studies, observational case-series data, standardized costing data and information on patient health-state values and preferences. This growing relevance of economic issues is reflected in the increasing number of randomized clinical trials (RCTs) that now include both economic and service use outcomes, alongside standard clinical outcome measure. However, it is likely that secondary economic analysis will remain a dominant evaluative methodology for some time, as trial-based economics outcomes, along with clinical outcomes, present real problems in their generalizability to other clinical settings.

The existence of such economic evaluations, with common measures of cost and benefit ratios, can provide a useful framework to support healthcare commissioners in comparing the relative 'value for money' of a variety of interventions, and to prioritize accordingly.

Structures for considering new treatments in the UK

The need to have a clear and structured evaluative process in support of healthcare commissioning decisions is being addressed by Health Technology Assessment (HTA) organizations world-wide, in order to provide an equity of care and to address the problem of legal challenges to decisions to withhold treatment. These organizations oversee the production of evidence-based reviews, which synthesize and critically evaluate potential clinical benefits and cost-effectiveness of new technologies.

In the UK, the evaluative role of national HTA programmes was previously supported through a series of independent regional development and evaluation committees (DEC). This role has now been co-ordinated on a national basis through a new government body, the National Institute for Clinical Excellence (NICE), as part of a move to provide more geographical equity to the decision process, and to provide much clearer guidance to commissioners, clinicians and, more importantly, to patients themselves.

Economic assessments of high dose chemotherapy

As part of this regional evidence-based review process, the Trent Institute for Health Services Research has produced reports examining the clinical effectiveness and cost-effectiveness of high dose chemotherapy (HDC) with bone marrow/autologous stem cell transplantation in three specific disease areas: non-Hodgkin's lymphoma (NHL), Hodgkin's disease (HD) and multiple myeloma (MM).[4,5]

The remainder of this chapter presents the economic results of these analyses of HDC, describing the methodology adopted and highlighting the key features relating to economic analysis of such treatments. The aim is to inform the reader of the specific results and provide a framework within which to judge similar economic evaluations of health care.

APPROPRIATE FORM OF EVALUATION

The term 'economic evaluation' encompasses a wide range of approaches that can be used to assess the economic implications of health technologies, both new and old. There are essentially four main types of full economic analysis

within which the costs and benefits of treatment alternatives can be compared and contrasted. These forms of analysis are cost-minimization, cost–benefit, cost-effectiveness and cost–utility (see Table 22.1).[6] All have a significant role to play in supporting healthcare commissioners to examine the most efficient and effective ways of allocating fixed health budgets.[7]

The majority of published economic reviews are conducted as either cost-effectiveness or cost–utility analyses. These two forms are most commonly used when comparing new interventions against current treatment options, particularly in cases where the new treatment may either increase overall or progression-free survival, or provide significant improvements in terms of quality-of-life measures.

We performed a series of cost-effectiveness analyses (CEA) for HDC, comparing the costs and life-year gained (LYG) survival benefits of treatment against standard chemotherapy regimens.

IDENTIFYING AND INTERPRETING EVIDENCE OF CLINICAL EFFECTIVENESS

Search strategy

The production of a credible health economic analysis of a new technology needs to be based upon high-quality clinical evidence. A clear and comprehensive search strategy should always be evident in support of an economic evaluation, in order to ensure that all potentially available trial data and clinical evidence have been captured.

Our analyses of HDC were based on evidence identified through a series of systematic literature searches of electronic databases including: MEDLINE, EmBASE, HEALTHSTAR, CANCERLIT, Cochrane Collaboration Library, HMIC (Department of Health, King's Fund, HELMIS), NHS CRD (DARE, NEED) and various health technology assessment databases. These electronic database searches covered the period January 1990 to December 1997. This was supplemented by information gained

Table 22.1 Forms of economic evaluation	
Form of economic evaluation	**Characteristics**
Cost-minimization	Considers the least-cost alternative to achieve a specific clinical outcome (e.g. minimum cost of treating a suspected broken limb). Provides information as to the most efficient way of achieving a chosen outcome
Cost–benefit	Considers the absolute costs and benefits of interventions compared with a 'do nothing' option. Values clinical benefit in purely monetary terms, via 'willingness-to-pay' and 'trade-off' techniques. Many economic analyses are wrongly labelled 'cost–benefit analysis'; in reality, they are difficult to perform and rarely conducted
Cost-effectiveness	Expresses overall cost-effectiveness of an intervention in terms of a cost per unit of clinical benefit. Benefits are typically measured in terms of life-years gained or quality-adjusted life-years gained, and used to calculate the marginal benefit compared with standard treatment
Cost–utility	Similar concept to cost-effectiveness, but values clinical benefit in terms of a patient's quality of life, assigning quality-of-life utilities to different health states

from internet web sites, personal contacts and other cancer-related literature databases.

The searches focused specifically on the role of HDC in the treatment of patients with HD, NHL or MM. In particular we looked for clinical trials comparing HDC treatment with the use of conventional first-line or salvage chemotherapy. Initially, RCTs were targeted as being 'gold standard' evidence, but due to a known lack of RCT evidence in these areas, data from large peer-reviewed case series were also considered. Other areas of 'grey' literature were also examined, including the draft NHS HTA report on Bone Marrow and Peripheral Blood Stem Cell Transplantation for Malignancy (now in full publication), and the European Bone Marrow Transplantation (EBMT) Registry guidelines.[8,9]

We limited the evaluation of potential cost-effectiveness benefits to those areas in which the clinical evidence for HDC, over standard treatment, appeared most convincing. These potential HDC groups covered:

- patients with untreated stage II/III MM,
- chemosensitive patients with relapsed intermediate/high-grade NHL, and
- chemosensitive patients with relapsed HD.

Whilst there are many other patient groups for whom HDC may eventually prove beneficial, the evidence was felt to be less convincing, and current EBMT guidelines recommend the ongoing participation in RCTs in these cases.[9]

There have been relatively few full RCTs considering HDC in these three specific patient groups. In fact we identified only one key RCT in each group. However, due to the level of clinical benefit suggested by a number of published case series, it may now prove unethical to enter such patients into further RCTs of HDC versus standard therapy. Therefore it is unlikely that further evidence from RCTs will become available in the future; ongoing trials are currently experiencing recruitment difficulties and previous trials have been stopped early due to strong patient preference in favour of HDC.

For these reasons, it was important for us to consider both randomized and non-randomized evidence in the form of published case-series data.

Identified HDC trials

We based our estimates of survival benefit for HDC in MM patients on the results of the trial reported by the Intergroupe Français du Myélome.[10] Examining the use of HDC in previously untreated MM patients, this remains the only published RCT in this specific patient group. There are also a number of ongoing RCTs examining the optimal timing of HDC and the potential role of double transplantation.[11-13]

The survival benefits for HDC in relapsed high/medium-grade HD patients were based on a single RCT reported by the British National Lymphoma Investigation (BNLI).[14] Forty patients were randomized to receive either subablative chemotherapy (mini-BEAM – BCNU, etoposide, Ara-C and cyclophosphamide) or ablative chemotherapy (BEAM) plus autologous bone marrow transplantation (ABMT). The study closed early because of poor recruitment; patients were requesting HDC and refusing randomization. A further randomized study comparing standard therapy with HDC from the EBMT closed early due to poor accrual.[15] Preliminary results showed no survival advantage for HDC, as the majority of patients who relapsed after standard therapy were then salvaged with HDC. Full details are not yet available, but the authors concluded that HDC is still the treatment of choice for patients with HD in first relapse.

For intermediate/high-grade NHL patients in first relapse, we used the survival benefits described in the Parma group study.[16] In total, 109 patients with relapsed intermediate/high-grade NHL were randomized to receive either induction therapy followed by HDC or to receive subablative therapy.

The survival differences between HDC and standard chemotherapy were statistically significant for NHL and MM. The survival advantage for HDC in relapsed HD[14] did not reach significance at conventionally held levels. This is likely to be due to underpowering of the study, as a direct result of the recruitment difficulties. However, a survival difference was further supported by consideration of observational retrospective case-series data of both HDC and standard chemotherapy.[17,18]

Interpreting the evidence of effectiveness

The use of both randomized trial and retrospective case-series data to support economic analysis requires many assumptions to be made regarding the interpretation of clinical outcomes and the generalizability of the trial experience. Patient groupings within trials are often very specific, excluding many types of patients that would typically be encountered within a general clinical setting. The selection of the comparative standard treatment may also be inappropriate for certain clinical settings. The level of resource use in supporting a treatment may also be felt to be over- or under-intensive, implying a different cost profile from that which would be normally be seen. The length of follow-up can be inadequate and patients lost to follow-up may not be included within analysis of results, thus biasing results further. The primary outcomes reported are often not directly applicable to economic evaluation, and assumptions may need to be made to convert specific outcome measures into, for example, quality-of-life utility scores.

These are all examples of potential study bias contained within the trial design itself, which can impose limitations on the generalizability

Table 22.2 Questions in evaluating evidence from randomized controlled trials
• Is the primary outcome measure directly applicable in an economic evaluation?
• Is the choice of alternative treatment representative of our clinical practice?
• Would the new treatment be applicable to our clinical practice?
• Was there an adequate period of follow-up?
• How were patients lost to follow-up represented in the results?
• Do the inclusion/exclusion criteria ensure a generalizable treatment population?
• Is the resource usage of patients typical of our own clinical practice?

of results into a local clinical practice context.[19] Therefore, careful interpretation of trial design and questioning of trial results is essential in developing any cost-effectiveness conclusions, as it is in evaluations of clinical efficacy (see Table 22.2).

The HDC trials reported on overall mortality, providing an appropriate unit of benefit for an economic evaluation. None of the trials provided outcome data on quality of life.

The HDC trials reported the outcomes for patients on an intention-to-treat basis (ITT), that is, outcomes were reported for all patients who were randomized to either treatment group regardless of whether they successfully completed treatment. This allows a realistic comparison of outcomes and is more reflective of clinical practice.

Taking all these aspects into consideration we accepted the published trial data as being an accurate representation of the likely marginal benefits for HDC treatment when administered within a UK context, for patients in the three disease states considered.

MEASUREMENT OF HEALTH BENEFIT

Choice of units of measure

Survival benefits can be expressed both quantitatively (i.e. in terms of improved survival) and qualitatively (i.e. improved quality of life). Although patient quality-of-life issues are an important consideration in the evaluation of any treatment, it is generally difficult to quantify such treatment benefits without access to primary research that includes a standard quality-of-life (QoL) indicator. QoL can be reflected within economic analyses using utility weightings. In the absence of such data for HDC, we therefore produced cost-effectiveness estimates based on the raw unadjusted overall survival outcomes derived from the identified RCTs.

In theory, event-free or progression-free survival can be used as a crude proxy for a quality-adjusted survival. It essentially values survival as worthwhile only up to the point at which progression occurs. However, this in effect ignores any survival after disease progression, a proportion of which may be spent in relatively good quality of life.

Survival advantages were calculated using area under the curve (AUC) estimates of benefit, taken directly from the published Kaplan–Meier survival curves. This process involves subtracting the estimated AUC for the conventional chemotherapy arm from the AUC for the HDC arm of each trial, providing an estimate of the incremental survival period (typically measured in months or years) gained by the HDC-treated cohort over the trial period (Fig. 22.1).

The main advantage of the AUC approach in estimating marginal benefits is that it provides an estimate of mean survival, based upon the experience of the whole cohort. For economic evaluation this is a more appropriate method than the use of the typically quoted median survival statistic, which estimates average survival at the time point reached by 50% of the initial cohort. Median survival will not allow for any significant differences between treatments in terms of long-term survival, effectively ignoring outliers towards the tail end of the curve.

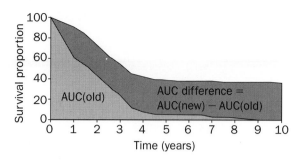

Figure 22.1
Example of area under the curve (AUC) estimation of marginal treatment benefit.

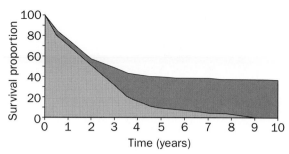

Figure 22.2
Example of median survival providing underestimate of benefit.

For example, if initial survival was not significantly different between the two arms (e.g. a median survival of 2–3 years), but a proportion of patients (e.g. 35–40%) achieved a long-term cure, the improved survival, which is clearly acknowledged using AUC methodology, is ignored using the median survival statistic (Figure 22.2). Similarly, if initial survival rates for the treated arm were significantly higher than for conventional treatment, but then survival rates gradually decreased more rapidly in the longer term, the median survival statistic would potentially overestimate the true survival advantage (Fig. 22.3).

Therefore when reviewing or conducting any such economic analysis of oncology treatments, care needs to be taken in judging which form of survival has been selected and exactly how it has been estimated. As HDC potentially provides a longer-term survival for at least some patients, we selected AUC-based estimates of mean survival, rather than using published median statistics (see Table 22.3).

Extrapolation of trial data

Any analysis of the survival benefits of HDC based upon the use of trial-period data alone is likely to provide an underestimate of the total potential cohort benefits. Restricting outcomes

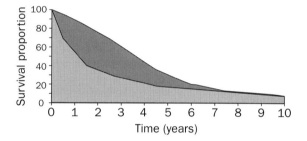

Figure 22.3
Example of median survival providing overestimate of benefit.

to the trial period effectively assumes that the survival advantages of the HDC arm will cease directly after the end of the study. In reality this is a very unlikely scenario, especially in those trials where a survival plateau appears to have been reached. Plateau duration is an important clinical end point. To address this issue in our HDC analysis, additional estimates of cost-effectiveness were made based on predicted long-term survival benefits. This was achieved by extrapolating the published survival data to a range of time horizons, informed where possible by evidence of longer-term benefits from reported non-randomized case series for both HDC and standard treatments (see Fig. 22.4).

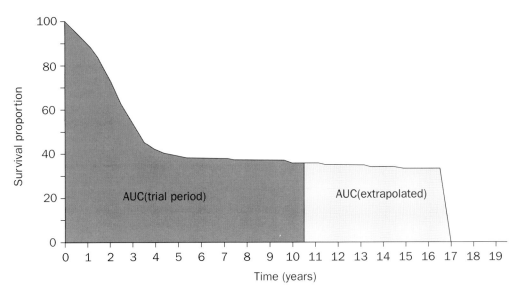

Figure 22.4
Extrapolation of trial outcome data.

Long-term survival for MM was estimated using non-randomized data from a single-centre study.[20,21] These data provided estimates of benefit for HDC at 6 and 10 years (i.e. 1 and 5 years after the IFM 5-year trial period). This was compared with a published estimate of 5% for overall survival at 10 years for conventional chemotherapy.[12] These data were used in the absence of RCT data. Comparison of benefits derived from non-randomized case studies is methodologically less sound than using long-term RCT data, due to differences between the patient groups and methods of these trials.

For HDC in relapsed NHL and relapsed HD, the survival curves appeared to reach a plateau and the 5-year trial-based survival curves were assumed to indicate a long-term cure. Survival cures were mathematically extrapolated to 5, 10 and 20 years, with long-term survival curves assuming no further lymphoma-related mortality, but including an underlying standard age-related mortality rate. Even when restricting extrapolations to 5 years only, we noted a marked impact in terms of the incremental cost-effectiveness of HDC (see Table 22.3). Given the

average age of these patient groups and the observed plateau in the published survival curves for HDC patients, a 5-year extension to survival benefits would seem reasonable.

ESTIMATING MARGINAL COST OF HDC

There are no standard published cost estimates available for patients undergoing conventional chemotherapy or HDC. We therefore calculated the costs of an average course of both HDC treatment and standard chemotherapy regimens using information from local clinical centres within the Trent region (see Table 22.3). The treatment costs were based on the costs of local NHS contract tariffs and were calculated to include the cost of drugs, staffing, inpatient stay and day visits.

It is possible that the high initial costs of HDC would be partially offset by the reduced likelihood of further chemotherapy following relapse and reduced palliative care costs. However, the costs included within this analysis were restricted to initial chemotherapy only

Table 22.3 Cost-effectiveness ratio – based on overall survival

Benefit period	Hodgkin's disease			Non-Hodgkin's lymphoma			Multiple myeloma		
	Survival benefit (months)	LYG*	Cost per LYG	Survival benefit (months)	LYG	Cost per LYG	Survival benefit (months)	LYG	Cost per LYG
Trial period only	10	0.8	£17 375	13	1.1	£12 636	8	0.7	£14 970
+5 years	28	2.3	£6043	27	2.3	£6043	20	1.7	£6160
+10 years	45	3.8	£3658	40	3.3	£4212	–	–	–
+20 years	78	6.5	£2138	66	5.5	£2527	–	–	–

LYG, Life-year gained.

and thus excluded the cost of follow-up or palliative care. As such, we adopted a conservative approach to costing in favour of the conventional therapy; that is, the likely true marginal cost of HDC was overestimated.

Significant additional costs for patients can also include blood transfusions, radiotherapy and analgesia, particularly in the case of MM patients. The cost of palliative treatment will vary considerably. In an attempt to quantify these costs the records of a small group of conventionally treated relapsed patients were reviewed. The patient records identified areas of resource use, including palliative chemotherapy, radiotherapy, hospital admissions, blood tests, scans, blood transfusions, antibiotics, etc. Based on these data it is calculated that the mean average cost of relapse treatment is typically around £9500, although it is clearly variable (range £4000 to £15 000).

The general costs of HDC procedures are considerably higher than those of conventional initial chemotherapy, due to the additional cost of the harvesting procedure and the need for inpatient stay. Costs for HDC were based on contract costings for the chemotherapy drugs, a 3- to 4-week inpatient stay, an additional six day visits and additional drug therapy. On this resource use basis it was estimated that HDC would typically cost between £12 500 and £16 000 per patient. Costs for standard chemotherapy were based upon six to nine courses of chemotherapy administered on a day-case basis for MM patients, costing £1980–2970 per patient. For the NHL and HD patient groups the cost included a CHOP chemotherapy regimen, including a 50% chance of admission for neutropenic sepsis. This was estimated at around £1710 per patient.

As the treatment costs included are almost exclusively placed in the first year of treatment, we did not include any element of discounting. The use of discounting is the recommended economic approach to valuing future costs and monetary health benefits. Typical UK cost discounting rates are recommended at 6% per annum. Discounting can also be theoretically applied to non-monetary LYG health benefits. However, this is a much more contentious issue and is generally not recommended or, if used, is applied at much lower rates (<3%) than with cost.

Overall, on the basis of this costing exercise, and accepting the assumptions taken, we estimated the overall marginal cost of HDC at £10 480 for MM and £13 900 for both relapsed

NHL and relapsed HD. Any differences in marginal costs between these patient groups are likely to be due to the variation in costs between centres, rather than any real significant cost differences.

RESULTS

Cost-effectiveness of HDC

The incremental cost-effectiveness ratio of an intervention is calculated by dividing the marginal (additional) costs of the new intervention by the marginal benefits of treatment (e.g. numbers of LYG, number of QALYs, progression-free survival). The use of common measures of benefit helps to create cost-effectiveness ratios that theoretically can be compared with one another, even where the treatments themselves may be for unrelated conditions and diseases.

Our analyses of HDC were based on cost-effectiveness ratios calculated using cost per LYG values. The results, based on the trial period data alone (representing a conservative view of survival benefits), show that the cost-effectiveness ratios for HDC remain in the region of £11 000–13 000 per LYG for NHL and MM patients, and are slightly higher at around £17 000–18 000 per LYG for HD patients (see Table 22.3). However, the impact of including extended benefits beyond the trial period, i.e. indicating potential life-time benefits of HDC, is marked. The cost-effectiveness ratios reduce by almost 50% after the inclusion of only an additional 5 years of extended benefit. Extending the benefits even further (up to a maximum of 20 years beyond the trial data), on the basis of the survival curve plateau for HD and NHL, these ratios reduce further to levels well below a £10 000 per LYG threshold.

While there is much controversy surrounding the use of league tables of cost-effectiveness,[22] there are guidelines as to figures which can be considered 'reasonable' in health commissioning terms.[23] A commonly adopted threshold for the general cost-effectiveness of new healthcare technologies in the UK is around £20 000–25 000 per LYG. Similarly quoted figures for the USA are in the region of $50 000 per LYG. Beyond this point, interventions are generally deemed as being 'high cost' and further evidence may be required before they are recommended for general commissioning. Our analysis indicates that HDC represents what would be considered a cost-effective treatment.

Sensitivity analyses

The majority of health economic evaluations are conducted as secondary analyses and as such are based on data derived from a wide range of possible sources, including randomized trials, case-series reports, clinical databases and clinical opinion. These data sources will always vary in terms of their overall quality, reliability and generalizability, necessitating the consideration of such uncertainty as part of the analysis.

Performing a series of formal sensitivity analyses is one approach that can allow us to deal with this type of inherent uncertainty, by attempting to define a confidence range to the baseline results, following the likely variations in the raw data. This generally involves examining a range of sensitivity scenarios in which each parameter is altered either individually (univariate or one-way sensitivity analysis), or in combination with other variables (multivariate or multi-way sensitivity analysis). This type of scenario approach can provide an indication of the scale and direction of potential changes in results under different key assumptions or conditions. For instance, there may be different choices of source data for health benefits or more intensive versions of treatment increasing resource usage.

Other forms of sensitivity analysis include threshold analysis, where the amount of variation in parameters is noted before the cost-effectiveness reaches a predefined limit, and extreme-scenario analysis, where all parameters are simultaneously taken to their extremes, providing a best and worst case view for the new technology or treatment. Extreme-scenario analysis is particularly useful for finding the widest potential range of values (even if this includes very unlikely combinations of data values).

The costs and health benefit assumptions made within our analysis are subject to a degree of uncertainty. Treatment costs will vary across regions, and between individual clinical centres, and are likely to differ if not restricted to initial treatment costs alone. Health benefits as observed in the randomized trials may not be truly achievable in clinical practice; patient groups may differ, treatment regimens may vary slightly or other adjuvant therapy may be given. In order to account for the effects of this potential uncertainty on the cost-effectiveness results, we performed a series of sensitivity analyses based on a variation of the extreme-scenario approach. We considered a ±50% range to the marginal benefits of HDC, as estimated from trial data, and explored a range of marginal cost difference between £10 000 and £20 000. These ranges of variation in both costs and health benefits were felt to be wide enough to include all reasonably expected differences,

whilst remaining meaningful. Importantly, we excluded all the extended trial benefits from this analysis, using trial-period benefits only, although the long-term benefits considered within our main analyses should be considered a form of sensitivity analysis due to the uncertainty inherent in the assumptions made regarding benefits.

Figures 22.5–7 present the results of this sensitivity analysis in a visual form, combining the cost and benefit variations for each disease area. Each shows the marginal cost of HDC along the x-axis, with the corresponding cost per LYG cost-effectiveness ratio values shown against the vertical y-axis. The figures each plot three separate data series, corresponding to alternative levels of marginal benefit for HDC. The middle data series on each graph represents the baseline health benefits, as taken from the relevant randomized trials for each disease area. The remaining data series correspond to the +50% and −50% LYG benefits limits.

The sensitivity graphs enable the reader to consider variations in costs and benefits, either separately or taken together, and allow the

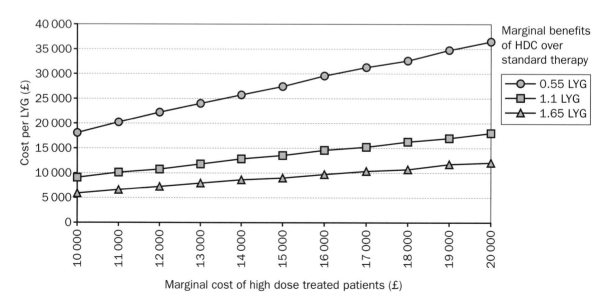

Figure 22.5
Sensitivity of cost-effectiveness (life-year gained, LYG) for non-Hodgkin's lymphomas.

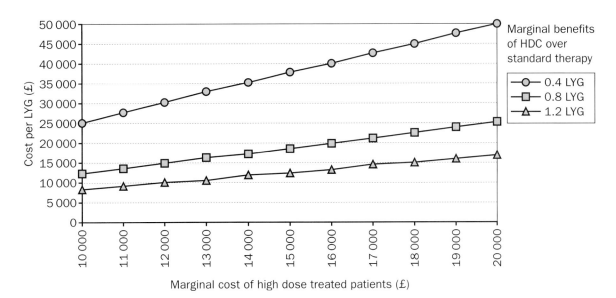

Figure 22.6
Sensitivity of cost-effectiveness (life-year gained, LYG) for Hodgkin's disease.

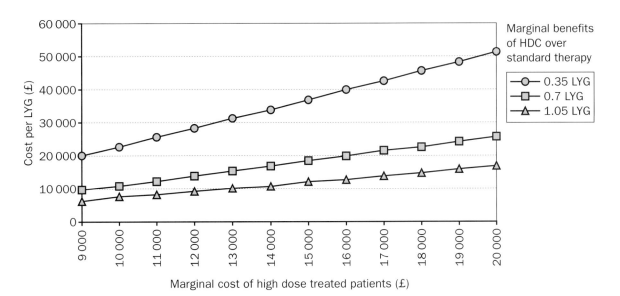

Figure 22.7
Sensitivity of cost-effectiveness (life-year gained, LYG) for multiple myeloma.

reader to make their own judgement as to where they feel the most likely combination of cost and benefit parameters lie.

The results show that, given the survival benefits as suggested by the identified RCTs (i.e. the middle data series), the cost-effectiveness ratios for HDC in all patient groups remain at levels below £27000 per LYG, irrespective of the range of cost variation considered. This threshold would only be exceeded if the marginal cost of HDC were to increase beyond £20000, which would seem unlikely. Even following our conservative costing approach, we only estimated marginal costs of around £13000. However, if the marginal health benefits from HDC were at levels of only half the values suggested by the RCTs, then this would naturally increase the cost-effectiveness ratios. For example, in the case of HD patients HDC would have a cost per LYG figure of £30000–35000, given the baseline marginal cost estimates. Nevertheless, the magnitude of the benefits is considered more likely to increase than decrease, as benefits will in reality extend beyond the published trial periods. Again, we leave the reader to make their own judgement on the reliability and generalizability of the health benefit data.

Finally, if we were to bring into the sensitivity analysis extended health benefits to 5 years beyond trial data, then effectively we would introduce a fourth data series to the sensitivity graphs. These lines would fall below the existing series, as the revised marginal health benefits would certainly be over 50% higher than the baseline values (see Table 22.3).

DISCUSSION

Clinical support from non-randomized studies of HDC in patients with myeloma, relapsed NHL and relapsed HD has led to the widespread use of HDC as a standard therapy, despite the limited number of RCTs in this area. As a result, further RCTs are unlikely on ethical grounds. Economic analyses within the published HDC trials were not considered a priori,

and as such there has been no readily available evidence for the cost-effectiveness of HDC. Similarly, there are currently no published UK studies providing cost-effectiveness estimates of HDC versus conventional chemotherapy for the three patient groups we have considered.

Using local costing data and results of the RCT evidence available, we have produced an estimate of the cost per life year gained of £11000–18000 depending on the disease and disease type. Underpinning our analysis was a conservative interpretation of both costs and benefits in favour of standard chemotherapy. Despite limiting costs to those of initial therapy alone and using conservative estimates of benefit based upon trial data alone, the cost-effectiveness ratios produced appear favourable. Extending treatment benefits out to reflect 10-year survival expectations, and including potential costs of palliative care, would suggest cost-effectiveness ratios of under £10000 per LYG, falling well below commonly quoted cost-effectiveness thresholds.

It is also important to acknowledge that the benefits of HDC cannot be measured solely in terms of overall survival advantages, as there are certainly issues of differences in patients' life quality. Further considerations of the cost-effectiveness of these HDC treatments should include adjustments for quality of life.

Although appropriate care should be taken in interpreting the results of these analyses, it would appear that the economic case for HDC is well grounded, given these levels of cost-effectiveness. Realistically, it is difficult to envisage a likely combination of variation in both costs and benefits that would lead to strongly negative impacts in terms of the commissioning of HDC for these three distinct patient groups. As such, our analysis supports the view that HDC should be considered as a cost-effective treatment for a carefully selected group, including patients with previously untreated MM, patients with relapsed HD or patients with NHL who have proven chemosensitive disease.

REFERENCES

1. Weinstein MC, Siegel JE, Gold MR et al. Recommendations of the Panel on Cost-Effectiveness in Health and Medicine. JAMA 1996;276(15):1253–8.

2. Siegel JE, Weinstein MC, Russell LB et al. Recommendations for reporting cost-effectiveness analyses. Panel on Cost-Effectiveness in Health and Medicine. JAMA 1996;276(16):1339–41.

3. Russell LB, Gold MR, Siegel JE et al. The role of cost-effectiveness analysis in health and medicine. Panel on Cost-Effectiveness in Health and Medicine. JAMA 1996;276(14):1172–7.

4. Beard SM, Lorigan P, Sampson F et al. The effectiveness of high dose chemotherapy with autologous stem cell transplantation in the treatment of non-Hodgkin's lymphoma and Hodgkin's disease. Guidance Note for Purchasers: 98/04. Sheffield: Trent Institute for Health Services Research, Universities of Leicester, Nottingham and Sheffield, 1998.

5. Beard SM, Sampson FC, Scott F et al. The effectiveness of high dose chemotherapy and bone marrow/autologous stem cell transplantation in the treatment of multiple myeloma. Guidance Note for Purchasers: 98/08. Sheffield: Trent Institute for Health Services Research, Universities of Leicester, Nottingham and Sheffield, 1998.

6. Drummond MF, O'Brien B, Stoddart GL, Torrance GW. Methods for the economic evaluation of health care programmes, 2nd edn. Oxford: Oxford University Press, 1997.

7. Drummond MF, Jefferson TO. Guidelines for authors and peer reviewers of economic submissions to the BMJ. BMJ 1996;313:275–83.

8. Johnson PW, Simnett SJ, Sweetenham JW et al. Bone marrow and peripheral blood stem cell transplantation for malignancy. Health Technol Assess 1998;2(8):1–187.

9. Goldman JM, Schmitz N, Niethammer D, Gratwohl A. Allogeneic and autologous transplantation for haematological diseases, solid tumours and immune disorders: current practice in Europe in 1998. Bone Marrow Transplant 1998;21:1–7.

10. Attal M, Harousseau JL, Stoppa AM et al. A prospective randomized trial of autologous bone marrow transplantation and chemotherapy in multiple myeloma. N Engl J Med 1996;335(2):91–7.

11. Barlogie B, Jagannath S, Vesole DH et al. Superiority of tandem autologous transplantation over standard therapy for previously untreated multiple myeloma. Blood 1997;89:789–93.

12. Vesole DH, Tricot G, Jagannath S et al. Autotransplants in multiple myeloma: what have we learned? Blood 1996;88:838–47.

13. Fermand JP, Ravaud P, Chevret S et al. High dose therapy and autologous peripheral blood stem cell transplantation in multiple myeloma: up-front or rescue treatment? Results of a multicenter sequential randomised clinical trial. Blood 1998;1992:3131–6.

14. Linch DC, Winfield D, Goldstone AH et al. Dose intensification with autologous bone marrow transplantation in relapsed and resistant Hodgkin's disease; results of a BNLI randomised trial. Lancet 1993;34:1051–4s.

15. Schmitz N, Sextro M, Pfistner B et al. High dose therapy followed by haematopoietic stem cell transplantation for relapsed chemosensitive Hodgkin's disease: final results of a randomised GHSG and EBMT trial (HD-R1). Available from the internet at http://www.asco.org/prof/me/html/99abstracts/all/m_5.htm

16. Philip T, Guglielmi C, Hagenbeek A et al. Autologous bone marrow transplantation as compared with salvage chemotherapy in relapses of chemotherapy-sensitive non-Hodgkin's lymphoma. N Engl J Med 1995;33(23):1540–5.

17. Chopra R, McMillan AK, Linch DC et al. The place of high-dose BEAM therapy and autologous bone marrow transplantation in poor-risk Hodgkin's disease. A single-centre 8-year study of 155 patients. Blood 1993;81(5):1137–45.

18. Longo DL, Duffey PL, Young RC et al. Conventional-dose salvage combination chemotherapy in patients relapsing with Hodgkin's disease after combination chemotherapy: the low probability for cure. J Clin Oncol 1992;10(2):210–18.

19. Jadad AR. Randomised controlled trials: a user's guide. London: BMJ books, 1998.

20. Cunningham D, Paz-Ares L, Gore ME et al. High-dose melphalan for multiple myeloma: long-term follow-up data. J Clin Oncol 1994;12:764–8.

21. Powles R, Cunningham D, Gore M et al. Long-term follow-up of myeloma patients treated with 140 mg/m^2 melphalan without autologous trans-

plantation. Bone marrow transplant 1998;21: S210.

22. Mason J, Drummond M, Torrance G. Some guidelines on the use of cost-effectiveness league tables. BMJ 1993;306:570–2.

23. Stevens A, Colin-Jones D, Gabbay J. Quick and clean: authoritative health technology assessment for local health care contracting. Health Trends 1995;27:37–42.

23

High dose chemotherapy in the new millennium

Thierry Philip and Ross Pinkerton

CONTENTS Introduction • High dose chemotherapy • Stem cell transplantation • Gene therapy • New directions • Growth factors • The future of high dose chemotherapy

INTRODUCTION

Dose intensification is the major rationale behind high dose chemotherapy;[1] bone marrow or stem cell transplantation is simply a tool to allow dose intensification.[2] It is clear at the beginning of the new millennium that despite some evidence that 'more is better',[1] no definitive proof of a role for high dose therapy can be found outside leukemia and lymphoma.[2]

HIGH DOSE CHEMOTHERAPY

The first European Bone Marrow Transplant (EBMT) group meeting in Granada 1985 was able to collect data on 100 cases of solid tumors where intensification with bone marrow transplantation was used. In 1998, more than 3000 cases were reported and 30% of autologous bone marrow transplant (ABMT) or peripheral blood stem cell (PBSC) transplants performed in Europe were in solid tumors, 50% of the 3000 cases of high dose chemotherapy were children and almost 50% were neuroblastoma. Among adult ABMT or PBSC, 50% were in breast cancer; other solid tumors comprised only 7.5% of the recorded cases.

Although lymphoma can be viewed as a link between leukemia and solid tumor, conclusions drawn from lymphomas cannot necessarily be used in other solid tumors. The current position of high dose chemotherapy in aggressive lymphoma is quite clear.

- Patients with primary refractory tumors are not good candidates for high dose chemotherapy regimens.[3]
- Partial response is considered an indication to intensify treatment despite the lack of convincing randomized studies.[3]
- Relapsed disease is an established indication for such therapy[4] Patients with sensitive relapse do significantly better than those with resistant relapse.[5]
- The question of optimal timing is still unresolved.
- No evidence exists for high dose therapy in first complete response (CR), with the exception of very high-risk patients.[3] Furthermore, a calculation for a group of 100 theoretical patients showed that to intensify in first CR will lead to a maximum

of 10 additional survivors for 70 additional ABMT or PBSCT procedures. Cost–benefit analysis favors BMT at relapse (T Philip, paper in progress)

There is limited evidence for a benefit from dose escalation in follicular lymphoma.[6] In relapsed patients, retrospective analysis demonstrated a better disease-free survival (DFS) for transplanted patients compared with conventional chemotherapy but a similar overall survival.[7,8] Benefit is also suggested for patients with tumors in histologic transformation. For patients in first remission, the benefit of autologous transplantation is currently under evaluation in a European Lymphoma Group (GELA) prospective randomized study (GELF 94).

The majority of pediatric patients with solid tumors who receive high dose chemotherapy do so for neuroblastoma. In adults, most data are available for breast carcinoma, but the results have been disappointing.[9–11] A number of prospective randomized trials have suggested that intensification of first-line therapy seems to be of benefit whereas consolidation is not effective. More data are needed using first-line protocols of high dose chemotherapy in this disease.

The concept of high dose chemotherapy is based on the Goldie–Coldman hypothesis.[12] Important observations in the Ridgway sarcoma in dogs[13] showed that a three-fold increase in dose may be enough to move from 0% cure to 100% cure. However, up to now, the optimum combination of drugs for high dose therapy has been unclear and the role (if any) of total body irradiation (TBI) is still a matter of debate.[2] There is a need for further pharmacokinetic studies of single and combined agents at high dose.

One firm conclusion from the last 20 years is that intensification with high dose therapy is not able to overcome resistant malignant clones.[2] High dose chemotherapy should not be used in patients with solid tumors or lymphoma where the tumor is resistant to conventional dose of the drugs. Only patients responding to standard therapy benefit from high dose chemotherapy.

An important question that remains in poor risk solid tumors is whether when CR is reached at conventional dose, is intensification necessary?[2] For testicular cancer the answer appears to be 'no'.

STEM CELL TRANSPLANTATION

We know how to collect PBSC effectively in the majority of cases, the exception being poor mobilizers and the elderly. There are differences between bone-marrow and blood-derived stem cell products. The number of CFU-GM necessary to obtain engraftment with PBSC was found to be at least 5×10^5/kg, significantly higher than for bone marrow.[14] Furthermore, there are differences in the expression of certain surface antigens, in particular the cell adhesion molecules (lymphocyte function associated molecule [LFA]-3, $\alpha L\beta 2$, integrins), which determine the stromal attachment, and of c-*kit*, which is involved in the regulation of migration-associated events.[15] Long-term culture initiating cells are the best approximation of stem cells, and their quantitation in limiting dilution analysis allows an estimate of the number of marrow repopulating cells. Interestingly, stem cells mobilized with chemotherapy and growth factors result in a lower number of long-term repopulating cells than that of bone marrow mononuclear cell suspensions, suggesting that the different mix of more committed progenitors may explain the difference in engraftment kinetics.[16]

Delayed or incomplete engraftment and late graft failures have been reported with small PBSC graft size. A clear dose–response correlation has been shown between the number of CD34+ cells infused and neutrophil and platelet recovery. The minimum number of CD34+ cells allowing sustained engraftment has been estimated to be 1×10^6/kg, although precise determination is confounded by a number of host and tumor factors that may influence engraftment.[17] The positive selection of

CD34+ cells results in purified cell suspensions which appear no different in their ability to generate sustained hematologic recovery compared with unselected marrow or PBSC.[18] In vitro cultures of CD34+ cells allow further enrichment for CD34+ cells without increasing the number of clonogenic epithelial tumor cells. Ex vivo expansion of as little as 1.1×10^7 peripheral CD34+ cells allows engraftment. This technology may significantly reduce the number of contaminating tumor cells.[19] However, the long-term reconstitution capability of cultured cells is not yet known; gene marking studies will provide definitive answers to this question.[20]

GENE THERAPY

Although many of the genetic events resulting in the development of cancer have yet to be identified, the rapidly emerging insight into its genetic basis has lead to strategies for gene therapy.[21,22] Anti-sense oligonucleotides are pharmacologic agents that can inhibit the synthesis of single proteins, and research to enhance their delivery is underway. That PBSC can be used as transfection targets for therapeutic gene transfer has been demonstrated in studies of gene replacement therapy to correct single genetic defects (e.g. adenosine deaminase [ADA]-deficiency, cystic fibrosis and *RevMl0* gene transfer in HIV-1 infections).[23] Experiments targeting the c-*myc* proto-oncogene to purge malignant cells have already been reported.[20] The genetic transfer into tumor cells of a pro-drug activation unit, for example the cytosine-deaminase transcription unit, can allow sensitization of malignant cells to the cell-cycle-independent cytotoxic effects of 5-fluorouracil, which is generated from 5-fluorocytosine. The transfer of the *MDR1* gene (multi-drug resistance) into hematopoietic precursor cells may provide a means to confer resistance to the toxic effects of chemotherapy.[24] Several other genes appear promising for gene transfer approaches to induce drug resistance in hematologic precursors.[25] Experiments using

drug sensitization genes in adenoviral vectors, which bind to integrin receptors poorly expressed on hematopoietic cells, may achieve a simple and selective elimination of contaminating epithelial tumor cells.[26]

Although safety concerns around gene expression in hematologic presursors remain, the successful use of this technology may soon broaden its clinical application.

NEW DIRECTIONS

New approaches will come with increased understanding of rare populations of stem cells, e.g. CD34+CD38−Thy+lin− cells or perhaps CD34−CD164+ cells, and with better knowledge of stem cell biology.

Malignant cells are present in autologous blood or marrow but despite work in leukemia and neuroblastoma, it remains unclear whether these cells are clonogenic. In breast cancer (node positive or negative) and in Ewing sarcoma, circulating occult tumor cells are detectable in bone marrow by immunohistochemistry or polymerase chain reaction (PCR) and may influence prognosis. These cells can be removed using positive or negative purging, but does it matter?[2] This will be one of the major questions to be answered in the next few years.

Allogeneic marrow transplant is not only an ablative procedure, but is also a way to manipulate the immune system after high dose chemotherapy. It is likely that allogeneic marrow transplant will re-emerge as an issue in solid tumors and lymphoma, when cellular therapy associated with high dose chemotherapy regimens will be a major area of investigation.

The new millennium should produce answers to questions that are obvious but remain unsolved outside lymphoma[4] and myeloma,[27] such as when to intensify for lymphoma (we believe at relapse) and in breast carcinoma (we believe at diagnosis). New ideas will also come in the area of new drugs. Novel combinations with novel targets will be explored and quality-of-life and cost–benefit studies will be prominent.

GROWTH FACTORS

Hematopoietic growth factors will continue to be important. While granulocyte colony stimulating factor (G-CSF) is routinely administered after autologous stem cell rescue following earlier uncontrolled reports of a clinical benefit,[28] the need for this and the optimal dose have not been defined.[29–31] In retrospective comparisons and in randomized studies, no consistent clinical benefit for the number of febrile days, septic episodes and transfusion requirements could be demonstrated although hospital duration of stay was shortened.[32,33] Differences with regard to the need for post-transplantation growth factor therapy may exist between marrow- or blood-derived stem cells. Multivariate analysis of parameters likely to influence engraftment of neutrophils and platelets has indicated that stem cell dose is the most important factor.[34]

Growth factor combinations have been explored in the hope of enhancing the quantity and quality of PBSC harvests and hastening engraftment. The use of granulocyte–macrophage colony stimulating factor (GM-CSF) plus interleukin-3 (IL-3) mobilizes more stem cells than G-CSF and although it does not shorten time to engraftment results in fewer infections and shorter hospital stay.[35] Combinations of either G-CSF or GM-CSF and stem cell factor (huSCF) for PBSC mobilization, and post-reinfusional G-CSF or GM-CSF, not only increase the PBSC yield but also significantly reduce the time to platelet recovery. Whether this improvement relates to effects on stem cell mobilization, on the hematologic recovery or on both has not yet been analyzed.[36] Interleukin-3 alone was no more effective than GM-CSF.[37] Combinations of G-CSF ± IL-3 accelerated multilineage recovery. The GM-CSF/IL-3 fusion protein PIXY-321 was comparable to GM-CSF for neutrophil recovery in a randomized trial, but platelets seemed to recover faster after PIXY 321 administration.[38]

Interleukin-6 and IL-11 alone or with G-CSF or GM-CSF have also been evaluated in small trials, with no noticeable improvement over G-CSF or GM-CSF alone.[39]

THE FUTURE OF HIGH DOSE CHEMOTHERAPY

Only new understanding of the mechanisms of drug resistance and the discovery of new drugs which avoid or overcome resistance will allow the 21st century to show any real breakthrough in this area. Research programs evaluating dose intensification are still needed, with emphasis on phase III prospective and randomized studies.

Because relapse remains the most significant problem despite very high rates of remissions following high dose chemotherapy, other approaches need to be explored to resolve the problem of refractory residual disease. Contributions from biological therapies, such as in vivo monoclonal antibodies, graft engineering by positive and negative selection, the manipulations of the cellular immune response in minimal residual disease by anti-tumor vaccines to stimulate an anti-tumor reactivity, as well as the rapidly emerging gene therapy tools are already resulting in new treatment strategies.

The activity of high dose chemotherapy in hematologic malignancies, in selected breast cancer patients and in pediatric tumors has been demonstrated in numerous non-randomized phase II trials involving highly selected patient populations. This has generated widespread use of this treatment modality. However, the results obtained in most studies cannot be readily compared with those from conventional treatments and may even be misleading due to patient selection or treatment selection bias. Few randomized trials with sufficient numbers of patients have been carried out and even less are mature enough to allow definitive conclusions regarding treatment efficacy. The cost and burden to patients can only be justified if firm data are produced from prospective randomized trials with meaningful numbers of patients to allow for stratification according to important prognostic indicators.

Many advances have been made by haematologists and oncologists with a special interest in high dose therapy and stem cell transplantation. It is through even closer interaction between clinicians and basic scientists that further progress will be made in coming years.

REFERENCES

1. Hryniuk W, Levine MN. Analysis of dose intensity for adjuvant chemotherapy trials in stage II breast cancer. J Clin Oncol 1986;4:1162–70.

2. Irle C, Philip T. High-dose chemotherapy and stem cell rescue. In: Souhami R et al. Oxford textbook of oncology 2nd edn. Oxford: Oxford University Press, 2001.

3. Philip T, Biron P. Role of high-dose chemotherapy and autologous bone marrow transplantation in the treatment of lymphoma. Eur J Cancer 1995;333:1540–5.

4. Philip T, Armitage JO, Spitzer G et al. High-dose therapy and autologous bone marrow transplantation after failure at conventional chemotherapy in adults with intermediate-grade or high-dose non Hodgkin's lymphoma. N Engl J Med 1987;316:1493–8.

5. Philip T, Guglielmi C, Hagenbeek A et al. Autologous bone marrow transplantation as compared with salvage chemotherapy in relapses of chemotherapy-sensitive non-Hodgkin's lymphoma. N Engl J Med 1995;333:1540–5.

6. Rohatiner AZ, Johnson PW, Price CG et al. Myeloablative therapy with autologous bone marrow transplantation as consolidation therapy for recurrent follicular lymphoma. J Clin Oncol 1994;12:1177–84.

7. Foran JM, Apostolidis J, Papamichael D et al. High-dose therapy with autologous haematopoietic support in patients with transformed follicular lymphoma: a study of 27 patients from a single centre. Ann Oncol 1998;9:865–9.

8. Freedman AS, Gribben JG, Neuberg D et al. High-dose therapy and autologous bone marrow transplantation in patients with follicular lymphoma during first remission. Blood 1996;88:2780–6.

9. Stadtmauer EA, O'Neill A, Goldstein LJ et al. Conventional dose chemotherapy compared with high dose chemotherapy plus autologous hematopoietic stem cell transplantation for metastatic breast cancer. N Engl J Med 2000;342:1069–76.

10. Baynes RD, Dansey RD, Klein JL et al. High dose chemotherapy and hematopoietic stem cell transplant for breast cancer: past or future. Semin Oncol 2001;28:377–88.

11. Lotz JP, Cure H, Janvier M et al. Intensive chemotherapy and autograft of hematopoietic stem cells for the treatment of metastatic cancer. Hematol Cell Ther 1999;41:71–4.

12. Goldie JH, Coldman AJ. A mathematical model for relating the drug sensitivity of tumors to their spontaneous mutation rate. Cancer Treat Rep 1979;63:1727–33.

13. Frei E, Canellos GP. Dose: a critical factor in cancer chemotherapy. Am J Med 1980;69:585–94.

14. To LB, Roberts MM, Haylock DN et al. Comparison of haematological recovery times and supportive care requirements of autologous recovery phase peripheral blood stem cell transplants, autologous bone marrow transplants and allogeneic bone marrow transplants. Bone Marrow Transplant 1992;9:277–84.

15. Simmons PJ, Leavesley DI, Levesque JP et al. The mobilization of primitive hemopoietic progenitors into the peripheral blood. Stem Cells 1994;12(suppl 1): 187–202.

16. Pettengell R, Testa NG, Swindell R, Crowther D, Dexter TM. Transplantation potential of hematopoietic cells released into the circulation during routine chemotherapy for non-Hodgkin's lymphoma. Blood 1993;82:2239–48.

17. Kiss JE, Rybka WB, Winkelstein A et al. Relationship of CD34+ cell dose to early and late hematopoiesis following autologous peripheral blood stem cell transplantation. Bone Marrow Transplant 1997;19:303–10.

18. Berenson RJ, Bensinger WI, Hill RS et al. Engraftment after infusion of CD34+ marrow cells in patients with breast cancer or neuroblastoma. Blood 1991;77:1717–22.

19. Alcorn MJ, Holyoake TL, Richmond L et al. CD34-positive cells isolated from cryopreserved peripheral-blood progenitor cells can be expanded ex vivo and used for transplantation with little or no toxicity. J Clin Oncol 1996;14:1839–47.

20. Williams CD, Goldstone AH, Pearce RM et al.

Purging of bone marrow in autologous bone marrow transplantation for non-Hodgkin's lymphoma: a case-matched comparison with unpurged cases by the European Blood and Marrow Transplant Lymphoma Registry. J Clin Oncol 1996;14:2454–64.

21. Gewirtz AM. Oligodeoxynucleotide-based therapeutics for human leukemias. Stem Cells 1993;11(suppl 3): 96–103.

22. Pierga JY, Magdelenat H. Applications of antisense oligonucleotides in oncology. Cell Mol Biol 1994;3:237–61.

23. Anderson WF. Human gene therapy. Science 1992;256:808–13.

24. Hesdorffer C, Ayello J, Ward M et al. Phase I trial of retroviral-mediated transfer of the human MDR1 gene as marrow chemoprotection in patients undergoing high-dose chemotherapy and autologous stem-cell transplantation. J Clin Oncol 1998;16:165–72.

25. Koc ON, Allay JA, Lee K, Davis BM, Reese JS, Gerson SL. Transfer of drug resistance genes into hematopoietic progenitors to improve chemotherapy tolerance. Semin Oncol 1996;23:46–65.

26. Sanchez FG, Pizzorrino G, Crystal R, Deisseroth AB. Receptor dependent uptake of the cytosine deaminase adenoviral vector into breast cancer but not hematopoietic cells for sensitization to 5-fluorocytosine induced cytotoxicity. Blood 1996;88(suppl 1) 1918 (abstract).

27. Attal M, Harousseau JL, Stoppa AM et al. A prospective, randomized trial of autologous bone marrow transplantation and chemotherapy in multiple myeloma. N Engl J Med 1996; 335:91–7.

28. Nemunaitis J, Singer JW, Buckner CD et al. Use of recombinant human granulocyte–macrophage colony-stimulating factor in graft failure after bone marrow transplantation. Blood 1990;76: 245–53.

29. Stahel RA, Jost LM, Honegger H, Betts E, Goebel ME, Nagler A. Randomized trial showing equivalent efficacy of filgrastim 5 micrograms/kg/d and 10 micrograms/kg/d following high-dose chemotherapy and autologous bone marrow transplantation in high-risk lymphomas. J Clin Oncol 1997;15:1730–5.

30. Bolwell B, Goormastic M, Dannley R et al. G-CSF post-autologous progenitor cell transplantation: a randomized study of 5, 10, and 16 micrograms/kg/day. Bone Marrow Transplant 1997; 19:215–19.

31. Bolwell BJ, Pohlman B, Andresen S et al. Delayed G-CSF after autologous progenitor cell transplantation: a prospective randomized trial. Bone Marrow Transplant 1998;21:369–73.

32. O'Day SJ, Rabinowe SN, Neuberg D et al. A phase II study of continuous infusion recombinant human granulocyte–macrophage colony-stimulating factor as an adjunct to autologous bone marrow transplantation for patients with non-Hodgkin's lymphoma in first remission. Blood 1994;83:2707–14.

33. Cortelazzo S, Viero P, Bellavita P et al. Granulocyte colony-stimulating factor following peripheral-blood progenitor-cell transplant in non-Hodgkin's lymphoma. J Clin Oncol 1995;13:935–41.

34. Weaver CH, Hazelton B, Birch R et al. An analysis of engraftment kinetics as a function of the CD34 content of peripheral blood progenitor cell collections in 692 patients after the administration of myeloablative chemotherapy. Blood 1995; 86:3961–9.

35. Lemoli RM, Rosti G, Visani G et al. Concomitant and sequential administration of recombinant human granulocyte colony-stimulating factor and recombinant human interleukin-3 to accelerate hematopoietic recovery after autologous bone marrow transplantation for malignant lymphoma. J Clin Oncol 1996;14:3018–25.

36. Moskowitz CH, Stiff P, Gordon MS et al. Recombinant methionyl human stem cell factor and filgrastim for peripheral blood progenitor cell mobilization and transplantation in non-Hodgkin's lymphoma patients – results of a phase I/II trial. Blood 1997;89:3136–47.

37. Nemunaitis J, Appelbaum FR, Singer JW et al. Phase I trial with recombinant human interleukin-3 in patients with lymphoma undergoing autologous bone marrow transplantation. Blood 1993;82:3273–8.

38. Vose JM, Pandite AN, Beveridge RA et al. Granulocyte–macrophage colony-stimulating factor/interleukin-3 fusion protein versus granulocyte–macrophage colony-stimulating factor after autologous bone marrow transplantation for non-Hodgkin's lymphoma: results of a randomized double-blind trial. J Clin Oncol 1997;15: 1617–23.

39. Lazarus HM, Winton E, Williams SF et al. Phase I multicenter trial of interleukin 6 therapy after autologous bone marrow transplantation in advanced breast cancer. Bone Marrow Transplant 1995;15:935–42.

Index